CLINICAL INTEGRATION

A Roadmap to Accountable Care

BRUCE FLAREAU, MD ◆ **KEN YALE, DDS, JD**
J.M. BOHN ◆ **COLIN KONSCHAK**

FOREWORD BY Michael Dudley

Edited by Rebecca J. Frey, PhD

Second Edition

D0557515

Praise for Clinical Integration: A Roadmap to Accountable Care

We are experiencing an unprecedented era in healthcare where our industry has a chance to get it right and significantly improve Health while we reduce cost. This will only happen through a collaboration of healthcare stakeholders who are innovative, visionary and willing to change. This book speaks directly to the infrastructure that will be needed to accomplish this change.

Steve Mason
President/CEO
BayCare Health System

This work is a concise evidence packed playbook for successful A.C.O. implementation with pivotal recommendations for obtaining effective physician alignment. The authors' delineation of desired governance and leadership competencies is a critical contribution to the literature on A.C.O's. This thoughtful and carefully researched book will be a resource to any leader challenged with an A.C.O. implementation.

Ann Chinnis, MD, MSHA, FACHE, FACEP
CEO Matrix Executive Coaching
Professor of Emergency Medicine
WV University School of Medicine

This book is a must read for those whose role is to provide leadership and direction to your healthcare organization. It's undeniable that the future of healthcare financing is gravitating towards a "value-based system" from the current "volume-based system". The authors have compiled the information and tools you will need to understand and succeed in the evolving environment, which includes examining how Accountable Care Organizations or Clinically Integrated Networks may change the status quo if designed properly.

Robert R. Sterling, CPA, CMPE
Executive Director
Mid-Atlantic Women's Care, PLC

In this increasing complex health care environment in which we try to operate, the Practice Administrator struggles to keep abreast of the ever-changing environment in which we are accountable for leading. It is necessary to surround ourselves with the tools to be successful. In the attempt to unwind and understand the complexities of the Accountable Care Organization I have found a terrific tool. "Accountable Care Organizations: A Roadmap for Success" has helped me to gain an acute knowledge of ACO's and how, I as an Administrator, needs to prepare my organization for the future. The ultimate outcome of ACO's has not been clearly defined. But I believe that some form of ACO will take shape over the coming year. This book clearly lays the groundwork so a health care administrator or physician can learn the basic principles and the new language that will be necessary to guide our organizations through this new challenge.

John E. Brown, CEO
Cardiology Consultants, Ltd.

An excellent contribution to the industry's literature on important health reform topics that will provide meaningful insights for C-level executives, researchers and policy makers alike.

Vickie Yates Brown, JD
President & CEO
Nucleus

With the ever-changing healthcare system in the U.S. it is more important now than ever to be unafraid of 'failure' in exploring clinical integration programs and ACO models given how they can transform value based healthcare. This comprehensive book highlights what we can learn quickly--what is working and challenges that lie ahead.

Joseph Steier, III, Ed. D., MBA, CPA
President/CEO
Signature HealthCARE

As a health care attorney, you must have a complete understanding of the changing landscape of health care and the emergence of clinically integrated networks and accountable care organizations. This book provides a very thorough discussion of all the pertinent issues giving the reader the knowledge base that he needs to navigate the shark infested waters facing health care providers and their advisors today. I would highly recommend it to all health care providers and their advisors so that they can succeed in the challenging environment in which they are currently operating.

T. Braxton McKee, JD
Partner & Health Care Chair
Kaufman & Canoles, P.C.

ISBN-13: 978-0-9834824-4-4
ISBN-10: 0-9834824-4-6

Convurgent Publishing, LLC
4445 Corporation Lane, Suite #227
Virginia Beach, VA 23462
Contact Information
Phone: (877) 254-9794, Fax: (757) 213-6801
website: www.convurgent.com; email: info@convurgent.com

Special Orders.
Bulk Quantity Sales: Special discounts are available on quantity purchases of 25 or more copies by corporations, government agencies, academic institutions, and other organizations. Please contact Convurgent Publishing's "sales department" at sales@convurgent.com or at the address above.

Library of Congress Control Number: 2011938568
Bibliographic data:

Flareau, Bruce
Clinical Integration. A Roadmap to Accountable Care / by Bruce Flareau, Ken Yale, J.M. Bohn, and Colin Konschak –2nd ed.
p. cm.
1. Healthcare administration. 2. Healthcare reform. 3. Healthcare quality. 4. Clinical integration. 5. Clinically integrated network. 6. Accountable care organizations. 7. Physician leadership. 8. Comparative effectiveness research.

ISBN: 978-0-9834824-4-4

Contributions:
Corresponding author, Colin Konschak (ck@divurgent.com)
Copy editor, Rebecca J. Frey, PhD (rebeccafrey@snet.net)
Cover design prepared by Steve Amarillo/Urban Design LLC
Formatting by Keri-Anne DeSalvo

About the Authors

Bruce Flareau, MD, FAAFP, FACPE, CPE, is the president of BayCare Physician Partners, and executive vice president of BayCare Health System, in Clearwater, Florida. As a family physician, Dr Flareau has served as a professor in two universities, has written and spoke nationally and internationally on a variety of health care topics. As an academic, president of the Florida Academy of Family Physicians, and physician executive, Dr. Flareau has over 20 years of healthcare experience.

Ken Yale, DDS, JD, is vice president of Clinical Solutions at ActiveHealth Management. Previously he built and launched innovative health technologies and business models for a variety of health organizations, including clinically integrated networks, patient-centered medical homes, accountable care organizations, health plans, medical management companies, and health information technology companies. Before building innovative health businesses, he was chief of staff of the White House Office of Science and Technology, served as a special assistant to the President and executive director of the White House Domestic Policy Council (DPC), was legislative counsel to the U.S. Senate, and a commissioned officer in the U.S. Public Health Service.

J.M. Bohn, MBA, is founder of Clinical Horizons, Inc. and focuses on communications, planning, and secondary research initiatives related to health care industry transformation and innovation. These fields include health information technology, health care provider, and academic research issues. Bohn's MBA is from the University of Louisville with a concentration in healthcare and economic studies.

Colin Konschak, MBA, FACHE, FHIMSS, is the managing partner of DIVURGENT, a healthcare management consulting firm. Mr. Konschak is a registered pharmacist, has an MBA in health services administration, is board-certified in healthcare management, and is a certified Six Sigma Black Belt. Colin leads DIVURGENT's advisory service consulting practice focused on operational and information technology strategies, including those related to accountable care organizations and clinically integrated networks.

PREFACE

Clinical Integration: A Roadmap to Accountable Care is the second edition of the book, *Accountable Care Organizations: A Roadmap to Success,* with timely updates on key changes affecting the industry as clinically integrated networks (CIN) and accountable care organizations (ACO) emerge in the United States (U.S.) healthcare industry. This work retains its focus on original literary research and reference material and incorporates new insights arising from the release of the Center of Medicare and Medicaid Services (CMS) notice of proposed rulemaking (Proposed Rule) on March 31, 2011 and the list of 33 quality measures from the Final Rule issued October 20, 2011. In addition, this second edition renews its focus on the formation of the clinically integrated network as well as adding:

- Operations of a Network.
- Comparative Effectiveness- Advancing the Model.

This second edition continues its presentation of important issues affecting hospitals, physicians, insurers, government agencies, and legal professionals on industry efforts to establish organizations with greater accountability for quality and value. The past decade has yielded numerous insights derived from demonstrations and pilot projects related to healthcare quality and payment reform, and has brought our nation to the present period of transition in the healthcare delivery system. Some issues from the Proposed Rule continue to be debated and have been incorporated in this update. In addition as CMS established an overarching framework with its Three Part Aim, a similar focus is used as a central theme throughout this second edition. Models and illustrations from the first edition have been kept throughout and provide the reader with visual aids that complement the most critical underlying issues.

Throughout this work you will see references to both accountable care organizations and clinically integrated networks. Many of the principles of design and implementation are identical and many would suggest a CIN is the necessary precursor to an ACO. The latter includes insurance risk-taking capabilities, while the former is more flexible in its payer relationships and may or may not take global risk, for example. In addition, we frequently refer to ACOs in the broader context but have made special efforts to clarify when we are using the more narrowly defined CMS point of view. Distinctions among these three business models (CIN, Medicare ACO, all payer ACO) will become clearer as the nation grapples with the complex issues of design and implementation.

Finally, we have placed roadmaps at the end of several chapters highlighting changes and new ideas to consider in your organization's journey toward formation of clinically integrated networks and implementation of accountable care organizations. In addition, tables are included at the end of Chapters 2 through 9 that highlight a set of challenges, risks and mitigation strategies. Risks are aligned to the challenges while mitigation strategies are presented as potential solutions to both challenges in the table as well as to broader issues addressed in the chapter. Overall, we have attempted to assemble a high-level guide to major activities and issues related to the development and establishment of CINs and ACOs, and delve into specific details where the industry has coalesced around best practices or consensus.

Our Goal

We offer this updated work as part of your tool kit to support strategic planning; provide a consolidated set of reference materials; and foster momentum for working toward clinically and financially integrated and accountable care organizations. A future edition will incorporate changes from CMS's recent final rule on the Medicare ACO program. As the industry moves forward with new legislative reforms, the health system in the United States is undertaking significant changes that will affect the availability of healthcare services. The accountable care model of delivery - and its corollary, the clinically integrated network - are each woven into the fabric of healthcare throughout the U.S. healthcare system and are part of the broader value-based purchasing focus designed to help improve quality care for all our citizens.

ACKNOWLEDGEMENTS

The authors wish to thank their families and colleagues for their patience and support in the time taken for the development of this book. In addition we wish to thank BDC Advisors' Dale Anderson, MD for the illustrations provided in Chapter 9. Greg Miller of Medicity, Inc. who contributed greatly to the development of material regarding health information exchange along with illustrations of the subject. We are most appreciative of Michael Dudley of Sentara Healthcare for providing the Foreword. The original authors would like to thank Ken Yale for joining the effort to prepare and improve this second edition. His contributions included not only writing the new chapter on comparative effectiveness research but also an extensive contribution to the full revision and updating of the original work, *Accountable Care Organizations: A Roadmap to Success.*

TABLE OF CONTENTS

FOREWORD

As the nation grapples with the transformation of its healthcare delivery system, a number of paradigm shifts are taking place. The authors of *Clinical Integration: A Roadmap to Accountable Care* have provided a succinct update and expanded version of their first edition. Recognizing the foundational aspect of clinical integration in the formation of accountable care organizations, Dr. Flareau and his co-authors built upon this earlier theme. They present multiple facets of its importance in delivering improved quality and value in the care provided by organizations embarking on the clinical integration journey as a precursor to accountable care models. The addition of co-author Ken Yale strengthened the team's insights throughout, especially with his knowledge of the legal system and his contributions to the new chapter on comparative effectiveness research.

The Center for Medicare and Medicaid Services issued their Notice of Proposed Rule Making (Proposed Rule) in the spring of 2011 regarding the new CMS Shared Savings Program. The authors also address the Pioneer ACO Model, which focuses on bundled payments and the opportunity for increased shared savings for those organizations that already have advanced capabilities and coordination across care settings in place. There are a multitude of references to the Proposed Rule throughout this refreshed work that integrate with and expand on original concepts in the first edition. The section on legal and regulatory matters summarizes a great deal of federal and state regulations along with opinions rendered by the Federal Trade Commission that anyone working in the field of clinical integration programs and future development of accountable care organizations must understand.

The quest to continue working toward the six aims of higher quality care set forth by the Institute of Medicine is embodied in the efforts of those striving to implement clinically integrated networks and accountable care organizations across the country. The authors have captured the importance of these goals in their opening chapter and underscore their importance throughout as the primary foundation of our mission in contemporary healthcare. The second chapter reinforces the importance of the patient-centered medical home as a basic element in all clinically integrated networks and accountable care organizations. The new chapter on network operations emphasizes the importance of patient-centered care as the nucleus of the network operation in establishing, supporting, and expanding the functions of a clinically integrated network or an accountable care organization.

At Sentara Healthcare we recognize the importance of these issues. We have moved forward in establishing strong ties with our regional physician communities to support the development of our own clinical integration program. Having initiated this program and the underlying transformation of administrative and clinical processes, we know the value of the messages conveyed in this work. The authors have expressed a deeper understanding of the continued evolution of the industry toward greater connectivity, interoperability, and efficient flow of information across all provider organizations.

Clinical Integration: A Roadmap to Accountable Care is a valuable new work that should be considered essential reading to help leaders open new pathways in planning; understand many of the factors impacting the healthcare services market; and set their course for navigating the future needs of patients and stakeholders of our nation's healthcare system.

Michael M. Dudley
President, Optima Health Plans
Senior Vice President, Sentara Healthcare

Chapter 1. History and Case for Action

Despite the cost pressures, liability constraints, resistance to change and other seemingly insurmountable barriers, it is simply not acceptable for patients to be harmed by the same health care system that is supposed to offer healing and comfort.[1]

To Err Is Human, 2000
Institute of Medicine

Introduction

The healthcare system in the United States (U.S.) is at a turning point in its history. The convergence of many factors—including experience with health maintenance organizations; shortages in the healthcare workforce; expansion of the uninsured segment of the population; rising healthcare costs, and challenges to the quality, affordability and accessibility of care—has led to enactment of major health reform. This process is not unprecedented; the recent history of American healthcare indicates that it has undergone major transitions every ten to twenty years. Specific examples range from the creation of Medicare in 1965 and passage of the Health Maintenance Organization Act of 1973 to the introduction of diagnosis-related group hospital reimbursement methodologies and the formation of physician-hospital organizations in the 1980s, as well as the Clinton Administration's efforts to reform healthcare in the 1990s. Each transition had various impacts on society and its requirements for healthcare services, and each transition resolved some—though certainly not all—issues in each reform initiative's respective decade.

The complexity of the challenges and attempts to overcome them has been further exacerbated by physicians' loss of power and autonomy. Physicians have seen changes not only in the field of medicine but also across society as Paul Starr explained so well in 1982.[2]

---

[1] Institute of Medicine, Committee on Quality of Health Care in America. Executive Summary. In: *Too Err is Human*. Washington, DC: National Academies Press; 2000. p. 2
[2] Starr P. The Social Origins of Professional Sovereignty. In: *The Social Transformation of American Medicine*. New York, NY: HarperCollins, 1982, p. 8.

In spite of major transitions and health reforms over the past 45 years, the problems of health care quality, affordability, and accessibility persist. The latest attempt at major health reform, the Patient Protection and Affordable Care Act of 2010 (hereinafter referred to as the Affordable Care Act), seeks to elicit new and innovative thinking to solve these problems. Of course, as Albert Einstein once said, "We can't solve problems by using the same kind of thinking we used when we created them." And so, given the persistence of many of these trends throughout the past decade and the drive for continuous improvement, it is no surprise that clinically integrated networks (CIN) and accountable care organization (ACO) delivery models have emerged as a way to think and act differently about healthcare finances, quality and delivery.

In 1999, the Institute of Medicine's (IOM) Committee on the Quality of Health Care in America issued its landmark report *To Err Is Human*, which increased awareness of the prevalence and impact of medical errors. The committee issued a second report in 2001 that noted the challenges confronting fundamental redesign of the U.S. healthcare system.[3] This report also outlined six aims to improve the quality of healthcare services provided throughout the United States. These six goals, provide a framework for many organizations seeking to improve the quality of contemporary healthcare.

Figure 1. Six Aims for Improvement in Quality Healthcare

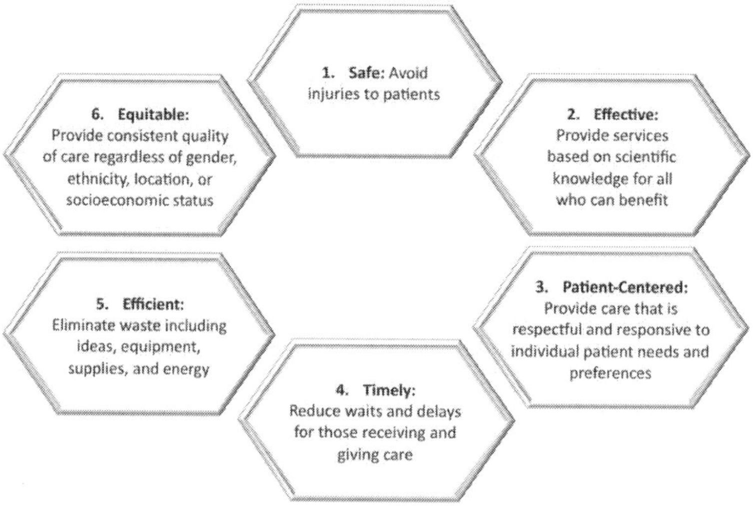

1. **Safe:** Avoid injuries to patients

2. **Effective:** Provide services based on scientific knowledge for all who can benefit

3. **Patient-Centered:** Provide care that is respectful and responsive to individual patient needs and preferences

4. **Timely:** Reduce waits and delays for those receiving and giving care

5. **Efficient:** Eliminate waste including ideas, equipment, supplies, and energy

6. **Equitable:** Provide consistent quality of care regardless of gender, ethnicity, location, or socioeconomic status

---

[3] Institute of Medicine, Committee on Quality of Health Care in America. Building organizational support for change. In: *Crossing the Quality Chasm: A New Health System for the 21st Century*. Washington, DC: National Academies Press; 2001, pp. 117–118.

The IOM's six aims have individually and collectively fostered numerous strategic initiatives across the healthcare industry since they were first published. These initiatives have attempted to address significant increases in the overall cost of medical care as well as the rate of growth in healthcare costs since the 1980s. They have also targeted quality and accessibility of healthcare services, which have improved for some diseases, conditions, geographic areas, and patient subpopulations. Patient satisfaction has also improved with the quality of services in recent years; however, medical errors still occur and inefficiencies still exist, leaving much room for further improvement.

One of the fundamental challenges facing health care in the United States is the reimbursement system. The fee-for-service payment system pays for each procedure, regardless of outcome, and has not led to optimal results. In fact, the IOM released a report in 2006 that called attention to problems with the fee-for-service payment system. The IOM maintained that the fee-for-service system "reward(s) excessive use of services; high-cost, complex procedures; and lower-quality care."[4] These incentives have resulted in a volume-driven system that contributes in many ways to reduced or stagnant quality of care in addition to concurrent rises in the cost of healthcare.

In recent years, healthcare expenditures in the United States have risen at an annual rate 2.4% faster than the rate of growth in gross domestic product (GDP).[5] In fact, the CMS stated in 2010 that total national health expenditures for 2009 reached $2.5 trillion—17.6% of GDP.[6] National health expenditures as a share of GDP are projected to increase to 19.3% by 2019,[7] given the historical trend from 1960 to 2008 as a percentage of GDP.[8] Many leading economists believe that expenditures above 20% of GDP will have a significant negative impact on the United States economy.

[4] Institute of Medicine, Committee on Redesigning Health Insurance Performance Measures, Payments, and Performance Improvement Programs. Summary. In: *Rewarding Provider Performance: Aligning Incentives in Medicare*. Washington, DC: National Academies Press; 2006, p. 4.
[5] Kaiser Family Foundation. Trends in health care costs and spending. March 2009.
[6] Center for Medicare and Medicaid Services. National health expenditures Fact Sheet. Accessed online July 20, 2011, at http://www.cms.gov/NationalHealthExpendData/25_NHE_Fact_Sheet.asp#TopOfPage.
[7] Center for Medicare and Medicaid Services. National health expenditure projections 2009-2019. Accessed online May 31, 2011, at : http://www.cms.gov/NationalHealthExpendData/25_NHE_Fact_Sheet.asp#TopOfPage.
[8] Kaiser Family Foundation. Industry trend charts. Accessed online July 20, 2011, at http://facts.kff.org/results.aspx?view=slides&topic=3&start=1.

Figure 2. National Health Expenditures as a Share of GDP, 1960-2008

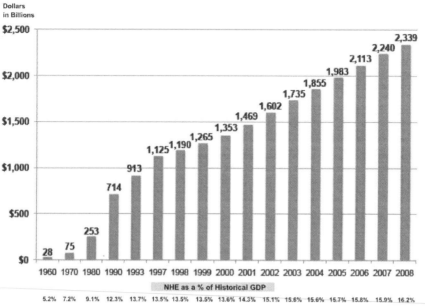

Source: Center for Medicare and Medicaid Services Statistics. Historical National Health Expenditures. Table 3. Accessed online at http://www.cms.gov/NationalHealthExpendData/downloads/tables.pdf

Because of the rapid and continuous escalation in the cost of delivering healthcare and its effects on the nation's economy, the 2006 IOM report recommended that the CMS move away from fee-for-service reimbursement and toward a pay-for-performance system. Pay-for-performance is intended to reward physicians and provider organizations for improving coordination of care, eliminating unnecessary tests and procedures, and improving overall quality of care as well as patient satisfaction with services received. In addition to the unsustainable nature of fee-for-service financing, another reason for making this recommendation may lie in the history of HMOs. Private insurer indemnity programs and health plans grew rapidly after 1973, when Congress passed the Health Maintenance Organization Act. While HMOs did in fact help reduce the rate of growth in national health care expenditures, they also used a gatekeeper approach, asking the physician to serve as a restrictive guardian of access to care. As a result physicians experienced a lowering of their professional reputation, as they appeared to put obstacles in the way of care delivery rather than serve their traditional role of patient advocates. Of course, if one looks closely at the graph representing national spending on healthcare, the only time the cost curve flattened occurred when HMOs and physician–hospital organization programs were put in place. Consequently, many observers argue from a financial perspective that HMOs and physician-hospital organizations were in fact successful. A few solid examples have survived, such as Kaiser Permanente and Geisinger Health System, which are well positioned in this new era.

Consumer Issues

Two issues that should be raised in the context of rising costs are consumer-directed health plans and the escalating premiums paid by consumers for health insurance coverage with private payers. Both issues involve the increasing percentage of care directly paid by the consumer.

Consumer-directed health plans were introduced after HMOs declined as a major vehicle for employers to reduce costs.[9] Consumer-directed health plans may be loosely defined as plans that give more responsibility to consumers to make decisions or set priorities regarding their healthcare needs. This is accomplished by funding an account controlled by the consumer, who then has responsibility for paying the bills and making choices about the care purchased. Some of the consumer-directed plans that have been developed and implemented include health savings accounts and high deductible health plans. These plans have opened a way to move consumers from an entitlement mindset ("if it's free it's for me") to an attitude of shared responsibility for decision-making. In these plans, the individual consumer must pay for some portion of healthcare service consumption from his or her "own" account. Consumers are more frugal in their consumption of healthcare resources when they are closer financially to the burden of expenses. The theory is that individual consumer choice should work better than physician gatekeepers or dictates from the health insurance company. The reality is that individual consumers may not have access to the clinical or financial information necessary to make the best choices, sometimes choosing to avoid necessary care to save money.

---

[9] Konschak C, Jarrell L. *Consumer-centric Healthcare: Opportunities and Challenges for Providers*. Chicago, IL: Health Administration Press; 2010.

A major distinction between health care systems in other countries compared to the system in the United States is in resource utilization. In Switzerland, for example, the public favors fiscal responsibility in the utilization of health care resources. In contrast, the indemnity approach to insurance in the United States encourages an entitlement mentality and the self-fulfilling "tragedy of the commons," in which each member of a group demands their immediate share of finite resources at the long-term expense of all. The more rapidly people consume limited resources, the higher the total spending curve. This problem is exacerbated by the fee-for-service reimbursement system, which pays more for higher utilization. Greater transparency of reporting through such available technologies as the Internet, coupled with the consumer movement and advocacy groups, have led to improved knowledge of health issues in the general population over time––resulting in conditions favorable to the growth of consumer-direct health plans that allow the consumer to be more aware of and responsible for resource utilization. On the other hand, consumer-directed health plans may have an adverse impact on health in some cases. Consumers given increased personal responsibility for healthcare decisions in the face of limited resources may make such unwise decisions as holding off necessary care due to cost considerations.

To give a specific example, the consumer may choose to forgo immediate care for acute symptoms; thus chronic diseases or conditions may present later when treatment costs are higher and outcomes poorer. While flexible spending accounts and health savings accounts are making a comeback, and many observers consider these plans a reasonable alternative to other insurance products as standard premiums become increasingly unaffordable, such consumer-directed health plans may have a long-term detrimental effect if they are decoupled from access to care for chronic disease management. In addition, these types of plans in the past were often available only to employers (who saw them as a means of offsetting the growing cost of employee healthcare) and not to self-employed individuals.

The second issue concerns rising insurance premiums, both in the aggregate as well as the portion required from consumers. The greater portion required of consumers is part of the trend toward increased consumer cost sharing for high- and low-value healthcare services.[10] The historical trend shows escalating out-of-pocket expenses for the consumer portion of healthcare expenditures with private insurers; which is a subset of the overall historical trend in out-of-pocket expenses.[11]

Figure 3. Annual Consumer Out-of-Pocket Expenses 1960-2008

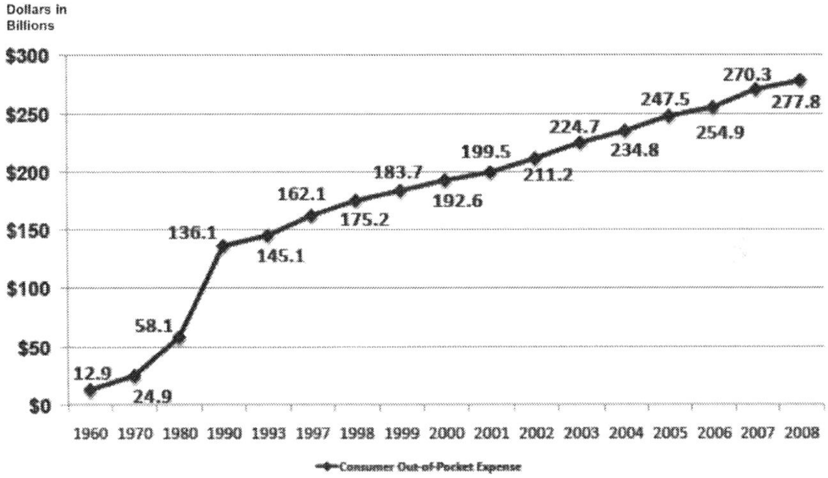

Source: Center for Medicare and Medicaid Services Statistics. Historical National Health Expenditures. Table 3. Accessed online at http://www.cms.gov/NationalHealthExpendData/downloads/tables.pdf

From the patient's perspective, rising premiums and out-of-pocket expenses are a significant concern. Value-based insurance design initiatives have been introduced to reduce the burden on consumers and curb rising healthcare costs;[8] however, these initiatives may still decrease utilization by consumers faced with choices regarding their healthcare needs based on out-of-pocket expenses. No matter who pays the invoice for healthcare services, whether employers or governments, consumers will still be responsible for some portion of insurance premiums, co-payments, and other out-of-pocket expenses for services rendered.

---

[10] Robinson JC. Applying value-based insurance design to high-cost health services. *Health Aff (Millwood)*. 2010;29(11):2009-16.

[11] Center for Medicare and Medicaid Services. Statistics. Historical national health expenditures. Table 3. Accessed online July 20, 2011, at http://www.cms.gov/NationalHealthExpendData/downloads/tables.pdf.

Up to this point we have reviewed historical patterns. Future projections of national health expenditures, along with their projected percent of gross domestic product, also raise concerns. Current CMS estimates forecast increases in private plans, Medicare, Medicaid, and out-of-pocket consumer expenses over the ten years between 2010 and 2019.[12] This trend is one of the reasons for the expansion of insurance coverage planned under the Affordable Care Act, as the population covered by Medicaid will expand significantly, causing the uninsured portion of the U.S. population is expected to decrease from 44.3 million in 2009 to 24.4 million by 2019. While overall out-of-pocket expenditures will still increase, the rate of acceleration in out-of-pocket expenses is projected to slow after 2014 when more consumers receive Medicaid coverage.[13]

Overall, there is a general trend toward marked increases in national health expenditures.[14] It is a known challenge for the United States and a major factor that has driven healthcare reform legislation over the last decade. There are many causes of the growth trend, some of which are uncontrollable, such as the impact of the baby boomer generation on Medicare and Medicaid's services for aging beneficiaries. Further evidence of financial challenges facing government-funded healthcare programs, given the forecasted increases in healthcare expenditures for Medicare is provided in Appendix A which contains an excerpt from the Medicare Board of Trustees August 2010 annual report.

---

[12] Centers for Medicare and Medicaid Services. National health expenditure projections 2009–2019 (September 2010), Table 2. Accessed online July 24, 2011, at
http://www.cms.gov/NationalHealthExpendData/downloads/NHEProjections2009to2019.pdf.
[13] Sisko AM, Truffer CJ, Keehan SP, Poisal JA, Clemens MK, Madison AJ. National health spending projections: the estimated impact of reform through 2019. *Health Aff (Millwood)*. 2010;29(10):1933-1941.
[14] Centers for Medicare and Medicaid Services. National health expenditure projections 2009–2019 (September 2010), Table 1. Accessed online July 24, 2011, at
http://www.cms.gov/NationalHealthExpendData/downloads/NHEProjections2009to2019.pdf.

Figure 4. Projected National Health Expenditures as a Share of GDP, 2010-2019

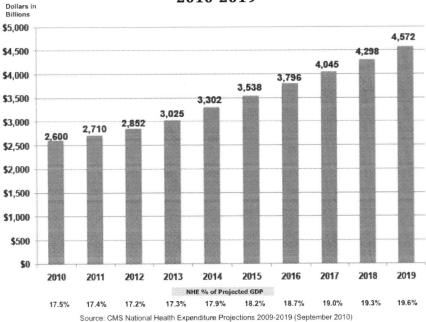

Source: CMS National Health Expenditure Projections 2009-2019 (September 2010)
Accessed online at http://www.cms.gov/NationalHealthExpendData/downloads/NHEProjections2009to2019.pdf

Figure 5 illustrates projected increases in consumer out-of-pocket expenditures as a subset of the overall escalation in healthcare expenditures.

Figure 5. Projected Consumer Out-of-Pocket Expenditures 2010-2019

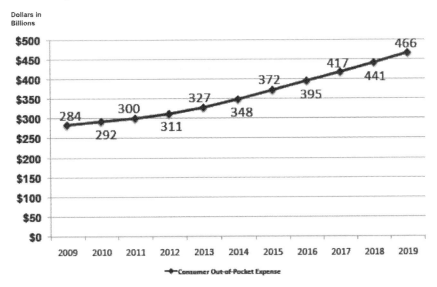

Source: Center for Medicare and Medicaid Services Statistics. Historical National Health Expenditures. Table 3. Accessed online at http://www.cms.gov/NationalHealthExpendData/downloads/tables.pdf

These inevitable increases in the growth of healthcare expenditures in the United States are some of the reasons such new business models, such as CINs and ACOs are being considered seriously as better ways to finance healthcare. Some of the new models that include bundled and global payment for reimbursing physicians and hospital organizations for healthcare services are described in Chapter 9. The need for these new models and other systemic changes is motivating industry stakeholders to adopt more advanced health information technology, meet stronger requirements for transparency in reporting, and improved the quality of patient care services. These new models have been and will continue to be tested by various stakeholder organizations across the industry.

Structural Issues and Delivery Model Innovation

The issue of business restructuring has been a very important factor throughout the history of modern medicine and in working toward the IOM's six aims of higher-quality care. As early as 1933, organization was one of the foundational recommendations for provision of medical care made by the Committee on the Costs of Medical Care (CCMC), a group of fifty economists, physicians, public health specialists, and major interest groups funded between 1926 and 1932 by eight philanthropic organizations that included the Rockefeller and Millbank Foundations. According to the CCMC's 1933 report, "Medical service should be more largely furnished by groups of physicians and related practitioners, so organized as to maintain high standards of care and to retain the personal relations between patients and physician."[15] The managed care organizations of the mid-1970s can be viewed as an attempt to implement the CCMC's recommendation.

Two organizational structures that emerged from the managed care era were the physician-hospital organizations and integrated delivery networks. These entities among others, will be discussed in more detail in Chapter 3. Physician-hospital organizations and integrated delivery networks emerged in the 1980s,

---

[15] Falk I, Rorem R, Ring M. A summary of the findings. In: *The Costs of Medical Care: A Summary of Investigations on the Economic Aspects of the Prevention and Care of Illness*. Chicago, IL: University of Chicago Press; 1933:582. Accessed online July 20, 2011, at http://www.deltaomega.org/costsof.pdf.

when hospitals and physician groups within specific geographic areas came together in a structured manner to achieve stronger alignment, economies of scale in contracting, and provision of better patient care required by their contractual relationships with HMOs.[16] A number of benefits and barriers resulted as these organizations evolved over the next thirty years. Benefits included better negotiating power with health insurance payers, while barriers included a lack of incentives to improve quality of care.[17] While these newer structures and arrangements helped the industry move in a positive direction, they were still challenged by issues raised on their contracts, limitations on patient choices, and antitrust laws imposed by the Federal Trade Commission (FTC) to ensure that competition in specific geographic markets was not restricted or negatively affected. These issues will be discussed in depth in Chapter 5.

Last is the issue of transitioning from a model of individual health management to population health management. During the era of HMOs and consumer-driven health plans, American healthcare focused on the individual patient, and in particular on persons with advanced chronic illnesses that could be easily identified through claims-based methods (reviewing claims to identify persons with specific codes indicating asthma, cardiac disease, diabetes, chronic obstructive pulmonary disease, and the like). This approach placed the emphasis on reactive medicine, sometimes when treatment was too late, rather than on proactive patient-centered care. One flaw in the individualized approach is that some advanced conditions are by definition terminal and cannot be treated without heroic or costly effort. Moreover, by focusing on disease management rather than total population health, healthcare providers overlook persons at-risk for chronic diseases who could have been identified through predictive modeling and other tools, and prevented from developing chronic conditions requiring high-cost interventions.

By contrast, a model that focuses on total population health (predictive

---

[16] Morrisey MA, Alexander J, Burns LR, Johnson V. Managed care and physician/hospital integration. *Health Aff (Millwood)*. 1996;15(4):62-73.
[17] Casalino LA, Devers KJ, Lake TK, Reed M, Stoddard JJ. Benefits of and barriers to large medical group practice in the U.S.. *Arch Intern Med.* 2003;163(16):1958-64.

modeling, risk stratification, patient-centered prevention, improved quality of care, and reduced cost), and care coordination returns responsibility for the health of a defined segment of the population to physicians who may be the best judges of better ways to intervene early to prevent disease and chronic conditions. Moving the United States toward greater population health management will require the use of health information technology by physicians to identify conditions early: provide better management of chronic conditions; and prevent multiple clinical conditions from becoming advanced chronic diseases. Putting such technology in place across the nation will in turn enable wider sharing of patient health data and information on clinical practices with all members of the care team.

The trends and lessons learned from the managed care era and earlier history of the healthcare industry has fostered a number of innovations in care delivery, quality improvement, and payment reform. One such innovation—the focus of this book—has been the emergence of such new business models as CINs and ACOs. The ACO concept originated from work done by policy researchers at the Dartmouth-Brookings Institute, and piloted in the Medicare Physician Group Practice Demonstration Project.[18] The demonstration and Congressional testimony provided sufficient interest for the federal government to support the formal advancement of the ACO model in the Affordable Care Act, and development of private payer ACO initiatives. Additional details on the results of the Group Practice demonstration are provided later in the present chapter; in the chapter on quality improvement; and in Appendix C.

The ACO model was first formally introduced to the Medicare Payment Advisory Commission (MedPAC) in November 2006[19] and by Dr. Elliott Fisher[20] in an article published in December 2006. Dr. Fisher described ACOs as partnerships between physicians and hospitals for coordinating and delivering healthcare services with greater efficiency and higher quality while lowering

---

[18] Centers for Medicare and Medicaid Services. Medicare Physician Group Practice Demonstration Project. Available at https://www.cms.gov/DemoProjectsEvalRpts/downloads/PGP_Fact_Sheet.pdf.
[19] Medicare Payment Advisory Commission public meeting November 8-9, 2006. p. 384. Transcript available at http://www.medpac.gov/transcripts/1108_1109_medpac.final.pdf.
[20] Fisher ES, Staiger DO, Bynum JP, Gottlieb DJ. Accountable care organizations: the extended medical staff. *Health Aff (Millwood)*. 2007;26 (1):w44–w57.

costs. ACOs accept ultimate accountability for clinical performance risk but are not responsible for overall insurance risk. Both public and private sector models strive to improve coordination and delivery of patient care as well as optimize the reimbursement system.

As public and private payer ACO models evolve, what are some of the key principles for their establishment? Drs. Fisher, McClellan, and colleagues summarized three key design principles for ACOs in a 2009 *Health Affairs* article illustrated below.[21]

Figure 6. Key Design Principles for Accountable Care Organizations

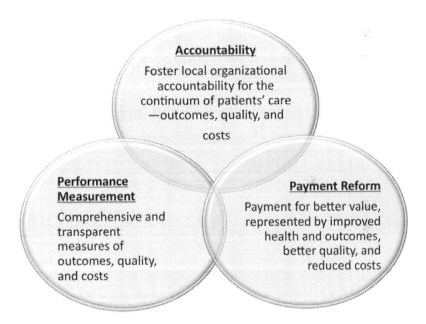

These three design principles have served as anchor points for industry leaders and government policymakers in their collaboration in crafting legislation and healthcare reforms to guide the development and implementation of ACOs. The principle of accountability, according to Dr. Fisher and his colleagues, includes returning the power and leadership of these organizations to physicians. The second principle, measuring performance to provide greater

---

[21] Fisher ES, McClellan MB, Bertko J, et al. Fostering accountable health care: moving forward in Medicare. *Health Aff (Millwood)*. 2009;28(2):w219-w231.

transparency to patients and other stakeholders who assess the value of the care provided, builds on the performance measurement requirements in the patient-centered medical home (hereinafter referred to as the medical home) discussed in Chapter 2. Third, payment reform builds on the pay-for-performance model, which relies on incentives for quality care, chronic disease management, and preventive care, rather than paying for such measures as episodic hospital stays to truly improve outcomes. If the industry moves from individual episodic pay-for-procedure to population-based pay-for-performance by managing patient cohorts (groups of patients with like conditions) with services ranging from primary prevention to chronic disease management, it is believed total healthcare expenditures will be lower.

The ACO can also be viewed from the perspective of consumer empowerment and the trend toward rising out-of-pocket premium expenses borne by consumers. One strategy described in the ACO literature regarding this issue is to offer consumers options on tiered premiums and tiered co-payments, depending on the ACO they select for their primary and specialty care services.[22]

ACOs and HMOs Compared

Given the influence of HMOs on the healthcare industry, a comparison of HMOs and ACOs (such as the Medicare Shared Savings Program), offers an interesting contrast.

---

[22] Sinaiko AD, Rosenthal MB. Patients' role in accountable care organizations. *N Engl J Med.* 2010;363(27):2583-2585.

Table 1. Historic HMOs vs. Public Sector ACOs

General Characteristic	HMO	ACO
Geographic coverage	Defined region determined by health services availability, responsible for services outside region	Primary coverage based on primary care provider coverage, also responsible for services provided outside the local area
Stakeholders	Hospitals, physician organizations, service suppliers, payers	Hospitals, physician organizations, service suppliers, and other organizations designated by CMS
Patient mix	Demographics vary based on plan	Medicare ACO: minimum of 5000 Medicare patients (mixed patient demographics) Private: varies according to payer plan
Care coordination	Restricted by contracting options, HMO responsibility	Increased flexibility, hospital/physician responsibility
Payment model	Fee-for-service shifting to pay-for-performance	Fee-for-service, pay-for-performance, partial capitation, full capitation, shared savings bundled payments[23]
Performance measure	HEDIS, shifting to broader set for pay-for-performance	Public: 65 quality measures (proposed) Private: HEDIS, NCQA, Premier, Joint Commission, AMA-PCPI
Locus of control	Payer organization	Physician-led

---

[23] de Brantes F, Rosenthal MB, Painter M. Building a bridge from fragmentation to accountability—the Prometheus Payment model. *N Engl J Med*. 2009;361(11):1033-1036.

This comparison shows the change in locus of control, which is one reason for the introduction of the Medicare ACO model (also called Medicare Shared Savings Program) and a major characteristic that differentiates it from the HMO model. When HMOs were launched in the 1980s, they became gatekeeper organizations for patients who needed access to appropriate healthcare services in a timely manner.[24] While there have been successful efforts by insurance payers and provider organizations to allow direct access, and the gatekeeper role is no longer an issue, high and unsustainable growth in costs continues. Moreover there is not enough flexibility in the current system of financing and delivery to meet the needs of physicians for greater accountability for care and of patients for responsibility for prevention. The continual rise in costs and lack of care options in HMOs in the 1990s led to dissatisfied patients and advocacy organizations; health reform efforts in the federal and state governments; and calls for greater physician engagement in controlling costs and improving quality. As a result, one of the key tenets for ACOs is to ensure that each is physician-led and physician-directed. In addition, CINs have emerged over the last decade as another provider-governed method of managing both clinical and financial risk.

Clinically Integrated Networks

Clinically integrated networks as allowed by the FTC are legitimate collaborations of otherwise competing providers (hospitals and/or physicians) organized in a way that improves efficiencies in care delivery (including quality improvement and cost reduction) in a way that outweighs any potential anticompetitive effects such as fixing prices among competitors). If providers meet specific criteria for clinical integration, they may not be prevented from collaborating and even negotiating prices with payers without running afoul of antitrust laws that prohibit competitors from price setting.

Clinical integration also provides a roadmap to accountable care because the infrastructure needed to meet the FTC criteria also provides many of the tools

---

[24] Mirabito AM, Berry LL. Lessons that patient-centered medical homes can learn from the mistakes of HMOs. *Ann Intern Med.* 2010;152(3):182-185.

and efficiencies needed to run a successful ACO. In addition, concurrent with release of the Proposed Rule, the FTC and Department of Justice (DOJ) Antitrust Division issued their Proposed Statement of Antitrust Enforcement Policy Regarding ACOs Participating in the Medicare Shared Savings Program. In that document, these two federal government agencies (who jointly enforce the federal antitrust laws) propose to treat Medicare ACOs similar to CINs and apply the existing guidance they use to determine whether collective activities by otherwise competing providers (such as negotiating or setting prices) are per-se illegal, or fall under more lenient "rule of reason" analysis, or certain "safety zones" where the providers' collective actions will not be challenged, absent extraordinary circumstances.

To fall under the "safety zones" providers need to share substantial financial risk and meet certain requirements for how much of the market for their services they control. Substantial risk sharing, the antitrust agencies believe, shows that the providers have a financial incentive to be efficient, control costs and improve quality. ACOs are designed to be responsible for the cost and quality of care, and therefore should fall under the safety zones, if properly established.

If a joint venture among providers does not qualify for a safety zone, for example they do not share substantial financial risk, they may still qualify for more lenient "rule of reason" scrutiny if the meet other requirements. The antitrust agencies generally require providers to establish an active and ongoing program to identify, evaluate and modify practice patterns by the physicians participating in the organization that also creates a high degree of interdependence and cooperation among the physicians to control costs and ensure quality.[25] If you consider the medical home as an effort to transform a physician office, the CIN is a medical home multiplied by many primary and specialty care physicians who collaborate to create a new service that benefits consumers, rather than trying to merely negotiate to increase prices.

---

[25] Federal Trade Commission. Statement #8. Paragraph 8(C)1: Examples of clinical integration. Available at: http://www.ftc.gov/bc/healthcare/industryguide/policy/statement8.htm.

According to the antitrust agencies, a legitimate clinically integrated network collaboration may include: "(1) establishing mechanisms to monitor and control utilization of health care services that are designed to control costs and assure quality of care; (2) selectively choosing network physicians who are likely to further these efficiency objectives; and (3) the significant investment of capital, both monetary and human, in the necessary infrastructure and capability to realize the claimed efficiencies."[26] The goal is to design a service that benefits consumers with lower costs and improved care that expands consumer choice and increases competition, and is therefore procompetitive.[27] Collective negotiation of prices with payers must be reasonably necessary and ancillary to these core goals.

Experience with clinical integration and meeting FTC/DOJ criteria leads to a number of areas of emphasis for an effective and efficient provider operation that meets the requirements for clinically integrated networks:

- Physicians: Physicians lead the development of quality, cost, and access initiatives, and are responsible for creating a new service that improves care and costs for consumers;
- Interdependence: collaboration, information sharing, and building physician affinity;
- Care coordination: primary and specialty care participation in coordinating care;
- Clinical protocols: used for a wide range of diseases and conditions;
- Clinician responsibility: ensure compliance with clinical protocols;
- Infrastructure: have appropriate systems and processes to meet the goals and objectives, and training available for everyone involved;
- IT integration: use of appropriate information technology and clinical decision support;
- Performance: monitoring and improvement of physician performance, including feedback and specific action taken;

---

[26] Ibid.
[27] Statements of Antitrust Enforcement Policy in Health Care, US Department of Justice and the Federal Trade Commission, August 1996. p. 71.

- Outcomes: measurable outcomes that demonstrate improved quality and affordability;
- Results: ability to report results, provide feedback, and improve poor performance.

Once an entity is legitimately clinically integrated, with appropriate infrastructure and processes to improve quality and lower costs, it can collectively negotiate to set prices for the new service developed. Specific requirements for clinically integrated networks will be covered in Chapter 5. In addition, in the Proposed Rule CMS has included clinical integration as an important element for Medicare ACOs.

Legislative Background

In light of the unsustainable economic trends and forecasts, concerns about quality identified by such organizations as the IOM, the Institute for Healthcare Improvement, and others, and the need to improve access to care, a number of new laws have been enacted in the last decade. Two key recently enacted laws for physician-led CIN and ACO business models include: The Health Information Technology for Economic and Clinical Health Act (HITECH), part of the American Recovery and Reinvestment Act (ARRA) enacted in 2009, and the Affordable Care Act. ARRA provided some of the foundation needed for new performance-based business models to exist. For example, ARRA authorized $25B in funds[28] and incentives to physicians and hospitals to stimulate the implementation and adoption of health information technology, a key infrastructure component for delivery models requiring monitoring and reporting of quality measures.

The Affordable Care Act is one of the most significant attempts to overhaul the U.S. healthcare system in the last 50 years. The intended effects of this legislation were summarized best in a 2010 article in the *Annals of Internal Medicine*:

---

[28] Kocher R, Ezekiel EJ, DeParle NA. The Affordable Care Act and the future of clinical medicine: the opportunities and challenges. *Ann Intern Med.* 2010:153(8):536-539.

[The law] guarantees access to health care for all Americans, creates new incentives to change clinical practice to foster better coordination and quality, gives physicians more information to make them better clinicians and patients more information to make them more value-conscious consumers, and change the payment system to reward value.[29]

As noted by Dr. Kocher and colleagues, Section 3022 of the Affordable Care Act is intended to encourage the formation of Medicare ACOs, leading to opportunities for physicians and other eligible participating organizations to operate within the rules of antitrust law, find new efficiencies, benefit from new health information technology, and acquire the managerial skills and resources necessary to move these organizations forward. With demonstration projects advancing the ACO model, Section 3022 of the Affordable Care Act, known as the Medicare Shared Savings Program, gives the Department of Health and Human Services (DHHS) the authority to establish new regulations for public sector ACOs on a broader scale. This section becomes operational by law on January 1, 2012, and its governing regulations are contained in the current Proposed Rule.

Entities eligible for the CMS Shared Savings Program under Section 3022 of the Affordable Care Act and the Proposed Rule are outlined in Table 2 below. It is important to note that private payers have been involved at the national level in the evolution of the ACO model through the Patient-Centered Primary Care Collaborative[30] the Premier ACO Collaborative, Dartmouth-Brookings ACO pilots, and so-called commercial ACOs. These entities continue to establish commercial ACO programs separate from the CMS Shared Savings Program, engaging providers and provider organizations in private-sector initiatives that turn health systems and physician group practices into insurance plans. In most cases, these initiatives are applying the ACO model to patient populations other than Medicare beneficiaries and usually to multiple populations that may include employer-based payers, Medicaid, and even Medicare.

---

[29] Kocher R, Ezekiel EJ, DeParle NA. The Affordable Care Act and the future of clinical medicine: the opportunities and challenges. *Ann Intern Med.* 2010:153(8):536-539.
[30] Patient-Centered Primary Care Collaborative members list. Accessed online June 5, 2011, at http://www.pcpcc.net/content/collaborative-members.

Many of these commercial ACOs find it important to include all payers to obtain the greatest economies of scale and economic benefits from quality improvement. One problem with applying ACO services only to certain populations is that the groups not officially included still benefit from improvements in physician care--a phenomenon known as the free-rider problem. If the goal of ACO and medical home programs is to transform medical practice to improve quality of medical care and lower costs, then the transformation of the practice affects all persons treated by the physicians and hospitals. But if only certain covered populations are paying for new services provided by an ACO, they are paying disproportionately for services received by others. As we will discuss throughout this book, the industry is working toward multi-payer medical home and ACO models in which the rules and requirements include all payers.

The CMS Proposed Rule was published April 7, 2011 in the Federal Register. It provides additional insights into Congressional and Executive Branch intent for the Medicare ACOs. Central to the Proposed Rule is the establishment of a Three Part Aim set forth by Administrator Berwick that serve as overarching principles for many of the new CMS programs.

Three Part Aim
1. Better care for individuals
2. Better health for populations
3. Lower growth in expenditures

Even though the rate of growth of healthcare expenditures is moderating, actually lowering increases in expenditures remains a top imperative for policymakers due to the unsustainable growth forecasts and concerns that health care will absorb an increasingly larger share of government budgets, leaving very little funding available for other important government programs.

In the Proposed Rule the CMS also stated eight goals[31] that should be embraced by all ACOs and clinically integrated networks:

- Put beneficiaries and families at the center of all activities;
- Coordinate care for all beneficiaries at any time and any location;
- Place strong importance on care transitions;
- Manage resources carefully and respectfully to reduce waste effectively and increase value for beneficiaries;
- Put in effect communication programs and initiatives that focus on helping patients with health maintenance;
- Collect, evaluate, and use data on healthcare processes and outcomes to measure what is achieved for beneficiaries;
- Be innovative in the service of the Three Part Aim;
- Ensure continuous development of workforce and affiliated physicians.

By maintaining a focus on these goals, an ACO will be strategically positioned to deliver improved patient care while also improving quality and lowering costs. Some of the high-level requirements for the Medicare ACO program, taken from Section 3022 of the Affordable Care Act and the Proposed Rule, are provided in the table below. The requirements for a Medicaid pediatric ACO are contained in Section 2706 of the Affordable Care Act. ACOs established for commercial populations by private payers may differ from these Medicare requirements.

---

[31] Fed. Reg. Vol. 76, No. 67. April 7, 2011. I.(C) Overview and Intent of Medicare Shared Savings Program. p. 19533.

Table 2. General Requirements for a Medicare ACO Program, Affordable Care Act Section 3022 and the Proposed Rule

Topic	Description
Number of Medicare beneficiaries	Minimum of 5,000.
Governance and legal structure[32]	**Governance**: Each ACO is to employ a shared governance and leadership structure responsible for receiving and distributing payments for shared savings to eligible participants. It will have responsibility for all financial, administrative, and clinical operations. **Legal Entity**: The Medicare ACO can be structured as a corporation, limited liability company, foundation, partnership or other organization based on the laws of the ACO's home state. **Clinical Management:** Each ACO must have a full-time board-certified physician serving at one of the ACO's locations as its senior-level medical director.[33]
Time commitment to venture	Each ACO must have an agreement with DHHS to participate in the ACO program for no less than 3 years.
Eligible entities[34]	◆ ACO professionals in group practice arrangements. ◆ Networks of individual practices of ACO professionals. ◆ Partnerships or joint venture arrangements between hospitals and ACO professionals. ◆ Hospitals employing ACO professionals. ◆ Such other groups of providers of services and suppliers otherwise recognized under the Act that are not ACO professionals or hospitals, as defined in §425.4. **Rural Area Services**: federally qualified health centers (FQHC), critical access hospitals (CAH) , and rural health centers (RHC) are proposed (in the Proposed Rule) for inclusion or participation for those ACOs providing health services in rural areas as part of the nation's safety net healthcare provider operations.

---

[32] Fed. Reg. Vol. 76, No. 67. April 7, 2011. II.(B)(b). Governance. pp. 19540-19541.
[33] Fed. Reg. Vol. 76, No. 67. April 7, 2011. §425.5. Eligibility and governance requirements. p. 19643.
[34] Fed. Reg. Vol. 76, No. 67. April 7, 2011. II.(B).(1). Eligibility and Governance. pp. 19537-19538.

Table 2. General Requirements for a Medicare ACO Program, Affordable Care Act Section 3022 and the Proposed Rule, cont.

Topic	Description
Health information technology	Care coordinated through the use of telehealth, remote patient monitoring, and other enabling technologies.
Patient-centeredness criteria	Patient and caregiver assessments or individualized care plans.
Defined processes	Promotion of evidence-based medicine and patient engagement.
Performance reporting	Sixty-five proposed quality measures across five domains to be reported on annually.
Benchmark setting	DHHS to establish a benchmark for each ACO's 3-year period with the most recent 3 years of per-beneficiary Parts A and B fee-for-service expenditures assigned to the ACO (Option 1).
Shared savings	ACOs that surpass the minimum savings rate (MSR) shall be eligible for savings distributions in line with the established maximum sharing cap and maximum sharing rate.

In addition to the Medicare ACO Program, the Affordable Care Act brought about several other major programs intended to generate transformative changes in the healthcare industry. Many of these new programs and initiatives affect key areas of the industry, including insurance markets, healthcare workforce education, safety net infrastructure organizations, and comparative effectiveness research. Table 3 offers examples.

Table 3. Sample of Affordable Care Act Reforms

Insurance Market Reform		
Section	**Topic**	**Action**
1311	Affordable choices among health benefit plans	Establishes new state-level health insurance exchanges
1511–15	New requirements on insurance for employers to offer employees	Changes to employer responsibilities for employees' insurance coverage

Table 3. Sample of Affordable Care Act Reforms, cont.

Insurance Market Reform		
Section	**Topic**	**Action**
1101	Immediate access to insurance for the uninsured with preexisting conditions	Mitigates challenges to segments of the population with preexisting health conditions
2718	Lowering the cost of health care coverage	Changes in medical care ratio threshold affecting payer organizations
10202	Incentives for states to offer home- and community-based services as long-term care alternatives to nursing homes	Qualified state Medicaid programs have opportunities for medical assistance incentive payments

Research and Healthcare Education Reform		
Section	**Topic**	**Action**
937	Dissemination of and building capacity for research	New grants to fund comparative effectiveness research and the dissemination of findings from Section 6301 initiatives
6301	Creation of a new patient-centered outcomes research institute	Establishment of a new nonprofit corporation, the Patient-Centered Outcomes Research Institute, along with a research agenda
5301	Training in family medicine, general internal medicine, general pediatrics, and physician assistantship	Establishment of a new 5-year grant program for primary care training programs ($125,000,000 total appropriated funds)

Other Reforms		
Section	**Topic**	**Action**
3002	Improvement of the physician quality reporting system	Requiring integration of physician quality reporting and electronic health record reporting
5601	Funding of federally qualified health centers (FQHC)	Increased appropriations for years 2010–2015 and beyond

Some of these reforms will interact with ACO initiatives. For example, the insurance-related reforms effect the relationships of employers, patients, and private payer organizations as well as payments to ACO participants for health services. Another insurance-related reform in the Affordable Care Act that could have a major impact on ACOs involves expansion of Medicaid coverage. This expansion of eligibility will likely result in millions of new Medicaid enrollees. State Medicaid programs have traditionally paid less than Medicare or commercial payers––in some cases paying as low as 63% of the Medicare rates.[35] As health reform is implemented and hospitals and physicians find themselves with a much larger Medicaid population, they need to carefully analyze carefully the impact of potentially low Medicaid revenues on their ACO plans, especially given budgetary pressures on the states.

As part of the agreement to expand Medicaid, the states were required to increase Medicaid reimbursement to 100% of Medicare fees for the first few years of the Medicaid program's expansion, partly to calm hospitals' and physicians' concerns that low reimbursement would not cover their costs. In addition, the federal government promised to cover the full amount of the difference between the state Medicaid rates and the Medicare rates for the first years of the program, after which the states would be responsible for their portion of the increase. There is no guarantee that the federal government will continue assisting states with the added expense of an expanded Medicaid population or the higher rates required, especially with government budget shortfalls at the state level and the federal budget deficit concerns.

A number of concerns have been raised about the Proposed Rule, including the retrospective attribution process, the sheer mass of reporting elements, and the inclusion of downside risk regardless of the option chosen. These issues and others are being actively debated as of the writing of this book. Proponents of retrospective attribution argue that physicians and hospitals should provide an appropriate level of service for all patients and not just ACO-related patients.

---

[35] States administer their individual Medicaid programs, setting their own reimbursement rates within certain parameters, resulting in Medicaid payment rates for services by physicians and hospitals that differ from Medicare. The overall budget of each state Medicaid program is financed in part with state tax revenues, with federal government matching funds paying the rest. State budget shortfalls have increasingly put pressure on the Medicaid payments, generally causing them to drop.

Others argue that it is difficult to manage or improve what one cannot proactively measure—such as Medicare Shared Savings Program beneficiaries you don't know are attributed to your practice until after the fact. Another issue is the 65 proposed quality measures required to be reported. They appear to be overwhelming, even for mature health systems. While many of the measures may already be collected, other questions remain, such as data definitions and data reporting complexities, not to mention the current state of affairs in which data collection remains a manual process. Technology will improve data collection over time as ACO and health information technology (HIT) initiatives advance in parallel. In the near term, however, some have advocated the use of fewer measures that can be increased over time as systems mature.

Finally, on the issue of downside risk, the program has both an immediate and delayed option for assuming this risk. Some observers would argue that this option is a disincentive to join the CMS initiative. This result is evidenced by the sparse number of reported applicants for the program, including the notable absence of several large and well-respected health systems that have declined to enter given the language of the current Proposed Rule. Nevertheless, hospital and physician interest in ACOs combined with the legislative mandate means the Shared Savings Program will continue moving forward toward implementation. The viability of the program, however, remains to be seen as details become clearer and the operational implications are worked out at the ground level.

Four specific programs from the Affordable Care Act are of particular relevance to the ACO program. We have provided a short summary of each program below; they will be referenced throughout the book.

I. Section 3021, "Establishment of Center for Medicare and Medicaid Innovation within CMS." This new center (hereinafter referred to as CMS Innovation Center) will provide opportunities to fund innovative projects through 2019 related to improvement in care coordination, implementation of medical homes, increased use of health information technology, and models for payment reform—all of which can support the advancement of ACOs. The Affordable Care Act currently calls for $10B to be appropriated between 2011 and 2019 to fund pilot projects at preliminary testing stages and provide follow-on funds for continued operation and demonstration when experimental models prove successful. In its early stage of operation as of this writing, the Innovation Center announced the Pioneer ACO Model project in May 2011. This model is an advanced Medicare ACO program for health systems with the capabilities and infrastructure already in place to move forward with advanced risk-sharing and payment reforms. Expect to see additional ACO activities from the CMS Innovation Center, as this is one of their major areas of emphasis. Moreover, the CMS Innovation Center is not constrained by many of the requirements in the Section 3022 Shared Savings Program.

II. Section 2706 of the Affordable Care Act establishes the Pediatric Accountable Care Organization Demonstration Project, scheduled to launch on January 1, 2012. This program follows the same rules established under Section 3022 but serves as a separate program for pediatric medical care providers and state Medicaid agencies.

III. Section 3502, "Establishing community health teams to support the patient-centered medical home." This new program allows the federal government to provide contracts and grants for the purpose of creating new interdisciplinary teams to support medical homes. The health teams are comprised of "medical specialists, nurses, pharmacists, nutritionists, dieticians, social workers, behavioral and mental health providers (including substance use disorder prevention and treatment providers), doctors of chiropractic, licensed complementary and alternative medicine practitioners, and physicians' assistants."[36] These teams are responsible for providing clinical support services to aid implementation of medical homes within their geographically defined areas. The teams will indirectly assist with the implementation of ACOs, as many medical homes will operate within or as part of ACOs. This section was designed to authorize community health teams required for the Multi-Payer Advanced Primary Care Practice demonstration.[37] Appendix B provides additional details

---

[36] H.R. 3590, Patient Protection and Affordable Care Act, §3502(b)(4), Eligible entities for community health teams to support patient-centered medical homes (2010).

[37] Center for Medicare and Medicaid Services. Multi-payer Advanced Primary Care Practice (MAPCP) Demonstration Fact Sheet. Accessed online August 12, 2011, at http://www.cms.gov/DemoProjectsEvalRpts/downloads/mapcpdemo_Factsheet.pdf.

regarding the clinical support services these teams are chartered to provide in the communities they serve.

IV. Section 3001, "Establishment of a Hospital Value-Based Purchasing Program." This section of the Act provides for a new demonstration program offering value-based incentive payments based on discharges during a three-year demonstration period. The program will become operative on October 1, 2012 (fiscal year 2013), [38] to hospitals that meet the performance standards based on selected measures. For fiscal year 2013 these measures will come from two areas: conditions and procedures; and the Hospital Consumer Assessment of Healthcare Providers and Systems survey, commonly referred to as HCAHPS. The five specific conditions or procedures used as measures will include acute myocardial infarction; heart failure; pneumonia; surgical care improvement project measures; and healthcare-associated infections. Second, measures of patients' experiences with nurses, physicians, and hospitals from HCAHPS will be part of the formula for determining hospital value-based purchasing incentives payments and will be determined through the federal rule-making process prior to the start of the program.

Total incentive payments made to hospital organizations consist of a base operating diagnosis-related group payment and a value-based incentive payment percentage for the hospital for the applicable fiscal year.[39] In addition, starting in 2014 the value-based measures shall include efficiency measures based on Medicare spending per beneficiary, adjusted for key patient population demographics. This program poses an interesting relationship to the ACO program, as it implements quality measures similar to those that may be used by an ACO to measure improvement in quality and performance.

---

[38] H.R. 3590, Patient Protection and Affordable Care Act, §3001(a)(1)(B), start date for hospital value-based purchasing program (2010).
[39] H.R. 3590, Patient Protection and Affordable Care Act, §3001(a)(6)(B), calculation of value-based incentive payments (2010).

Figure 7. Benefits Alignment: ACO and Value-based Purchasing (VBP)

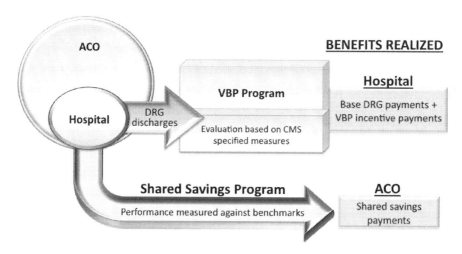

Figure 7 illustrates that when a hospital is part of an ACO (various potential models are discussed in Chapter 3), the entity could benefit financially from the ACO shared savings, base diagnosis-related group payments, and value-based purchasing incentive payments. While only the hospital can receive the value-based purchasing program and diagnosis-related group incentive payments as they are designated for inpatient hospital services,[40] one can see how the structure created by the ACO's formation with governance, leadership, and health information technology elements could yield opportunities for these rewards to support the ACO's structure and mission.

ACO Pilot Programs and Demonstrations

A number of pilot projects and demonstrations related to ACOs have been and are being conducted across the country. We shall discuss these efforts in two separate categories: public sector-related ACO projects and private sector-related ACO projects.

---

[40] Fed. Reg. Vol. 76, No. 6. January 13, 2011. Medicare Program; Hospital Inpatient Value-Based Purchasing Program. pp. 2454-2491.

Public Sector Projects

The original public sector demonstration, the Medicare Physician Group Practice Demonstration Project launched in 2000 is ongoing as of early 2011.[41] The program was initially established as a five-year program involving ten different physician groups. Its purpose is summarized in the 2009 CMS program fact sheet:

> The demonstration creates incentives for physician groups to coordinate the overall care delivered to Medicare patients, rewards them for improving the quality and cost efficiency of health care services, and creates a framework to collaborate with providers to the advantage of Medicare beneficiaries.[42]

The physician groups participating in the demonstration include the Dartmouth-Hitchcock Clinic, Geisinger Clinic, Marshfield Clinic, Park Nicollet Health Services, Forsyth Medical Group, Middlesex Health System, St. John's Health System, Billings Clinic, the Everett Clinic, and the University of Michigan Faculty Group Practice. Thirty-two ambulatory and preventive care measures were selected to evaluate improvement in outcomes in the demonstration. These quality measures were identified for three diseases and conditions (diabetes mellitus, congestive heart failure, and coronary artery disease) and preventive care as fourth priority area for the demonstration project.

[41] Centers for Medicare and Medicaid Services. *Roadmap for Implementing Value-driven Healthcare in the Traditional Medicare Fee-for-Service Program*, Physician PGP Demonstration. p. 13. Accessed online July 20, 2011, at http://www.cms.gov/QualityInitiativesGenInfo/downloads/VBPRoadmap_OEA_1-16_508.pdf.

[42] Center for Medicare and Medicaid Services. Physician Group Practice Demonstration Program. (December 2010). p. 1. Accessed online July 20, 2011 at https://www.cms.gov/DemoProjectsEvalRpts/downloads/PGP_Fact_Sheet.pdf.

Table 4. Physician Group Practice Demonstration Quality Measures[43]

Diabetes Mellitus	Congestive Heart Failure	Coronary Artery Disease	Preventive Care
HbA1c Management	Left Ventricular Function Assessment	Antiplatelet Therapy	Blood Pressure Screening
HbA1c Control	Left Ventricular Ejection Fraction Testing	Drug Therapy for Lowering LDL Cholesterol	Blood Pressure Control
Blood Pressure Management	Weight Measurement	Beta-Blocker Therapy – Prior MI	Blood Pressure Control Plan of Care
Lipid Measurement	Blood Pressure Screening	Blood Pressure	Breast Cancer Screening
LDL Cholesterol Level	Patient Education	Lipid Profile	Colorectal Cancer Screening
Urine Protein Testing	Beta-Blocker Therapy	LDL Cholesterol Level	
Eye Exam	ACE Inhibitor Therapy	ACE Inhibitor Therapy	
Foot Exam	Warfarin Therapy for Patients HF		
Influenza Vaccination	Influenza Vaccination		
Pneumonia Vaccination	Pneumonia Vaccination		

As a result of improved outcomes—all ten participants surpassed their goals for 28 measures—five of the physician groups shared in $78.1M of incentive payments out of $97.9M in total savings for improving quality of care based on the specified ambulatory care and preventive care measures over the four-year performance period from 2006 through 2009.[44] It is interesting to note that the other five physician groups did not obtain any incentive payments. The 2010 report noted a number of factors that contributed to achievement of the program goals including:

---

[43] Centers for Medicare and Medicaid Services. Physician Group Practice Demonstration Program (December 2010). p. 3. Accessed online July 20, 2011, at https://www.cms.gov/DemoProjectsEvalRpts/downloads/PGP_Fact_Sheet.pdf.
[44] Centers for Medicare and Medicaid Services. Physician Group Practice Demonstration Program. (December 2010). pp. 4-5. Accessed online July 20, 2011, at https://www.cms.gov/DemoProjectsEvalRpts/downloads/PGP_Fact_Sheet.pdf.

- Having clinical champions (doctor or nurse) responsible for quality reporting at each practice.
- Redesign of clinical care processes.
- Investment in health information technology, electronic health records, and patient registry improvements that allow practices to better identify gaps in care; alert physicians to gaps during patient visits; and provide feedback on performance.

Appendix C provides an additional summary of these ten organizations, their individual approaches, and benefits derived from their demonstrations. Chapter 7 will also touch on some specific performance measure results from their efforts.

A second public sector example is related to Section 2706 (Pediatric Accountable Care Organization demonstrations). Because of the focus on a specific population, pediatric patients--these projects will be different from the Medicare shared savings program, even though they will be governed by the same rules. An illustration of an existing pediatric ACO is the Nationwide Children's Hospital organization in Columbus, Ohio.[45] Already organized as a pediatric accountable care organization under their Partners for Kids physician hospital organization, this organization has over 760 physicians caring for over 285,000 pediatric patients across central and southeastern Ohio. Payments are arranged through capitated Medicaid fees for pediatric Medicaid patients from three Medicaid programs.[46]

While most of the literature surrounding ACOs focuses on initiatives related to adult patients, a key point regarding these Medicaid pediatric ACOs should be made—each state has its own Medicaid laws and the state can influence the focus and mandate the operations of these ACOs separately from the Medicare- or private payer-based ACOs.

---

[45] Nationwide Children's Hospital Accountable Care Organization. Accessed online July 20, 2011, at https://www.nationwidechildrens.org/accountable-care-organization.
[46] ACO discussions begin; pediatricians will play a role. *Hospitalist News* [serial online], September 9, 2010. Accessed online July 20, 2011, at http://www.ehospitalistnews.com/news/practice-trendsleaders/single-article/aco-discussions-begin-pediatricians-will-play-a-role/38db10d39d.html.

As federal rules are defined, state rules will emerge from state Medicaid offices that may differ from the federal rules in such areas as pediatric-specific quality measures.

Private Sector Projects

In the private sector, a number of organizations have led efforts to prepare physician practice groups and health systems for ACO implementation. The Premier ACO Collaboratives[47] and the Accountable Care Organization Learning Network,[48] a joint initiative between the Brookings Institute and the Dartmouth Institute for Health Policy and Clinical Practice, are two of the leading programs. These programs meet industry needs to understand and prepare for implementation of the ACO model. First, they facilitate forums for participants to share lessons from similar organizations that have started the process of implementing an ACO. Second, the collaboratives provide opportunities for those organizations further down the path of implementation to help with guidance and serve as valuable case studies of early adopters.

The Premier Collaborative has 24 health systems engaged in their implementation collaborative[49] and 49 health systems in their ACO Readiness Collaborative[50] as of September 24, 2010. The Dartmouth-Brookings collaborative has engaged three different health systems for pilot ACO projects: Carilion Clinic in Roanoke, Virginia; Norton Healthcare in Louisville, Kentucky; and Tucson Medical Center in Tucson, Arizona.[51] Each organization in these demonstration projects is at a different stage in its ACO readiness or implementation. Norton Healthcare is partnering with Humana. Tucson Medical Center with United Healthcare, and Carilion Clinic with Aetna.[52,53]

---

[47] Premier Accountable Care Organization Collaboratives. Accessed online July 20, 2011, at http://www.premierinc.com/quality-safety/tools-services/ACO/index.jsp.
[48] Brookings-Dartmouth ACO Learning Network.
[49] Premier ACO Implementation Collaborative Participants (as of 9/24/10).
[50] Premier ACO Implementation Collaborative Participants (as of 9/24/10).
[51] Taylor M. The ABCs of ACOs. Accountable care organizations unite hospitals and other providers in caring for the community. *Trustee*. 2010;63(6):12-14.
[52] Tucson Medical Center picked to pilot program to improve patients' health, reduce costs. *Tucson Business* 3/12/10. Accessed online July 20, 2011 at http://www.azbiz.com/articles/2010/03/12/news/doc4b9a74a555d04943487875.txt; Norton, Humana involved in pilot program emphasizing wellness, preventive care. *Courier Journal* 11/21/10; Roberson J. Growing an ACO—easier said than done. *Physician Executive*, September-October 2010.

Part of the ACO concept is the ability to maintain flexibility. Case studies of organizations participating in the CMS Physician Group Practice Demonstration Program showed that each organization focused on improving different aspects of their clinical processes and programs (Appendix C). Likewise, as early adopters evolve, the industry will learn about benefits realized and lessons derived from innovations implemented by these participating organizations in such different areas as governance, infrastructure, leadership, technology, decision support, and cultural change as well as payment model reform. In addition, each ACO participant may concentrate on such different technical challenges as advanced application of electronic health records and health information exchange to strengthen care coordination, medical home initiatives and meeting CMS meaningful use requirements.

An example of the formation of an ACO-like arrangement in the private sector is the Blue Cross/Blue Shield of Massachusetts Alternative quality contract program.[54] While not an ACO by definition, it demonstrates novel payment arrangements that could be considered by ACOs. Launched in 2009, this program focuses on implementing an "innovative global payment model that uses a budget based methodology, which combines a fixed per-patient payment (adjusted annually for health status and inflation) with substantial performance incentive payments (tied to the latest nationally accepted measures of quality, effectiveness, and patient experience)." This is a hybrid medical home shared-savings program for those providers who agree to participate. As of early 2010, Blue Cross/Blue Shield of Massachusetts had contracted with nine provider groups in its network to engage in the program, which provides participants support with training, metrics dashboards, reporting, regular communications, and best-practice sharing. While not established as identical to the ACO concept and not specifically calling for a hospital or physician-led provider entity as is the case with the ACO model, the program is set up as a five-year arrangement for participating providers. It focuses on payment reform and performance measurement, looking at both ambulatory and hospital-based measures.

---

[53] Aetna and Carilion Clinic Announce Accountable Care Collaboration, March 10, 2011, accessed online August 10, 2011 at http://www.carilionclinic.org/Carilion/CC+Aetna.
[54] Blue Cross Blue Shield of Massachusetts Alternative Quality Contract Program. Accessed online July 20, 2011, at http://www.qualityaffordability.com/solutions/alternative-quality-contract.html.

Summary

The foundation for change is in place with the strategic direction set by the Institute of Medicine, Department of Health and Human Services, and Centers for Medicare and Medicaid Services, and other key industry stakeholders. Public and private ACO models are being implemented and are evolving separately. Given the challenges and complexities of working with the federal government, it is very important for a public ACO to keep a long-term perspective and work toward a multi-payer ACO model[55] that allows the ACO to reap the benefits of increased reimbursement in exchange for improved population health management, reduced cost of care, improved reporting, and strong accountability. In May 2011 the CMS Innovation Center announced the establishment of the Pioneer ACO Model.[56] Organizations engaging in this advanced model will be able to demonstrate they already perform advanced care coordination for patients across multiple sites and have the infrastructure and systems in place to move forward at an accelerated pace in transitioning out of fee-for-service payment toward a "value-based model" that works to incorporate a multi-payer approach to performance, benchmark setting and shared savings evaluation. The notion of this advanced ACO model will be addressed again in later chapters.

A concept from the first edition of this book retained in this edition is the roadmap for the path to CIN and ACO establishment. These roadmaps are strategic and present a set of ideas for "functional streams" (not all-inclusive) that need to be engaged by resources from ACO and CIN participants to drive their healthcare finance and delivery models forward. While similar to a "value stream" map, these maps are not intended to show all interlocking paths. They should be used instead to generate ideas of the various critical actionable elements necessary for executive physician, clinician, and administrator action. Three chronological phases are placed across the top of each map. This arrangement is to provide a notion of progress over time, which may vary for

---

[55] MedPAC Report to Congress: Improving Incentives in the Medicare Program (June 2009), Chapter 2: Accountable Care Organizations. p. 55. Accessed online July 20, 2011, at www.medpac.gov/documents/Jun09_EntireReport.pdf.
[56] Fed Reg. Vol. 76 No. 98. Request for Applications to Medicare Pioneer ACO Model. May 20, 2011 pp. 29249-29250.

each organization based on its resources and infrastructure in place. The first map presented is one that is overarching with eight functional streams identified that are typical functional areas across many healthcare organizations.

Figure 8. Roadmap 1: CIN and ACO- Advancing Care Delivery

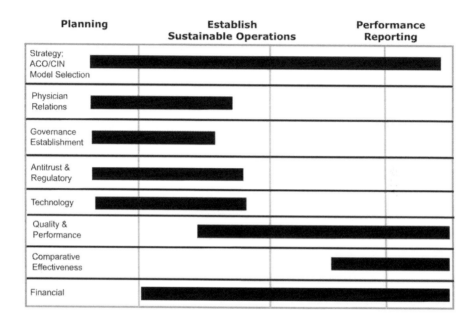

Other maps throughout this book will identify additional unique functional stream areas pertinent to the topic being discussed in the chapter. These streams highlight key topics covered throughout the book.

Assessing and reaching consensus on implementation strategies and choosing whether to embark on a CIN or ACO path is a key threshold issue at the start of any program. As resources and goals shift over the life of the entity, the strategy should be revised annually and updated to set a new baseline for all stakeholders and evaluators of organizational progress, including consumers and patients in the organization. To drive the CIN or ACO forward, recruiting key regional primary care and specialty care physician groups as participants, are needed. Each plays a significant role in the development and management of every CIN and ACO.

The United States faces tremendous challenges in providing needed healthcare services as well as managing their cost and continuing to improve the quality of care. Many physicians practicing in the field are skeptical of the changes that lie ahead. A 2010 survey conducted with over 100,000 physicians after the release of the Affordable Care Act found strong sentiments expressed regarding anticipated increases in patient volume that must be handled with resources already stressed. Other respondents were even more concerned that the legislation will lead to the closing of more private practices.[57] Even amidst these challenges, ACOs, the shift to pay-for-performance, value-based purchasing, population health management, rising consumer expectations, and other agents of change are already affecting our nation's healthcare services.

[57] Physicians Foundation. Health reform and the decline of physician private practice. p. 45. Accessed online June 15, 2011, at: http://www.physiciansfoundation.org/uploadedFiles/Health%20Reform%20and%20the%20Decline%20of%20Physician%20Priv ate%20Practice.pdf.

Chapter 2. Primary Care Engagement: The Foundation

A physician is obligated to consider more than a diseased organ, more even than the whole man - he must view the man in his world.

Harvey Williams Cushing, M.D.
Father of modern neurosurgery
(1869-1939)

Background of the Patient-Centered Medical Home

The medical home is a major industry initiative for the primary care sector that was first introduced in 1967 by the American Academy of Pediatrics. Initially a program designed to aggregate all paper records of a child in one practice, it has gained significant momentum in the past ten years. A basic element of the contemporary medical home is the chronic care model that emerged in 2002.[58] This model provides components of care intended to meet major challenges for redesigning the healthcare system, as described in the Institute of Medicine's 2001 report titled *Crossing the Quality Chasm*.[59] These challenges are illustrated in Figure 9 below, and represent both the need to reform primary care services and the advancement of such other care delivery transformation initiatives as the CIN and ACO.

---

[58] Bodenheimer T, Wagner EH, Grumbach K. Improving primary care for patients with chronic illness: the chronic care model, Part 2. *JAMA.* 2002;288(15):1909-1914.
[59] Institute of Medicine, Committee on Quality of Health Care in America. Formulating new rules to redesign and improve care. In: *Crossing the Quality Chasm: A New Health System for the 21st Century.* Washington, DC: National Academies Press; 2001:61–62.

Figure 9. IOM's Six Challenges for Redesign (2001)

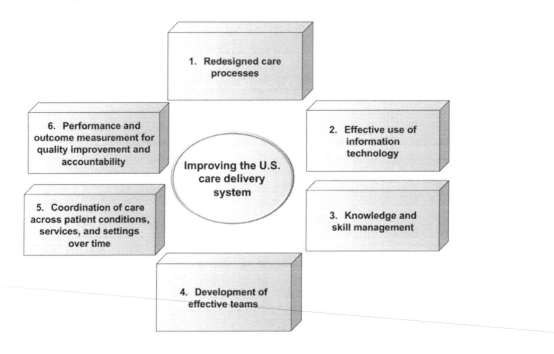

Looking at the IOM's redesign challenges for healthcare organizations, all six are addressed in the central design principles for a CIN and the ACO as well as the foundational elements and principles of the medical home model. The medical home is based on a set of principles approved jointly by the American College of Physicians, the American Academy of Family Physicians, the American Academy of Pediatrics, and the American Osteopathic Association in 2007 (Joint Principles). These principles are:

- Physician-directed medical services
- Quality and safety
- Personal physician
- Whole-person orientation
- Payment reform
- Coordinated and integrated care
- Enhanced access to care

The medical home is essentially a transformation of the practice of medicine, involving both cultural and workplace changes in the practice of family medicine. With so much change occurring in the past decade, however, practicing physicians are challenged to keep up. One thing that has become clear, however, is the need for change in the medical school curricula to support future physicians in understanding the medical home and other changes occurring in healthcare. To improve the training of family physicians the nation's medical schools have made great strides at incorporating elements of the Joint Principles into the didactic training and experiential curricula, covering such critical topics as population health management, engaging in and adopting health information technology, and the use of disease registries.[60] But as the medical home model and its incorporation into CINs and ACOs continues to evolve, it will be increasingly important for medical educators to refine curricula for their students. They need to understand how practicing physicians and physician leaders in the field are overcoming challenges to transform the physician community culture to improve care coordination for effective population health management in the CIN and ACO models of care delivery.

Medical home implementation focuses on practice transformation by improving coordination and integration of care; strengthening partnerships among physicians, patients, and their families; adopting and using electronic health records and other health information technologies; and implementing methods of tracking performance measures based on industry-recognized requirements. Improving patients' access to care through open-access and flexible scheduling, appropriate use of the team concept, and proactive management between office visits are only a few of the activities conducted in the medical home. For many physicians, however, these changes represent disruptive innovations to traditional office practice. The uncertainty of moving to on-demand same-day appointment scheduling or corresponding with patients electronically are challenges that must be met. True roll-up-your-sleeves work is required to overcome older embedded patterns. This task parallels the substantial changes that ACOs will require of hospitals and hospital systems.

---

[60] David A, Baxley L. Education of Students and Residents in Patient Centered Medical Home (PCMH): Preparing the Way. *Ann Fam Med.* 2011 May-Jun;9(3):274-5.

While certification as a medical home is not the only measure of success, it is one way to obtain recognition and begin the transformation.

The National Committee for Quality Assurance (NCQA) is recognized as the primary industry certification and recognition program for the medical home model. Physician Practice Connections®–Patient-Centered Medical Home (PPC-PCMH™) is the present name of the NCQA program and certification. It has nine standards for physician practice reward and incentive payment eligibility. Attaining this certification supports key tenets for a CIN and in 2011 the NCQA is establishing the first accreditation program for ACOs. We will mention three topics central to the NCQA PPC-PCMH™ program, including some of which are specifically addressed in the committee's guidance for physician practices: program standards; steps to achieving recognition; and program scoring. First, in 2011 the NCQA refined its previous nine standards for attainment of PPC-PCMH™ recognition to a set of six "must-pass elements."

Figure 10. PPC-PCMH™ Standards[61]

Standards and Sections	Points	Standards and Sections	Points
Standard 1: Enhance Access/Continuity		**Standard 4: Provide Self-Care and Community Support**	
a. Access during office hours **	4		
b. Access after hours	4	a. Self-care process **	6
c. Electronic access	2	b. Referrals to community resources	3
d. Continuity	2		9
e. Medical home responsibilities	2		
f. Culturally and linguistically appropriate services	2		
g. Practice organization	4		
	20		
Standard 2: Identify and Manage Patient Populations	3	**Standard 5: Track and Coordinate Care**	
a. Patient information	4	a. Test tracking and follow-up	6
b. Clinical data	4	b. Referral tracking and follow-up **	6
c. Comprehensive health assessment	5	c. Coordinate with facilities / Care transitions	6
d. Use of data for population management **	17		18
Standard 3: Plan and Manage Care		**Standard 6: Measure and Improve Performance**	4
a. Implement evidence-based guidelines	4	a. Measures of performance	4
b. Identify high-risk patients	3	b. Patient/family feedback	4
c. Manage care **	4	c. Implements continuous quality improvement **	3
d. Manage medications	3	d. Demonstrates continuous quality improvement	3
e. Electronic prescribing	3	e. Performance reporting	2
	17	f. Report data externally	20

** Indicates "must pass" elements

---

[61] New PCMH 2011 Content and Scoring Summary. Accessed online June 1, 2011 at http://www.ncqa.org/tabid/631/Default.aspx.

Six must-pass elements are included within the six standards. By meeting these must-pass elements, a primary care practice can be set up to achieve improved chronic care management and patient compliance on prescribed interventions; stronger performance reporting; and the adoption and competent use of health information technology. As primary care practices provide part of the foundation for an ACO and CIN network model, applying for and achieving the PPC-PCMH™ certification serves as a strong indication that systemic processes are in place to aid physician leaders, clinical care groups, and administrative teams in the launching of an ACO or CIN.

Second are seven "Steps for the Physician/Practice" to achieve National Committee for Quality Assurance recognition.

Table 5. Steps to Recognition[62]

Step No.	Description
1	Review program information
2	Participate in a standards workshop
3	Obtain a survey tool
4	Participate in a WebEx ISS demonstration of the survey tool
5	Use survey tool to self-assess current performance
6	Submit completed application, agreements, fee, and results to NCQA
7	Receive final recognition decision and level in 30-60 days

The survey tool is central to the certification process and achieving required scores on the nine standards. This instrument helps a practice assess its progress in preparing to submit an application and is required for recognition.

The third concern is program scoring. The NCQA established a three-level qualification model based on the six-certification standards.

---

[62] NCQA Standards Workshop. Physician Practice Connections—Patient-Centered Medical Home, 2009. Slide 94. Accessed online July 20, 2011, at http://www.ncqa.org/.

Table 6. NCQA PCMH 2011 Scoring by Level[63]

Level of Qualifying	Points	Must Pass Elements at 50% Performance Level
Not Recognized	0-34	< 6
Level 1	35-59	6 of 6
Level 2	60-84	6 of 6
Level 3	85-100	6 of 6

Physician practices that apply to the program make an investment through the purchase of the survey tool, application fees, and costs associated with the transformation of the practice's workflow, tools and culture. By progressing through the three levels of recognition, physician practices are better positioned to take advantage of and capture private and public financial incentives based on achieving and maintaining improvements in quality of care and operational performance.

Common Ground: Medical Home and ACO

The medical home model has been identified as a starting point for successful implementation of the ACO, and with the focus on improving access to care; coordination of care; and performance reporting, they also strengthen initiatives for successful CIN implementation. In fact a close alignment can be illustrated between the seven joint principles of the medical home and the three core principles of the ACO.

---

[63] NCQA Patient-Centered Medical Home Standards Workshop 2011. Part 1: Standards 1-3. Slide 9. Accessed online July 2, 2011 at http://www.ncqa.org/tabid/1316/Default.aspx.

Figure 11. Alignment of PCMH and ACO Principles

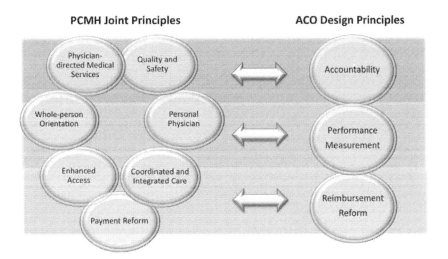

Each of the three ACO design principles is considered in relationship to the medical home principles to provide perspective on this common ground. As noted earlier an additional area of commonality is with the new ACO accreditation; however our focus here is with the medical home and the core ACO design principles.

The medical home model follows a three-level certification and recognition process based on standards and elements to be met by all physician groups applying to the NCQA for recognition. In the case of ACOs, industry experts and the National Committee for Quality Assurance have explored the issues related to qualification and certification. In two articles published in 2010. Shortell and colleagues proposed a three-tier qualification model for CMS to consider adopting and adding to the federal rules on structuring public sector ACOs.[64] In the article from the *Journal of the American Medical Association*, the authors recommended a three-level qualification process for ACOs that could be combined with a set of characteristics set forth in their article in the May 2010 issue of *Health Affairs*.[39]

---

[64] Shortell SM, Casalino LP, Fisher ES. How the center for medicare and medicaid innovation should test accountable care organizations. *Health Aff (Millwood)*. 2010;29(7):1293–1298. Fisher ES, Shortell SM. Accountable care organizations: accountable for what, to whom, and how. *JAMA*. 2010;304(15):1715–1716.

Table 7. CMS ACO Qualification Levels and Characteristics

Level	Qualification Level[65]	Characteristics[66]
1	ACOs without electronic health records: could rely for the near term on key measures derived from claims data	◆ Legal entity with basic health information technology and performance reporting capabilities ◆ Shared savings for meeting quality and cost targets without downside risk ◆ Adoption of core starter set measures: quality, efficiency, and patient experience
2	ACOs with site-specific electronic health records and registries: expected to add more advanced measures (such as patient-reported health outcomes for selected conditions)	◆ Strong infrastructure in place with advanced health information technology and care coordination staff ◆ Larger shared savings with accountability for cost performance ◆ Adoption of core starter set measures: quality, efficiency, and patient experience
3	ACOs with comprehensive electronic health records across all sites: may be used to test and implement measurement systems to drive practice improvement and accountability in areas that challenge the industry (such as informed patient choice and health outcomes for a variety of conditions)	◆ Advanced infrastructure, full complement of services, and reserve requirements ◆ Risk-adjusted partial capitation coupled with performance bonuses ◆ Strongest performance and reporting targets

These qualifications and characteristics were only proposals based on recommendations from industry experts. They show an increasing capability to identify actions that improve quality and assume greater risk and reward as the medical home infrastructure and experience evolve. While the Proposed Rule does not contain a specific "three-level certification program," guidance was included to evolve from a one-sided to a two-sided risk-sharing model. One-sided

---

[65] Fisher ES, Shortell SM. Accountable care organizations: accountable for what, to whom, and how. *JAMA*. 2010;304(15):1715-1716.
[66] McClellan M, McKethan AN, Lewis JL, Roski J, Fisher ES. A national strategy to put accountable care into practice. *Health Aff (Millwood)*. 2010;29(5):982-990.

risk puts an ACO at risk for potential upside rewards based on shared savings, while two-sided risk allows the ACO to benefit from dollars saved, but also puts the entity 'at risk' for lesser performance or missed expense reductions. The decision to participate in the Medicare ACO model should be based on the participant organization's willingness to take risk, and the existing ability of the organization to manage that risk both clinically and financially. As ACOs are formed, more unified requirements will emerge allowing physicians and hospitals to better understand the infrastructure needed to both improve quality and reduce costs––thereby enabling them to manage risk and obtain greater rewards. Until such experience is accumulated, it will be impossible to determine whether certification can effectively predict success. Next we consider how each of the ACO design principles is aligned with the joint principles of the medical home.

Accountability

Accountability is central to the business success of the ACO. For the healthcare industry to move away from the fee-for-service system and the HMO-dominated private insurer market, placing physicians as the leaders of ACOs and assuring their accountability for results is of paramount importance. In terms of the model depicted in Figure 11, one can draw an immediate parallel between physician-directed medical services, having a personal physician, and an emphasis on quality and safety on the one side, and the ACO element of accountability for clinical and financial results on the other side. All three themes in the medical home can be directly related to the importance of having physicians in leadership roles in an ACO.

Accountability extends beyond the single encounter or episode of care. From this perspective we are moving toward measures of ongoing health and health maintenance across the entire population. Last, no discussion of accountability is complete without considering the patient. The health care team can accomplish much but they cannot do it alone. Personal responsibility and patient self-management are integral to obtaining good results. The ACO is designed to better equip patients to take ownership of their healthcare. Reminder notices, follow-up visits, simplified navigation of complex health care systems—all better enable patients to help their physician obtain the results that both expect. Thus, engaging patients in their own care and partnering with them are essential features of both the medical home and the ACO. Surprisingly, the Medicare shared savings program did not require some level of accountability or personal responsibility from the patients.

Performance Measurement

Defining benchmarks for ACO evaluation are important in establishing the performance measures of structure, process, outcomes, and cost. The central principles of whole-person orientation, coordinated and integrated care, and enhanced access to care provide a framework for specific performance measures. Chapter 7 will address benchmark setting in greater detail. Two other important areas in the Proposed Rule related to performance measurement are processes to promote patient engagement and promote coordination of care. Patient engagement in the management of personal healthcare starts with understanding preventive activities that patients can use to improve their own health, and continues with enabling better access to care providers when needed. Evaluating efforts to improve the coordination of care is, in part, hinges in part on the adoption of such new technologies as remote monitoring, telemedicine, EHRs, and predictive modeling tools to better coordinate care within and beyond the defined geographic boundaries of an ACO.[67]

Reimbursement Reform

Reimbursement reform is central to success for both the medical home and the ACO. As discussed above, moving away from the fee-for-service/episode-of-care model of reimbursement in the direction of adoption of advanced methods— including bundled service payments, partial capitation, value-based purchasing arrangements, and shared savings incentives—is critical to success. More specifically, paying the physician and the care team to provide care between

---

[67] Fed. Reg. Vol. 76, No. 67. April 7, 2011. II.(B)(9) Process To Promote Evidence-Based Medicine, Patient Engagement Reporting, and Coordination of Care. p. 19546-19547.

episodes of treatment is essential to making the model work. Some of these methods have already been tested previously and will be used in new models under both Section 3021 of the Innovation projects and Section 3022 Shared Savings Program.

There is one significant difference between the medical home and ACO worth mentioning. A 2009 report by the American Academy of Family Physicians Task Force. noted:

> The Accountable Care Organization model mainly differs from the Joint Principles of the PCMH in that the medical home focuses on physician practice structure and processes improvements (e.g. electronic health records, patient registries, same-day appointments, etc.) and not on accountability for cost and quality for a defined patient population.[68]

While there are differences between medical homes and ACOs, these are not a shortcoming or inconsistency. Rather, the medical home provides many foundational elements that are essential to the formation of ACOs and clinical integration, evidence of the ongoing evolution of the healthcare delivery system.

Successful Medical Home Models Leading to ACO Industry Initiatives

Two examples of successful medical homes that could form the foundation for future ACO initiatives are the Vermont Blueprint for Health and the Geisinger Medical Home Initiative.[69]

Vermont Blueprint for Health

The Vermont Blueprint for Health Project[70] began in 2006 as a state-based health care reform program with two phases: the first, an enhanced medical home

---

[68] AAFP Accountable Care Organization Task Force Report, October 2009. Accessed online July 20, 2011, at http://www.aafp.org/online/etc/medialib/aafp_org/documents/policy/private/healthplans/payment/acos/acotfreport.Par.0001.File.d at/AAFP-ACO-Report-NoRecs-20091010.pdf.
[69] Fields D, Leshen E, Patel K. Analysis and commentary. Driving quality gains and cost savings through adoption of medical homes. *Health Aff (Millwood)*. 2010;29(5):819–826.

model; and the second, implementation of an ACO-like shared savings program. The state of Vermont provides a unique payer environment, as it has only three commercial payers and a history of collaboration on reform initiatives. Vermont's model "creates a shared savings incentive pool based on projected medical expenses, which is distributed on the basis of agreed-on quality measures and population health targets." By end of 2009, three enhanced medical home community pilot programs were established with five components.

Table 8. Components of the Vermont Pilot Program[71]

Component	Description
Financial reform	Private and public payers agreed to make changes that included monthly per capita payments to each practice and funding of a community health team, similar in nature to the new program required by Section 3502 of the Affordable Care Act.
Community health teams	Multidisciplinary clinician teams focused on providing direct services to support the program's physician practices.
Health information technology	Each practice uses a web-based patient data tracking system called DocSite Registry, mapped to EHRs and state-driven health information exchanges to provide population-based reports.
Community activation and preventive care	Three tasks assigned to the community health teams include: development and management of community risk profiles; setting priorities for preventive care interventions; and design and implementation of a "local prevention plan in coordination with the delivery system."
Evaluation	Program effectiveness is evaluated over a period of 20 months for the patient population based on "NCQA Patient-Centered Medical Home scores, clinical process measures, health status measures, cost and utilization measures from a multi-payer claims database, and population health indicators." Results will be compared to matched samples of patients outside the program's area.

The first phase of the program lays the foundation for the second phase and the implementation of the shared savings program. A central feature of the planning for the Vermont Pilot Program was a focus on the Institute for

---

[70] Hester J Jr. Designing Vermont's pay-for-population health system. *Prev Chronic Dis.* 2010;7(6):1-6. Accessed online July 20, 2011, at http://www.cdc.gov/pcd/issues/2010/nov/pdf/10_0072.pdf.
[71] Hester J Jr. Designing Vermont's pay-for-population health system. *Prev Chronic Dis.* 2010;7(6):6. The reader is referred to the section titled "Phase I: Enhanced Medical Home."

Healthcare Improvement's Triple Aim Project.[72] The three tenets of this project are 1) control of total per capita medical costs; 2) improvement of population health; and 3) improvement of consumers' healthcare experience. While the shared savings portion of the project is still in the planning stage as of January 2011, the foundation is in place and the state's positive collaboration with payers should provide valuable insights for future implementations.

Geisinger Health System

The second medical home model is that implemented by the Geisinger Health System (hereinafter referred to as Geisinger). Geisinger is an integrated delivery system headquartered in Danville, Pennsylvania, with three acute care hospitals along with nearly 61 clinical practice sites that provide adult and pediatric primary and specialty care. Geisinger serves a population of over 2.6 million patients as of early 2011. The system is recognized as an industry leader for innovation in delivery system initiatives; is one of ten participants in the CMS Physician Group Practice Demonstration Project; is a member of Premier's ACO Collaborative Implementation Workgroup; and is a recipient of a BEACON Community Grant from the Office of National Coordinator for Health Information Technology.

Two pioneering innovations that have contributed to Geisinger's successful medical home implementation and ACO model preparation are its Personal Health Navigator and Geisinger Proven Care®.[73] The Personal Health Navigator system and its services include 24/7 access to primary and specialty care; a nursing care coordinator at all community practice sites; predictive tools to identify risk trends; virtual care management support; and evidence-based care to reduce hospitalization.

---

[72] Institute for Healthcare Improvement (IHI). The Triple Aim Project. Accessed online July 20, 2011, at http://www.ihi.org/IHI/Programs/StrategicInitiatives/TripleAim.htm.
[73] Paulus RA, Davis K, Steele GD. Continuous innovation in health care: implications of the Geisinger experience. *Health Aff (Millwood)*. 2008;27(5):1235-1245.

Additional features of the Geisinger medical home model include access to electronic health records for physicians, patients, and care managers; practice-based payments that include base monthly payments to physicians, a stipend for each practice, and incentive payments shared by physicians and care teams; and performance reports that are jointly reviewed by members of each community practice in concert with their payer group.

Another innovation that strengthens Geisinger's position as an industry leader of early ACO implementation is their acute-episode care program called Geisinger ProvenCare.® This program, which focused initially on coronary artery bypass graft procedures, has three primary elements: putting best practices in place across the full episode of care; creation of risk-based pricing with an up-front discount to the payer for the historical readmission rate; and establishment of a path to patient engagement. Given the success of these programs and others at Geisinger, the system is a leader to watch for best-practice implementation as it evolves towards an ACO model.

As health reform legislation shed light on ACOs over the last few years, Dr. Shortell, a leading proponent of integrated delivery, provided a set of must-haves for all ACOs in 2009.[74] The parallels between these must-haves for ACOs and the existing requirements for medical homes shows why the medical home is viewed as a foundational element of ACOs.

---

[74] Shortell SM. Organizing healthcare for higher quality and lower cost. Slideshow presented at: Capstone Conference; May 14, 2009; Menlo Park, CA. Accessed online July 20, 2011 at http://www.slideshare.net/capstoneconference09/stephen-shortell-organizing-health-care-for-higher-quality-and-lower-cost-1456226.

Table 9. ACO Must–Haves...

No.	Element
1	Have a governance structure that is the focal point for accountability
2	Able to measure costs, productivity, quality, and outcomes of care
3	Able to aggregate data from individual units
4	Have a sufficient number of patients to detect statistically significant differences in performance from established targets
5	Able to report data to external groups
6	Have the information technology and work process design capability to improve care on a continuous basis

This list embodies several of the key tenets of ACOs already described. In addition to these six tenets, a seventh must-have is proposed:

Relentless drive to achieve new levels of integration for the benefit of improving quality of care across targeted patient populations.

This seventh tenet focuses on creating efficiencies, critical for ACOs and CINs to be successful, but also highlights the relentless effort needed to achieve these new levels of integration and efficiency. Maintaining a relentless drive will require determined and motivated teams and physician leaders who work closely with practicing physicians, nurse leaders, administrators, and staff to make the difficult changes necessary to improve quality of care. These first six elements, while originally proposed for ACOs, are also critical for the success of CINs. All these principles and the CMS Three Part Aim should be integrated into the objectives of future ACOs and CINs.

One final medical home example that has emerged from CMS is the Multi-Payer Advanced Primary Care Practice (MAPCP) Demonstration. This program, announced by Secretary Sebelius in 2009 and awarded to eight states in late 2010, provides an opportunity for the selected states to participate in an advanced medical home program that will take a multi-payer approach to medical home services designed to improve care for a broad population.[75] The states are required to coordinate all payers including Medicaid, Medicare and private payers. A central focus of the program is to create medical homes using health information technology and practice transformation. To avoid overlapping programs and potentially confounding results, the organizations involved in an MAPCP demonstration will be allowed to participate in ACOs "...as long as the payment under the MAPCP demonstration does not involve a shared savings component."[76] The MAPCP is a three-year demonstration started in 2011. As the demonstration moves forward, it will be interesting to monitor lessons and best practices obtained from the demonstration participants' experiences.

INFOCUS: Challenges Ahead

Understanding the common objectives and infrastructure shared by the medical home, CIN and ACO models enhances their ability to meet the challenges ahead and develop strategies for success. As noted earlier, Section 3502 of the Affordable Care Act establishes new interdisciplinary community health teams, a key ingredient for the MAPCP. As demonstration grants are released and these teams start work in communities across the country to help primary care practices with disease prevention, chronic disease management, and care transitions,[77] it will be important for CIN and ACO governance boards to recognize potential synergies with these teams. We have discussed key elements of the medical home, the medical home as a building block for CINs and ACOs, and presented examples of medical home model organizations that are also leaders in ACO adoption and implementation. So what are some of the challenges for CINs and ACOs in collaboration with medical homes?

---

[75] Center for Medicare and Medicaid Services. Multi-payer Advanced Primary Care Practice (MAPCP) Demonstration Fact Sheet. Accessed online July 2, 2011 at http://www.cms.gov/DemoProjectsEvalRpts/downloads/mapcpdemo_Factsheet.pdf.
[76] Center for Medicare and Medicaid Services. Multi-payer Advanced Primary Care Practice Demonstration Questions & Answers- Updated April 12, 2011. Accessed online July 2, 2011 at http://www.cms.gov/DemoProjectsEvalRpts/downloads/mapcpdemo_QA.pdf.
[77] Fed. Reg. Vol. 76, No. 67. April 7, 2011. I.(D)(4) Community Health Teams. p. 19535.

Table 10. Chapter 2 Challenges and Risks

Challenges	Risks
Implementing an integrated performance reporting system.	Revenue lost in transition to new reimbursement models.
Achieving consensus across ACO participant medical homes on clinical guidelines.	Without consensus on clinical guidelines, unintended adverse consequences may be experienced in patient care services due to a lack of standardization during the shift to population-based disease condition management.
Aligning advanced medical home objectives with ACO qualification level criteria.	Lost opportunity to further solidify the linkage between primary care and hospital organizations.
Attribution of patients to specific providers in ACOs.[78]	Loss of required beneficiaries and inability to hold an ACO accountable for a patient's care received outside their region.[79]
Having sufficient resources to manage large-scale complexity, overcome tradition, and change activities required for a multiyear ACO implementation.	Emergence of barriers and silos; slower rates of adoption; and loss of efficiency and achieving economies of scale for all ACO participants.
Managing the impact on revenue cycle for hospitals when chronic disease management has been optimized but payment methods have not caught up.	Negative economic impact on consumers related to potentially higher out-of-pocket expenses and increased cost of navigating the care system.

---

[78] Luft HS. Becoming accountable—opportunities and obstacles for ACOs. *N Engl J Med*. 2010;363(15):1389-1391.
[79] Luft HS. Becoming accountable—opportunities and obstacles for ACOs. *N Engl J Med*. 2010;363(15):1389-1391.

Table 10. Chapter 2: Challenges and Risks, cont.

Potential Mitigation Strategies
√ **Impact on patient care**: Use of predictive modeling tools[80] for identification of chronically illness population segments, and drilling down to individual patients for targeted prevention efforts.
√ **Impact on patient care:** Implement ambulatory care and disease management programs[44] to meet the patient's needs following inpatient treatment, and interventions, and between physician office visits.
√ **Lack of investment 1:** Engaging resources to establish financial plans that identify options for securing needed investments to cover capital, training, and expenses of the formation, ramp-up, and transition periods.
√ **Lack of investment 2:** Encouraging physicians in need of capital infusion to consider partnering with health systems and such large entities as health plans.
√ **Mitigating financial impact**: Physicians and providers negotiate rapid-cycle implementation of new payment methods to compensate for new and improved models of healthcare services.
√ **Organizational transformation**: Utilize change management and process improvement methodologies to minimize risk and facilitate adoption.

---

[80] Boland P, Polakoff P, Schwab T. Accountable care organizations hold promise, but will they achieve cost and quality targets? *Manag Care*. 2010;19(10):12-6, 19.

Chapter 3. The Lens of Leadership

I find the great thing in the world is not so much where we stand, as in what direction we are moving.

Oliver Wendell Holmes Sr., M.D.
Dean and Professor
Harvard Medical School
(1809–1894)

Establishing the governance, infrastructure, and leadership of each CIN and ACO is critical to their success as these transformative models of care delivery evolve. The issue of putting an appropriate governance and leadership structure in place from the onset, regardless of whether the organization is public or private payer-focused, is a critical early-stage development issue.

ACO/CIN Organization

Chapter 1 listed the kinds of organizations ("participants") that CMS has identified as potentially eligible to become Medicare ACOs. For purposes of the Section 3022 Medicare Shared Savings Program, ACOs are generally defined as organizations of ACO professionals, or their joint arrangements with hospitals, that provide services and supplies to Medicare recipients. ACO professionals are physicians, physician assistants, nurse practitioners, or clinical nurse specialists who accept accountability and responsibility for the quality and cost of care. If they meet certain requirements set forth in the Proposed Rule, they may participate in the Section 3022 Medicare Shared Savings program.

Several organizations critical to providing health services to Medicare recipients were not listed as ACO participants in the legislation and proposed rule, including: nursing homes, skilled nursing facilities, home healthcare providers, and long-term care hospitals.[81]   Other important groups include providers of community pharmacy services and palliative care services. Medicare

---

[81] Fed. Reg. Vol. 76, No. 67. April 7, 2011. II.(B)(1) Eligible Entities. p. 19528.

recipients need the services of these ancillary healthcare professionals and organizations; and Medicare ACOs can draw on them to meet the needs of the populations they serve. It is up to the ACO and CIN to determine how best to use the services of these organizations in cost-effective ways. In time, as CINs and ACOs evolve they will determine which services of these providers are appropriate, and provide the greatest value. Other critical participants in a Medicare ACO include payer organizations (private and public); and under certain circumstances federally qualified health centers, rural health centers, and critical access hospitals may be included as ACO participants.[82]

ACO professionals and hospitals aligned as legal entities are eligible to participate in the CMS Section 3022 Shared Savings Program. A number of different healthcare organizations, hospitals and physician practice arrangements can fit into this Medicare ACO model. According to some industry observers there are seven potential entities that may independently or collectively form ACOs and/or be involved in CINs. The following table outlines these entities; the actual organizations allowed to participate in Medicare ACO formation will depend on the outcome of the CMS Proposed Rule.

Table 11. Provider Organizations That May Participate in CMS Shared Savings Program[83]

Independent practice association (IPA)	Hospital medical staff organization (MSO)[84]	Integrated delivery network (IDN)
Multispecialty physician group (MSPG)	Physician-hospital organization (PHO)	Primary care physician practice
Extended hospital medical staff[85]		Clinical integrated network (CIN)

[82] Fed. Reg. Vol. 76, No. 67. April 7, 2011. Section 425.7. Payment and treatment of savings. pp. 19645–19647.

[83] Devers K, Berenson R. Can accountable care organizations improve the value of health care by solving the cost and quality quandaries? Robert Wood Johnson policy analysis paper, October 2009. Accessed online August 26, 2011, at http://www.rwjf.org/files/research/acobrieffinal.pdf.

[84] Smithson K, Baker S. Medical staff organizations: a persistent anomaly. *Health Aff* (*Millwood*). 2007;26(1):w76–w79.

[85] Fisher ES, Staiger DO, Bynum JP, Gottlieb DJ. Creating accountable care organizations: the extended hospital medical staff. *Health Aff* (*Millwood*). 2007;26(1):w44–w57.

A survey was conducted of healthcare leaders across the industry in April 2011 following release of the CMS Proposed Rule. Eighty-four percent of those surveyed belonged to hospital, physician organizations, or integrated delivery networks. As the industry prepares for this next step in ACO implementation, there are several results to note from this survey. Seventy-two percent of the respondents recognized the need for stronger clinical integration programs, and 57% recognized the importance of market competition driving the need for integration as a key factor in establishing ACOs. This growing interest in integration and ACO formation along with the push to find new ways to do business in an increasingly competitive environment has spawned formation of CINs and ACOs outside of the Section 3022 Shared Savings Program. While a Medicare ACO will be focused on a designated Medicare patient population, there are also Medicaid and private-payer ACOs being formed that cover other populations and may have different contractual relationships with ancillary provider organizations.

Although all ACOs operate under the same basic principles of ensuring accountability and payment reform, each type of ACO may have different performance measurement requirements based on its payer and patient population. Such other requirements as patient self-management, patient-provider communications, the ability of the information system to collect and track data, physician agreement on measurements, and clinical workflow processes that enhance patient satisfaction may also be defined differently and must also be taken into account. Each type of ancillary provider organization will relate to patients at different points across the continuum of care. The long-term goal of the ACO is forming an entity that will meet all patients' needs effectively, efficiently, at the lowest cost, and at the highest level of quality. It is up to the ACO to determine which ancillary health providers to use and how best to use their services to obtain the highest value for the resources expended.

An example of how an ACO might be structured appears in a 2006 *Health Affairs* article co-authored by Dr. Elliot Fisher, widely recognized as one of the originators of the ACO concept. Dr. Fisher describes the extended hospital medical staff as "essentially a hospital-associated multispecialty group practice that is empirically defined by physicians' direct or indirect referral patterns to a hospital."[86] This definition is based on the notion that physicians, groups of physicians, and their ancillary providers who operate separately from an IDN or other hospital-type organization as independent practices can actually be viewed as part of an extended single virtual organization. Dr. Fisher's study was based on quantitative analysis of Medicare claims data that showed referral patterns and revealed ways to better organize delivery of care. The article also identified a number of challenges and barriers to integration along with more efficient care delivery that included local market structures, physician-community cultural issues, legal hurdles, physician practice-hospital organization alignments, and performance measurements and evaluation. A number of these issues are noted in the *INFOCUS* section at the end of this chapter; they are also being addressed across the industry with ongoing reform efforts.

Leadership

Engaging the right persons in governance and leadership of CINs and ACOs is critical to long-term success. This section will cover two key topics: first, styles of leadership to fit the goals and culture of each CIN and ACO; second, a discussion of why physician leadership is central to the CIN and ACO's success. Leaders of healthcare organizations have confronted challenges in the past. The present transformation of the healthcare industry resulting from health reforms and the search for higher-quality care and greater economic gains has compounded the challenges inherent in our current health finance and delivery methods. Some of these challenges include:[87]

- A highly professional workforce concentrated in silos;
- Traditional physician training that tends to inhibit collaboration;
- Lengthy and demanding training to develop clinical skills and knowledge that may delay the development of leadership skills;

---

[86] Fisher ES, Staiger DO, Bynum JP, Gottlieb DJ. Creating accountable care organizations: the extended hospital medical staff. *Health Aff (Millwood)*. 2007:26(1):w44–w57.
[87] Stoller JK. Developing physician-leaders: a call to action. *J Gen Intern Med*. 2009;24(7):876–878. Accessed online September 7, 2011, at http://www.ncbi.nlm.nih.gov/pmc/articles/PMC2695517/pdf/11606_2009_Article_1007.pdf.

◆ An increasingly complex external environment (such as insurance and payer reimbursement, state licensing requirements, and antitrust laws) requiring a high level of astuteness and business acumen to function in the primary/specialty care or hospital environment.

There are several specific aspects of the transformation toward CINs and ACOs, such as the accelerated movement toward collaboration and integration that requires new leadership styles. Because each community and its complement of healthcare providers are unique, the leadership required from physicians to achieve the goals of CINs and ACOs to improve population health and lower cost of care has never been greater. In addition to dealing with the challenges described at the close of Chapter 2, the CIN and ACO carry with them an increased need for skills and knowledge related to managing change. Large-scale organizational transformations require leaders who understand the emotional turmoil their personnel may undergo, and the complex interdependencies that will develop among participants as innovations are introduced by the ACO to enhance the ability to deliver care at the right time in the right place.

A 1996 quote from Dr. Donald Berwick may serve as a theme for this section: "Effective leaders challenge the status quo both by insisting that the current system cannot remain and by offering clear ideas about superior alternatives."[88] Along with implementing change and addressing the challenges, current and future leaders of CINs and ACOs must welcome innovation in order to challenge the status quo. We now turn to leadership style issues that can assist in the development of these care delivery models.

Favorable Leadership Styles

There are a number of foundational skills and traits needed for future physician leaders to support CIN/ACO development. Though not all-inclusive, the model presented here for CIN/ACO leadership represents a set of core skills and traits

---

[88] Berwick DM. A primer on leading the improvement of systems. *BMJ*. 1996;312(7031):619-622. Accessed online August 17, 2011, at http://www.ncbi.nlm.nih.gov/pmc/articles/PMC2350403/pdf/bmj00532-0035.pdf.

required of leaders in advancing these new organizational models in the healthcare systems of the twenty-first century.

Figure 12. Leadership Skills & Traits Needed for CIN/ACO Leaders

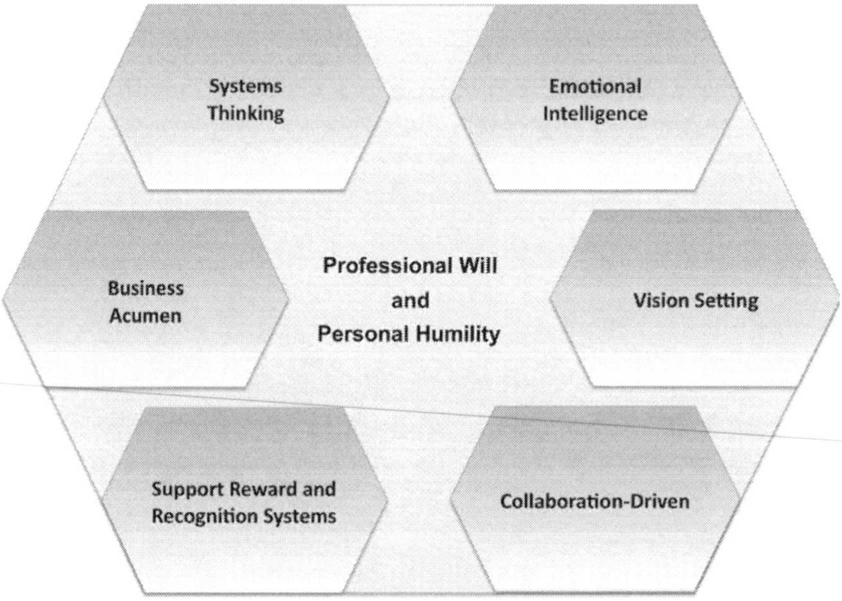

Each physician leader will bring his or her own clinical expertise to the CIN/ACO based on background and the specific disciplines involved in training, residency, and practice. Nonetheless, Figure 12 illustrates seven key traits and skills that will enable CIN/ACO leaders to forge the partnerships required by these new care delivery models to bring about collective and effective improvement of population health across the communities they serve.

1. **Systems thinking**. Originating in the field of engineering, systems thinking pertains to understanding the interrelationships of complex entities and the ways in which individual components affect the functionality of the whole. Systems thinking is part of the foundation of the learning organization theory[89] applied in Chapters 9 and 10 to illustrate the future progression of the CIN and

---

[89] Pisapia J, Reyes-Guerra D, Coukos-Semmel E. Developing the leader's strategic mindset: establishing the measures. *Leadership Review*. 2005;5:41-68. Accessed online August 31, 2011, at http://www.leadershipreview.org/2005spring/PisapiaArticle.pdf; Senge P. *The Fifth Discipline: The Art and Practice of the Learning Organization*. Knopf Doubleday Publishing Group:New York, NY, 1990,2006.

ACO models. Future systems will emerge as CINs and ACOs are formed through new partnerships. Within these organizations, a systematic approach to problem solving oriented to people, process, and technology will be a powerful tool for physician leaders to confront these challenges.

2. **Business acumen**. CIN/ACO leaders will need core skills derived from the business world to manage the spectrum of legal, fiscal, and strategy-related issues that arise daily.

3. **Support reward and recognition systems**. The IOM noted in its 2001 report, *Crossing the Quality Chasm*, that physician leaders should have a strong understanding of incentive systems. Leaders will need to motivate their CIN/ACO physicians, administrative, clinical, and technical teams along with maximizing the effect of economic stimuli to be gained from the public shared savings programs, private initiatives, and pay-for-performance incentives.

4. **Collaboration-driven**. A passion for effective collaboration across multiple organizations will be a necessity, given the inertia in moving traditional models of practice forward towards ACO and CIN integration. Strong communication skills will help reinforce this trait along with diplomacy to secure consensus rather than imposing decisions. This is a particularly challenging skill for physician leaders to adopt, as they are generally trained to make quick decisions and take personal action in life-or-death situations.

5. **Vision setting**. The ability to describe the future of an organization and convey it in a meaningful way to physician peers, clinical team members, and other stakeholders is necessary if they are to have a clear vision of the outcome and motive to collaborate in establishing and operating a CIN or ACO.

6. **Emotional intelligence**. Beyond the intelligence quotient or IQ, emotional intelligence or EQ is defined as "how leaders handle themselves and their relationships."[90] This trait is considered a must-have in the formation of clinically

---

[90] Serio CD, Epperly T. Physician leadership: a new model for a new generation. *Fam Pract Manag*. 2006;13(2):51-54. Available at: http://www.aafp.org/fpm/2006/0200/p51.pdf.

integrated networks or accountable care organizations. People and their relationships will determine whether a CIN or ACO is a success or a failure. Physician leaders must have a firm grip on their own emotions each day, along with the awareness and empathy to support and meet the needs of others in their organizations.

7. **Professional will and personal humility**. James Collins identifies these traits as central to what he calls Level 5 Leaders.[91] Physician-executives leading CIN/ACO initiatives will need both of these traits. Leaders in the twenty-first century healthcare system will have a greater need for engaging in and driving collaborative multidisciplinary groups that involve of highly talented team members and other strong leaders. To maximize effectiveness, an undying will to succeed coupled with a degree of empathy will be needed.

These seven skills and traits may serve as a set of management indicia for CIN/ACO leaders. All these skills will be required to meet leadership requirements in a new operating environment shaped by reforms and the changing culture in the United States. Some of these requirements will include:[92]
+ Managing expanded physician relations;
+ An expanded focus on community and population health;
+ A new integration of financial modeling and quality/performance measurement with the new care delivery model focus on compensation for the value of care delivered.

Leaders typically subscribe to a particular style based on their own traits, strengths and experiences. Given the challenges in healthcare, with the constant changes and industry shifts, several leadership styles may be considered by physicians and other healthcare leaders to help move CIN and ACO organizations forward. Three styles to consider include situational, transformational, and servant. Each of these is applicable to healthcare organizations—especially those on the way to forming CINs and ACOs. Leaders of these new organizational

---

[91] Collins J. Level 5 Leadership. In: *Good to Great: Why Some Companies Make the Leap and Others Don't*. New York, NY: Harper Business, 2001. pp. 17–40.
[92] Jarousse, LA. On the Agenda. *Trustee*. 2011 Feb;64(2).

models must bring management expertise to their positions along with an unwavering commitment to quality and excellence, and dynamic skills that allow them to conform their style to the current challenges. While each organization and community will have its particular features and requirements that shape its goals and objectives, it can reach a higher level with the help of a leader who understands how to apply the different leadership styles as they are needed.

Table 12. Leadership Styles and Successful ACO/CIN Implementation

Situational[93]	Transformational[94]	Servant[95]
Adaptable to specific situations	Influences subordinates to move toward "ethically inspired goals transcending self-interest"	Engages in active listening
Leader assumes one of four roles: coaching, supporting, delegating, or leading		Demonstrates empathy for workers and peers
	Four central components: "idealized influence, inspirational motivation, intellectual stimulation, and individualized consideration"	Strong communicator of concepts
Understands need for workers' empowerment and recognition		Possesses strong persuasive abilities
Leader knows his or her strengths but adjusts when needed	Facilitates team growth through individualized mentoring or coaching relationships	"Exerts a healing influence on individuals and institutions"
Recognizes the need for change		Establishes a community in the workplace

Each leadership style can prove beneficial to a CIN/ACO's development. The transformational style of leadership, however, may be the best approach where such new challenges are faced as balancing the investments needed for better patient-centered, population health management against the economic needs of

---

[93] Chaudry J, Jain A, McKenzie S, Schwartz RW. Physician leadership: the competencies of change. *J Surg Educ.* 2008;65(3):213–220. Accessed online July 20, 2011, at http://www.uthscsa.edu/gme/documents/PhysicianLsp-CompetenciesofChange.pdf.

[94] Xirasagar S, Samuels ME, Curtin TF. (February 2006). Management training of physician executives, their leadership style, and care management performance: an empirical study. *Am J Manag Care.* 2006;12(2):101–108. Accessed online July 20, 2011, at http://www.ajmc.com/media/pdf/AJMC_06febXirasagar101to108.pdf.

[95] Schwartz RW, Tumblin TF. The power of servant leadership to transform health care organizations for the 21st-century economy. *Arch Surg.* 2002;137(12):1419–1427. Accessed online July 20, 2011, at http://archsurg.ama-assn.org/cgi/reprint/137/12/1419.

the workforce and the greater good of the community. Different leaders will bring their respective talents and backgrounds; however, understanding the importance and skills of transformational leadership will enable them to implement ACOs successfully and reduce risk across clinical, administrative, financial, regulatory, and information technology domains.

Who Drives the Bus?

One of the most important components in establishing governance for a CIN or ACO initiative is the element of physician leadership. Meeting the requirement of accountability means that CINs and ACOs must be led by physicians. The American Medical Association (AMA), Institute for Healthcare Improvement, NCQA, Medicare Payment Advisory Commission, and other organizations have all endorsed this requirement. Ensuring that physicians are the source of medical decisions and leadership is critical to ensuring that patient safety and quality-of-care goals are met across the continuum of care. This insistence on physician leadership is related in part to past experiences with HMOs in the 1990s.

In contrast to the HMO model, in which payers primarily used various utilization management methods to control costs, the physician-led CIN or ACO model maintains that physicians who are focused on patient care clinical outcomes are far better positioned to help patients achieve or maintain their best state of health and therefore to indirectly lower the total cost of care. An associated change is the shift from the utilization review metrics of the past to the quality outcomes measures of the present and future.

It is important to note that leadership of these new models of healthcare delivery bears further study and analysis.[96] As our health system evolves, different organizations emerge and new relationships lead to changing dynamics in the industry. Following our discussion of leadership styles, we shall turn to

---

[96] Shortell SM. Challenges and opportunities for population health partnerships. *Prev Chronic Dis.* 2010;7(6):1–2. Available at: http://www.cdc.gov/pcd/issues/2010/nov/10_0110.htm; Shortell SM, Casalino LP, Fisher ES. How the center for medicare and medicaid innovation should test accountable care organizations. *Health Aff (Millwood).* 2010;29(7):1293–1298.

some of the possible organizational configurations for establishing CINs and ACOs.

A clinically integrated network or CIN, compared to an ACO, is a narrower term, encompassing collections of physicians and hospitals working together as an integrated unit. A CIN typically forms to achieve economies of scale in care delivery, enable joint contracting initiatives with insurers, and launch programs designed to increase the quality and coordination of patient care while reducing the cost of that care. Clinical integration is a necessary building block of an ACO. This integration is especially important in situations where the majority of physicians are not employed by the ACO entity. It is an attractive model for independent physicians who wish to retain their autonomy while engaging with a larger organization collectively focused on quality, integration, collective negotiation, and health care value to the consumer.

Figure 13. Forming the Clinically Integrated Network[97]

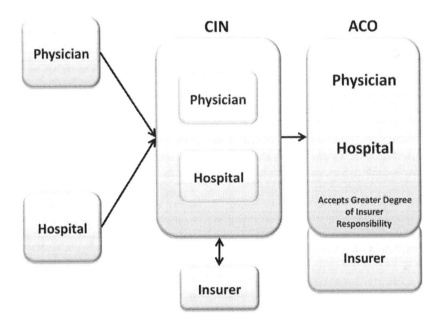

[97] Illustration developed based on BDC Advisors presentation to VHA on Clinical Integration (slide 2). Accessed online June 29, 2011, at http://bdcadvisors.com/presentations.asp.

As the physicians and hospitals come together formally through various types of joint venture arrangements, new opportunities emerge through integration to achieve stronger clinical services, economic incentives, and economies of scale in shared services. The FTC has enabled the development of CINs by allowing hospitals and physicians to integrate and negotiate collectively, without running afoul of monopoly and anti-competition laws, as long as they meet certain criteria. How to form a CIN is one of the topics in Chapter 4, while Chapter 5 discusses antitrust legislation, regulatory issues and safe harbors related to the formative requirements for ACOs and CINs. The next illustration shows the potential combinations of ACO participants[98] as they have emerged and been analyzed by industry experts in recent years.

Figure 14. Potential Models of ACO Development

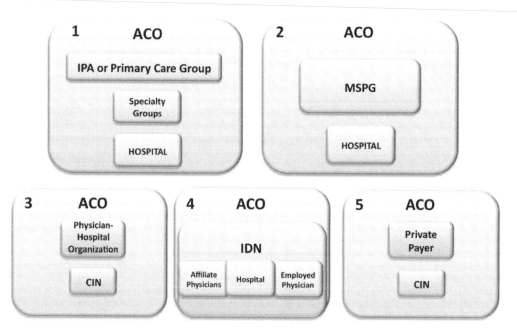

[98] H.R. 3590, Patient Protection and Affordable Care Act, §3022(b)(1)(A-E); Rittenhouse DR, Shortell SM, Fisher ES. Primary care and accountable care—two essential elements of delivery-system reform. *N Engl J Med.* 2009;361(24):2301–2303; Devers K, Berenson R. Can accountable care organizations improve the value of health care by solving the cost and quality quandaries? Robert Wood Johnson policy analysis paper, October 2009. Accessed online August 27, 2011, at http://www.rwjf.org/files/research/acobrieffinal.pdf.

Additional configurations are possible, including academic medical centers in the position of the integrated delivery network, and virtual models[99] that combine health systems, physician groups, and payer organizations that provide collaborative care coordination. Hence these models are intended as representative examples rather than an inclusive list of all the types of arrangements that exist or will take shape in the future. Each model has a different partner taking the lead in the formation and management of the ACO. Let us now take a closer look at these five possible configurations and their major characteristics.

1: The IPA-directed ACO. This first model positions the IPA, or primary care physician group in the leadership role of the ACO, with specialty groups and hospitals in a subordinate position. This model also brings the medical home model, already noted as the foundation of the ACO, to the forefront in establishing the newly structured entity. This model allows physicians, both primary care and specialists, flexibility in assigning exclusive or nonexclusive contracting rights. An alternative to this approach is to have primary care physicians operate under exclusive contract rights but allow specialists to work across multiple ACOs within the community.

2: The MSPG-directed ACO. In this second model the multispecialty physician group (such as the Mayo and Cleveland Clinics) directs the ACO with the hospital subordinated to the MSPG. Here physicians (primary care and specialists) work in an ACO with nonexclusive contracting rights, and the ACO partners with hospitals and ancillary service providers (laboratories, skilled nursing facilities, rehabilitation clinics, and the like) to support clinical integration needs.

3: The PHO-directed ACO. The third model places the physician-hospital organization at the center of the ACO. The PHO creates partnerships with the physician practices that will serve as a collective risk-bearing organization. The PHO will also negotiate the contracts for the physician practices (primary or specialty care) when they join the ACO as part of clinical and financial

[99] Blue Shield of California press release. Blue Shield of California, Catholic Healthcare West and Hill Physicians Medical Group to pilot innovative new care model for CalPERS; April 22, 2009. Accessed online July 20, 2011, at
http://www.hillphysicians.com/Documents/common/press%20releases/press_rel_CalPERS_announce_042209.pdf.

integration. Sutter Health and Scripps Health in California and Advocate Health in Chicago are representative examples of this model.[100] As this third model evolves, the clinically integrated network or PHO (CIN/PHO) has the potential to expand beyond a single ACO.

4: The IDN-directed ACO. The fourth model places the IDN at the forefront of the ACO. In this position the IDN has the option of exclusive or nonexclusive contracting with primary care practices and specialty care groups regardless of whether they are affiliated or unaffiliated with the IDN. In addition, the IDN has control over hospital medical staff organizations, which could be under exclusive contracts to the IDN to support the required level of beneficiaries needed for care under the ACO. Examples of these types of arrangements are Kaiser Permanente, Intermountain Healthcare in Utah and southeastern Idaho, and the Henry Ford Health System in Michigan.

5: The private payer-directed ACO. The fifth model is based on a private payer's forming a direct partnership with physicians, creating a physician-only CIN that would subcontract for hospital or other services. This ACO model could also be formed with IPAs or MSPGs, as it intends the private payer to serve as the partner to provide needed financial support for such infrastructure development of the ACO as health information technology, population data aggregation, and training. As the purpose of the ACO is to improve population health in the communities it serves, it would contract separately with hospitals and ancillary service providers to provide services when needed for inpatient procedures, tests, rehabilitation, and other elements of patient care. Contracting with physicians may be more rigid; that is, the ACO may require more exclusive relationships. This is particularly important for the Medicare ACO that requires a specific number of beneficiaries needed to support the ACO model. Even though the payer serves as a principal partner under this model, accountability for patient care would still reside at the local level with a governance board headed by physician leaders.

---

[100] Boland P, Polakoff P, Schwab T. Accountable care organizations hold promise, but will they achieve cost and quality targets? *Manag Care*. 2010;19(10):1--6, 19; Shortell SM, Casalino LP, Fisher ES. How the center for medicare and medicaid innovation should test accountable care organizations. *Health Aff* (*Millwood*). 2010;29(7):1293–1298.

One issue that should be highlighted is the way in which patients are assigned or "attributed" in ACOs. Attribution is important because it designates which physician gets assigned patients for purposes of accountability and reimbursement. The concept of patient attribution is complex and often worked out by using computer algorithms based upon the last physicians seen. Beyond the technical aspects, in the Medicare ACO there are public policy reasons that drive these calculations in the Medicare ACO. In the Medicare ACO, assignment of patients is done retrospectively, based upon the patient's visit history. The history is contrasted against a prospective selection or assignment process in which either the patient selects or the plan or network assigns the physician(s) in most private ACO and commercial insurance plans. While controversial and under debate with the proposed rulings, CMS has focused on the retrospective attribution methodology. The public policy rationale is that retrospective assignment avoids discrimination in level of service against persons who are not assigned. It is believed by some government policy makers that physicians should improve quality of care and reduce costs across the board with regard to whether a patient is part of a particular group. The practical reality, however, is that if you don't know who is attributed to your ACO population, you will not be able to properly direct additional resources you may obtain from participation in an ACO.

It will be interesting to see how CMS implements the attribution rule. With the publication of their Proposed Rule, however, we can begin to offer some clarification. According to the Proposed Rule, the following points will determine beneficiary assignment under the proposed Medicare ACO program:[101]

Assignment will be made based on beneficiary utilization of primary care services and the affiliation of those primary care service providers with a specific ACO. Specifics on the proposed attribution methodology from CMS include:

---

[101] Fed. Reg. Vol. 76, No. 67. April 7, 2011. Section 425.6. Assignment of Medicare fee-for-service beneficiaries to ACOs. p. 19645.

- Identification of all primary care physicians who were ACO participants for a given performance year;
- At year-end for each performance year, identification of all beneficiaries that who received services from these primary care physicians;
- Establishment of the total allowed charges for primary care services received by these beneficiaries during the performance year;
- Compilation of allowed charges for primary care services provided under each ACO per beneficiary;
- Assignment of a beneficiary to an ACO based on the primary care ACO participant from who the beneficiary received a plurality of his or her primary care services in the performance year.

When a single ACO is held accountable for the quality of care and outcomes experienced by a patient, however, attribution becomes complicated when healthcare services are needed outside the ACO. If a patient receives care outside an ACO's geographic market or service area, the ACO may have little or no authority over the orders made for the patient's care, whether the orders are related to inpatient, outpatient, or ancillary care. This possibility may lead to the ACO being held accountable for a patient's outcomes over which the ACO has no control. The handling of these issues varies between public and private payers. In addition, there are many different attribution formulas. It is expected that these differences will reconcile over time as the industry gains more experience and as it moves toward multi-payer models in which all payers are participating and patients are given increased flexibility to access care when and where they need it. The national debate around Medicare ACO patient attribution methods will widen as ACO stakeholders increasingly understand both the complexity and the implications of this methodology. Lobbying efforts are already underway by many large national healthcare trade groups asking for prospective attributions to better enable the ACO to manage their beneficiaries. Stay tuned as this issue plays out at the national level.

Governance

Governance is a critical factor in maintaining effective collaboration and strategic oversight of operations for the ACO's financial, quality and safety, and legal compliance objectives of the ACO. The AMA released a set of 13 principles to guide ACO establishment in November 2010; one of which is an ACO governance principle.[102] The ACO governance principle, the AMA identifies four elements necessary for effective governance of an ACO:

- Medical decisions should be made by physicians;

- The ACO/CIN should be governed by a board of directors elected by the ACO professionals;

- ACO/CIN physician leadership should be licensed in the state in which the ACO operates and licensed for the active practice of medicine in the ACO's service area;

- When an ACO has a hospital, the ACO's governing board should be separate from and independent of the hospital's board of directors.

These principles have particular relevance to integrated health systems considering establishment of a CIN/ACO. The governance of an ACO is such that it will not be business as usual. Table 2 in Chapter 1 lists a few highlights of the governance structure of the Medicare ACO Program, but there are additional details. Additional guidance from the Proposed Rule on governing a Medicare ACO include the following:

- Report the taxpayer identification number (TIN) of each ACO participant;
- Coordinate antitrust agency reviews;
- Inform CMS of receipt of any antitrust agency letters;
- Obtain CMS approval of any ACO marketing material;

---

[102] Interim meeting of the American Medical Association House of Delegates. Accountable care organization (ACO) principles; November 2010; San Diego, CA. Accessed online July 20, 2011 at http://op.bna.com/hl.nsf/id/bbrk-8b5szv/$File/ACOandAMA.pdf.

- Certify that the ACO is a recognized legal entity in the state in which it was established;
- Elect to operate under one of two tracks:
  - One-sided risk model for two years, then the two-sided risk model for the third year;
  - Two-sided Risk Model to share in losses and savings for all three years;
- Have a physician-directed quality assurance and process improvement committee;
- Implement an evidence-based medical practice;
- Have an information technology infrastructure with the ability to collect and evaluate data and provide feedback to ACO participants.

Once these governance elements are in place, the ACO board must have contracting oversight of the entire ACO and assume the functions typically performed by a health system or health plan board. Having a physician-led board and governance structure represents a substantial transition for many health systems. Ensuring that comprehensive clinical transformation is undertaken for the merged organizational activities regardless of the conceptual model or configuration should be the primary oversight activity of the ACO governing body, and may be a substantial transition for the physicians involved. The healthcare industry has experienced significant changes since the early 2000s with the influx of electronic health records in large- and small-scale organizations alike; and just as strategic governance and oversight have proven to be critical to success in these initiatives, so will it be crucial to have strong governance boards to provide similar strategic oversight over ACO implementation efforts. Transformation in clinical practice will require effective investment in infrastructure technologies and staff, clinical and administrative process redesign, improved preventive care initiatives and coordination, and better management of chronic disease.[39]

An example of the importance of effective governance in assisting the organizational integration of physician and hospital entities comes from the St. Jude Health System in Fullerton, California. A 2009 article published in *Trustee* summarizes the importance of shared governance in achieving the system's positive results over the years:

Hospital and health system boards can improve the odds. Our experience with a successful 15-year-old hospital-physician partnership demonstrates the value of shared governance in creating effective integrated systems. It creates opportunities to reconcile competing interests, formulate long-term goals and strategies, and provide the long-term support that such ventures require to succeed.[103]

The authors of the article also cite six principles that were central to the success of the integration spearheaded by their governance.

Figure 15. Principles of Successful Integration

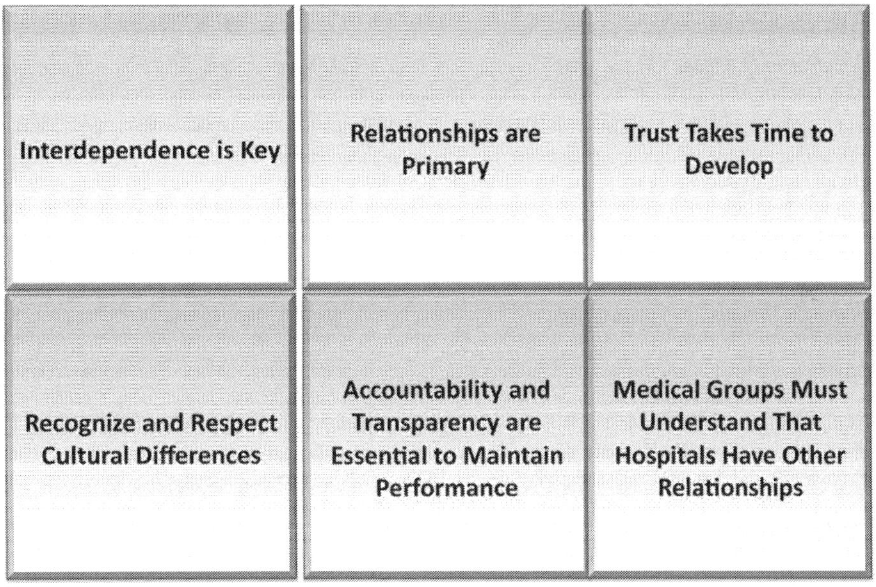

Interdependence is Key	Relationships are Primary	Trust Takes Time to Develop
Recognize and Respect Cultural Differences	Accountability and Transparency are Essential to Maintain Performance	Medical Groups Must Understand That Hospitals Have Other Relationships

These principles and the necessity for overseeing such multiyear initiatives as CINs and ACOs lead to the subject of both financial and clinical integration.

---

[103] Fraschetti R, Sugarman M. Successful hospital-physician integration. *Trustee*. 2009;62(7):11–12, 17–18.

Clinical and Financial Integration of the CIN/ACO

Clinical integration of the clinician and hospital participants in a CIN is a major goal that must be accomplished to reach an advanced level of cooperation to achieve efficiencies in administrative operations, clinical processes, and most importantly for operational transformation. In the June 2009 MedPAC Report to Congress, the authors recommended the ACO as a new model to improve clinical and financial integration and accountability for the healthcare of a defined population of Medicare beneficiaries.[104] The MedPAC report went on to describe the elements of two hypothetical ACO models. The first model is based on voluntary participation; in this model, physicians would join with little downside risk but greater potential for upside rewards through a shared savings program similar to the CMS Physician Group Demonstration Project. The second model would require mandatory participation (with CMS assignment of physicians to the ACO), and both penalties and rewards would be based on the ACO's performance. The benefits and importance of clinical integration between hospitals and physician practices were noted for both models.

The significance of clinical integration has grown over the past seven years with review by the Federal Trade Commission (FTC) of many clinically integrated networks. These networks are allowed when they avoid violations of Sherman Act, other antitrust laws and pertinent FTC laws to be addressed in Chapter 5. Examples of the FTC opinions and rulings in specific cases will also be discussed. Based on the body of evidence from antitrust evaluation of procompetitive benefits and anticompetitive effects of clinical integration, the Proposed Rule calls for all providers and suppliers who wish to participate as an ACO in the CMS Shared Savings Program to be committed to clinical integration.[105] CMS goes on to propose that participants in the ACO share a substantial financial burden of risk and demonstrate the establishment of necessary interrelationships as

---

[104] MedPAC Report to Congress: Improving Incentives in the Medicare Program (June 2009), Chapter 2: Accountable Care Organizations. p. 55. Accessed onlne July 20, 2011 at www.medpac.gov/documents/Jun09_EntireReport.pdf.
[105] Fed. Reg. Vol. 76, No. 67. April 7, 2011. II.(B)(c)(3). Leadership and Management Structure. pp. 19542-19543.

required by the FTC, to collectively realize improvements in the cost and quality of care.

There are a number of issues and challenges to be resolved for each Medicare ACO to achieve the heightened level of functionality of a clinical integration program. A few of the most important issues include:

- Ensuring that integrated evidence-based practices are in place;
- Ensuring that an adequate number of primary care professionals are available to provide services;
- Meeting patient-centeredness criteria specified by the DHHS, which include patient and caregiver assessments or using individualized care plans.[106]

Financial integration of the ACO is part of payment/incentive reform (such as pay-for-performance, payment bundling, gain sharing or value-based payments) along with tying the financial processes, reward evaluation processes, and risk sharing into the operation and funding of a single new legal entity. These issues will be discussed in more detail in Chapter 9.

Alignment Strategies

Successful alignment of all participants is the lifeblood of the CIN or ACO. Moving traditionally competitive organizations in a community to become a high-performing team of collaborators is an important objective requiring tact, diplomacy, and a sense of mission on behalf of leadership as well as the members of the CIN/ACO's governance board. This section of the chapter will touch on several topics that leaders should consider in planning for their CIN/ACO regardless of whether they are at an early stage of development or have been operating as an integrated entity for some time.

---

[106] H.R. 3590, Patient Protection and Affordable Care Act, §3022(b)(2)(G). ACO Requirements (2010).

A major issue for all healthcare organizations involved in establishing CINs and ACOs is the cultural as well as organizational transformation that takes place when multiple institutions are required to become interdependent and to cooperate. Two issues to address are: the importance of cross-functional teaming activities in large-scale transformation initiatives; and issues related to organizational change management that will be important for CINs and ACOs as they move forward. A study identified a number of practices critical to coordination and improved outcomes--an issue called "high performing work practices to relational coordination."[107] A key strategic objective for the CIN/ACO previously noted is improving coordination of care. Dr. Jody Gittell and her colleagues summarized a number of practices proven to bring about better relational coordination and improved outcomes. Below is an illustration of these practices.

Figure 16. "Relational Model of How High-Performance Work Systems Work"

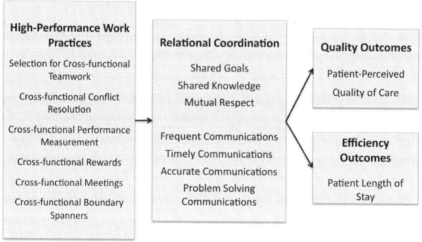

Source: Model from the work of Dr. Jody Gittell on Relational Coordination in Healthcare Organizations. http://www.jodyhoffergittell.info/content/rc2c.html

---

[107] Gittell J, Seidner R, Wimbush J. A relational model of how high-performance work systems work. *Organization Science.* 2010;21(2):490-506; additional material available at: http://www.jodyhoffergittell.info/content/rc2c.html.

So what can we derive from this model? First, with the transformation initiatives required by CINs and ACOs to integrate previously disparate entities into a cohesive organization, the establishment of multiple cross-functional practices can improve opportunities for greater care coordination and evaluation of the impacts on community or population-level economic and health outcomes. From the author team's collective experience, the importance of these cross-functional and collaborative practices cannot be overemphasized. It has been demonstrated that utilizing a number of cross-functional multidisciplinary committees and councils to strategically guide EMR implementation for large integrated delivery networks can lead to mitigating risks, highlighting successes, and removing long-standing barriers and silos that inhibit collaboration. This approach has the potential to yield similar or greater rewards when applied to CIN/ACO development, in view of the transformation that takes place during clinical integration of the CIN/ACO participants and the opportunity to improve quality of patient care.

Another finding of Gittell and her colleagues is the importance of sharing of goals and knowledge together with establishing of multiple paths of communication. Increased use of health information technology and electronic health records by CIN/ACO helps support knowledge sharing and better communication, which underscores the critical nature of these factors as elements that leading to improved efficiency and quality of care for the organizations.

Managing Organizational Change

There are several concepts from the field of organizational change management that are critical for successful implementation of a CIN or ACO. The importance of clinical integration in the ACO model requires ensuring that physicians are heavily involved in the leadership, formation, and operation of the ACO. For this reason there are a number of change management factors to be considered followed by a sample model based on the work of an industry expert on effective management of cultural and organizational change. To begin, what are some of the issues to consider?

- **Resistance to change**: Virtually all organizational transformations are affected to some degree by resistance to forthcoming changes. This resistance may lower efficiency and effectiveness in operations if not managed appropriately, thereby affecting the quality and cost of care delivered by the CIN or ACO.

- **Importance of communication**: There are many channels for sending and receiving messages in contemporary healthcare delivery systems. One of the most critical tasks in the management of major organizational change is ensuring that stakeholders receive needed information on a timely and regular basis.

- **Recognizing tolerance for change**[108] **and having situational awareness**: Physician leaders must pay attention to their team's ability to deal with, accept, and respond to changes that come with CIN and or ACO implementation. In addition, the leaders themselves must possess a high level of situational awareness that will enable them to foresee both positive and negative developments for participants in their implementation.

- **Participation in decision making and enlisting**[109] **support**: Involving physicians (whether employed, affiliated, or unaffiliated) and clinicians in the joint decision making process will be critical to ensuring adoption of new policies and new attributes of the CIN or ACO as changes are implemented. By enlisting the support of the ACO's physician and clinician population, its physician leaders will secure needed expertise for major decisions as clinical processes are integrated and redesigned across traditionally disparate organizations with the goal of achieving improved population-based health outcomes.

- **Evaluating progress**: Each CIN and ACO needs to select metrics to evaluate operational performance (discussed further in Chapter 7) in clinical quality and cost of care. Ensuring transparency and visibility of

---

[108] Kotter J, Schlesinger L. Choosing strategies for change. *Harvard Business Review*. 1979;57(2):106-114.
[109] LeTourneau B. Communicate for change. *J Healthc Manag*. 2004;49(6):354-357.

these metrics so that all stakeholders understand the pace of progress is important in diffusing resistance to change and helping the CIN or ACO perform on a positive level.

Presented below is a simple model for managing change and moving an organization along a program adoption curve based on the principles of John Kotter's eight-step change model as presented in his book *Our Iceberg is Melting.*[110] The model illustrates a three-stage approach to managing change as a CIN or ACO moves forward.

Figure 17. CIN/ACO Change Management and Program Adoption Model

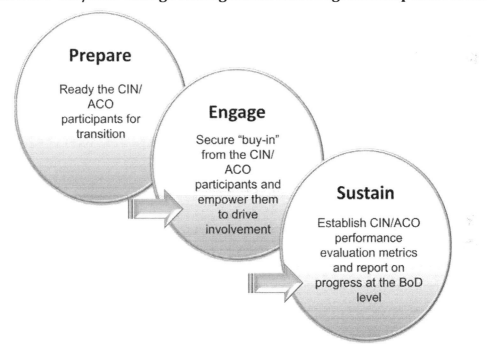

This three-stage model starts with a **preparation** stage. In this stage physician leaders must set the tone for the organization by defining and communicating a clear vision of the organization's future while acknowledging challenges and risks to be confronted. Second is the **engagement** stage. Ensuring that clinicians and administrators buy into the CIN/ACO at this point is critical, along with empowering physicians and other key personnel to take action in and serve as

---

[110] Kotter J, Rathgeber H. *Our Iceberg Is Melting*. New York,NY: St. Martin's Press, 2005. pp. 130–131.

champions of redesigning clinical and administrative processes. Third is the **sustaining** stage. In this phase the CIN/ACO redesign effort has been completed, cross-functional teams are moving forward, and key resources are in place. Required reporting of clinical quality and operational performance measures are initiated in this stage for both the CIN and public or private-payer ACOs. Periodic evaluation of progress at all levels of the organization helps to reinforce gains and support management changes needed for midcourse corrections.

There are many other workable models of change management, including Kurt Lewin's, which consists of four elements: field theory, group dynamics, action research, and three steps to implement change.[111] Our intention here is to bring the issue to the reader's attention as one to be considered in operational planning to ensure long-term success in implementing a CIN or ACO. Adopting a strategic approach to managing change in any large-scale organizational transformation will help to mitigate risks that can affect the quality of care delivered to the patient populations served by the CIN/ACO participants.

Many Routes, One Goal

An important consideration for those moving toward CIN/ACO implementation is to recognize that there is not a one-size-fits-all option in the path to implementation. With so many different potential organizational combinations, legal structures, models of reimbursement and incentives for physicians and hospitals, as well as the different stages organizations find themselves in their adoption of health information technology and electronic health records there will be different routes to setting up and achieving the goals of ACOs and CINs.

The second roadmap illustrates a number of elements that are necessary to ensure and stabilize a general path for planning and rolling out a CIN or ACO from the perspective of governance and leadership issues. As the functional areas are not linear in nature or totally dependent on one another to be initiated, they

---

[111] Suc J, Prokosch HU, Ganslandt T. Applicability of Lewin's change management model in a hospital setting. *Methods Inf Med.* 2009;48(5):419–428.

focus on the core requirements for a strong launch of these new models of care delivery.

Figure 18. Roadmap 2: Governance and Leadership

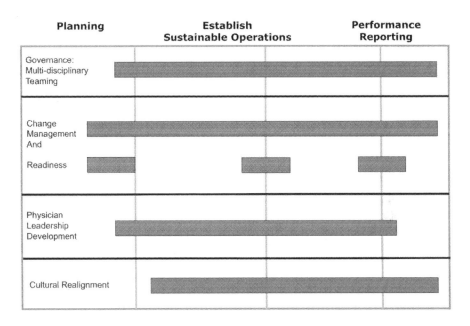

Five key functional streams are identified in this second roadmap. First is the issue of establishing multidisciplinary teams for the long-term governance of the new organization. Perhaps the most critical early task is engaging physicians in the design and formation of a clinically integrated network. From the outset, physicians must not only be involved but also openly asked to lead the initiative to realize the proposed benefits. With the physicians on board together with administrators and other personnel, the group can turn to designing the functional processes necessary to manage the CIN and or ACO. After the basics of the design and its functional elements are complete, the organization's formal governance can be put in place.

Due to the complexity of delivering healthcare services and the integrated elements of the participants in the organization, jumpstarting a CIN or ACO cannot happen without the involvement of many participants and stakeholders from across the multiple entities required for success. Multidisciplinary teaming was discussed earlier; however, engaging physicians, nursing, pharmacy, health information technology, finance, legal, and risk management professionals in a collaborative and cohesive manner will be an ongoing requirement. At the executive level, a strong board of directors providing collaborative governance ensures oversight of all the elements of clinical and financial integration.

The second functional area may be new for some organizations. Change management has become an increasingly important topic for organizations, not only at the beginning of their journey but also across throughout the course of any organizational transformation. Installing champions, identifying and acknowledging barriers and challenges, and finding the path to speed adoption will be necessary at various points in the life cycle of every organization given the rapid pace of change and reform issues affecting the launch of these new models of care delivery. Assessing readiness at key stages in the life cycle of the program or entity when major transitional points are reached is another important factor in all CIN and ACO startups.

Next is development of physician leaders. Physician recruitment is critical to establishing a successful CIN or ACO and to securing the participation of independent or unaffiliated community physicians in the CIN or ACO. Recognizing that these new models of care are to be physician-led and that the core focus of any clinical integration program will involve deepening the relationships with the physician community, establishing a strong leadership development program for physicians should be a priority for those entities in the vanguard of these new models of care.

Last is the function of cultural realignment. In the realm of governance and alignment strategies, it is imperative to recognize the cultural transformation that will occur with the implementation of these care delivery models. The culture of every organization is grounded in its values and the people that actually deliver the care every day.

Such leading organizations as Geisinger, the Mayo Clinic, and the Intermountain Health System already have many of these advanced capabilities in place for launching an ACO. Organizations that choose to apply for the Pioneer ACO Model will also certainly be further along the implementation and adoption curve and likely have many of these high -level requirements in place. In addition, to meet the health information technology and interoperability requirements the exchange of health information and data aggregation are critical to a large-scale CIN and the success of an ACO. Section 3022 of the Affordable Care Act calls for having a leadership and management infrastructure that includes clinical and administrative systems.[112] These systems are key to the infrastructure and communication requirements for ACOs and CINs. Many organizations are at Stage 1 of the three-stage meaningful use program that runs through 2016. Eligible hospitals and physicians across the country are working to meet those requirements and prepare for stage 2, to be introduced in the future by the Office of the National Coordinator for Health Information Technology (ONC-HIT).

Regardless of the path and participants engaged in the creation of an ACO, the Proposed Rule identifies a number of assumptions and uncertainties to be considered. Some of the uncertainties include:[113]

- The ACO participant's degree of integration to support improving quality and efficiency of health services delivered;
- The total pool of providers and suppliers that will be available to participate in the CMS ACO program in light of many organizations that may choose to participate in other models tested through the CMS Innovation Center;
- The full array of savings for participating ACOs in first three years of the ACO program;
- Local variations in projected beneficiary Part A and B cost growth in comparison to projected national averages and benchmarks.

While identified for the Medicare ACO program, these uncertainties, along with others that include the degree of risk a group of ACO participants are willing to accept, can also impact private payer ACOs. Much of the uncertainty raised by

---

[113] Fed. Reg. Vol. 76, No. 67. April 7, 2011. V(C)(1)(a). Assumptions and uncertainties. p. 19635.
[113] Fed. Reg. Vol. 76, No. 67. April 7, 2011. V(C)(1)(a). Assumptions and uncertainties. p. 19635.

the Proposed Rule will have universal applicability and provide additional support for the need for multi-payer models.

Joint Venture Legal Structures: Options for Formation

CINs and ACOs can pursue a number of possible legal structures. For Section 3022 Medicare ACOs, the Affordable Care Act states: "The ACO shall have a formal legal structure that would allow the organization to receive and distribute payments for shared savings under subsection (d)(2) to participating providers of services and suppliers."[114] While this issue of legal structure is discussed in depth in the chapter on antitrust issues, the requirement set forth in the Affordable Care Act and Proposed Rule ensures that these organizations will have a mission-oriented focus and legitimate business purpose for clinical and financial integration. Some types of mergers may include:

- Horizontal: an integrated delivery network merging with another hospital or CIN;

- Horizontal: a primary care medical home practice merging with a multispecialty group practice;

- Vertical: an integrated delivery network or CIN merging with one or more medical homes and multispecialty physician group practices.

There are two examples of the legal structure mandated by the Affordable Care Act. First is the *hospital direct employment model,* which would apply to an integrated delivery network vertical merger. In this model the physician practice essentially joins the hospital, forming an operating division of the integrated delivery network. The second model is the *health system parent-subsidiary legal entity model*, in which two or more legal entities are maintained with separate governance boards while the parent health system retains some authority in critical issues involving the subsidiary. The parent or the subsidiary may employ

---

[114] H.R. 3590, Patient Protection and Affordable Care Act, §3022(b)(2)(C). ACO requirements (2010).

physicians, and financial statements are prepared separately for each entity to help ensure financial transparency for stakeholders and regulatory concerns.[115]

In this second model the physicians are not necessarily employed directly by the ACO, although they can be. The clinically integrated network model using an integrated delivery network subsidiary corporate structure brings employed and affiliated physicians together within a common CIN provider network. Traditionally, the primary care physicians in the network are exclusive to that network and the specialists are not––or at least not at first. For nonprofit health systems this is one vehicle by which to set up an ACO in an environment with an open medical staff model. When forming these structures and others, ACO participants should adhere to guidance by the Department of Justice and Federal Trade Commission Statements of Antitrust Enforcement Policy in Health Care.[116]

INFOCUS: Challenges Ahead

Establishing the appropriate governance structure with so many different possible configurations of physician practices and hospital organizations presents a number of challenges in the early stages of CIN/ACO formation. Identifying physicians who are willing to participate in a network offering to a community is a formidable task.

Another important perspective for leadership to consider, however, is how patients feel about existing models and these new models of care. Patient experiences and satisfaction are critical to success.[117] Satisfaction includes a wide range of issues, from patient surveys to accounting for cultural values and beliefs that may impact or influence patients' ability to accept physician care recommendations. From a leadership perspective both the CIN and ACO models shift the way we approach care toward a greater focus on quality and value. This

[115] Johnson B, Christiansen J. Integrated delivery system legal and organizational structures. MGMA Health Care Consulting Group and Faegre & Benson LLP. Accessed online July 16, 2011, at http://64.27.92.85/files/IDS%20legal%20and%20organizational%20structures.pdf.
[116] Federal Trade Commission. Guidance on antitrust policy enforcement. Accessed online July 16, 2011, at http://www.ftc.gov/bc/healthcare/industryguide/policy/index.htm.
[117] Pourshadi KM. Putting Patient-Centered Care Into Perspective. *HealthLeaders Media.* May 2, 2011. Accessed online June 1, 2011 at http://www.healthleadersmedia.com/print/FIN-265604/Putting-PatientCentered-Care-Into-Perspective.

shift may prove challenging for patients accustomed to volume-based, fee-for-service care in which they obtain the care they want when they want it. In a value-based system, patients may get only what they need, when they need it. For leadership, periodically evaluating the patient's perspective must be a high priority.

Patient Perspective on Leadership in the Future of Healthcare

Where does the patient stand in regards to leadership for the future accountable care organizations? The patient's primary interface with each healthcare organization is with their physician first and foremost. In situations in which this relationship breaks down then those physicians and executives in leadership positions may be sought out to resolve any adversarial situations. A few points to consider, however, in planning for leadership of ACOs in regards to the patient's perspective may include:

- Ensuring that their care is coordinated across the efforts of physicians from multiple provider organizations can be an essential need that is a high priority for the patient.

- Ensuring that the organization provides patients with accurate information regarding both clinical decision-making as well as financial data in support of their treatments/interventions received is an imperative.

Ultimately the power, authority and position of leadership held by the physician executive derive from caring for the patient first and foremost. It is this focus that serves as the essence of patient-centered care. In concluding this chapter a number of challenges, risks, and potential mitigation strategies have been identified that are applicable to CIN and ACO development.

Table 13. Chapter 3 Challenges and Risks

Challenges	Risks
Engaging physicians to develop and participate in a network initiative and gaining their "buy-in."	Hospital systems may develop networks in isolation or from the top down and fail to maintain a sufficient number of providers to adequately manage the patient population.
Determining whether an ACO will be physician practice-led or hospital-led.	Selection of a suboptimal leadership model that doesn't maximize improvement in quality and cost of care.
Establishing a strong clinical integration program that meets the Medicare ACO requirement for participants.	Hospitals that create true cooperation and interdependence and move from a focus on inpatient to outpatient services may lose revenue in the near term.[118]
Securing seed funding for an ACO startup.	Lack of investment will strain CIN/ACO participant's ability to secure necessary infrastructure, processes, and talent.
Securing competent leadership to ensure the success of the CIN and/or ACO and mitigate risk of failure.	Continued fragmentation and lack of synergy across the ecosystem resulting in setbacks and inability to achieve goals.

Potential Mitigation Strategies

√ **Engaging Physicians**. Provider organizations should consider bolstering their physician network development initiatives to strengthen early physician engagement in the development and management of the CIN or ACO.

√ **Who Drives the Bus.** Regardless of whether the ACO is led by a physician practice or hospital, its stakeholders should elect the board of directors from participant organizations and it should establish a shared governance approach.

√ **Collaboration**. CIN and ACO participants should collaborate with payers early in planning an ACO startup to ensure alignment with risk sharing models, contracts and incentives to mitigate loss of revenue during the transition period.

√ **Funding.** Leaders should proactively seek grant opportunities for startup funds through the CMS Innovation Center and other entities sponsoring ACO demonstration projects.

---

[118] Kocher R, Sahni NR. Physicians versus hospitals as leaders of accountable care organizations. *N Engl J Med.* 2010;363(27):2579–2582.

Chapter 4. Operations of a Network

In the realm of ideas, everything depends on enthusiasm; in the real world, all rests on perseverance.

Johann Wolfgang von Goethe
(1749–1832)

Thus far we have discussed health system history, reform, leadership, governance, alignment and the collaboration necessary for the start of CINs and ACOs in the twenty-first century health system in the United States. Primary care physician practices provide the underpinnings of patient-centered care. In the contemporary health system they are increasingly called upon to improve effectiveness and efficiency, coordinate care, and manage care transitions. Getting an ACO or CIN off the ground requires a great deal of coordination within a network of providers to effect change and align participants with the vision of the new organization. In the last chapter we described a number of different models, each with its own unique network of participants focusing on a designated patient population. When the CIN or ACO reaches a multi-payer model, the complexity of the process typically increases as providers care for multiple patient populations with new ways of delivering, evaluating, and receiving compensation for care. In this chapter we discuss a number of tactical issues to consider in establishing the CIN/ACO network.

CIN/ACO: The Tactical Framework

Creation of a CIN or ACO requires a new operational infrastructure. As the Medicare ACO model takes shape under the Proposed Rule and private payer initiatives continue to flourish, we have identified a number of common infrastructural elements. Eleven elements are illustrated for consideration in Figure 19 regardless of the CIN/ACO model implemented.

Figure 19. Elements of the Network Operation

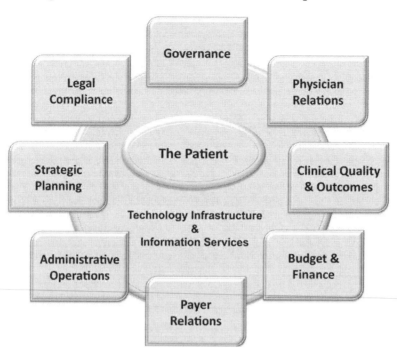

Establishing a CIN or ACO is essentially the creation of a new business entity comprising of multiple organizations brought together to participate in the administration, management, and delivery of healthcare services in a specific geographic region. We have identified 11 elements that are essential for any CIN or ACO. At the center of these elements is the patient. The following sections provide some details of the issues to consider in establishing this infrastructure.

The Patient

The ultimate purpose of every CIN, ACO, physician, and healthcare worker is improving the health of patients. The IOM identified patient-centered care as one of its six aims to improve the U.S. health system. To put a CIN or ACO into operation, network participants must put policies, procedures, rules and guidelines in place that ensure the delivery of patient-centered care. Many, including CMS, have suggested having a patient on the CIN or ACO board to bring this perspective. Other observers, including the medical home initiative and the

IOM, have published principles of patient-centered care. The IOM identified six elements of patient-centered care.[119]

Figure 20. Elements of Patient-Centered Care

Respect for patient's values, preferences, and expressed needs	Coordination and integration of care	Information, communication, and education
Physical comfort	Emotional support-Relieving fear and anxiety	Involvement of family and friends

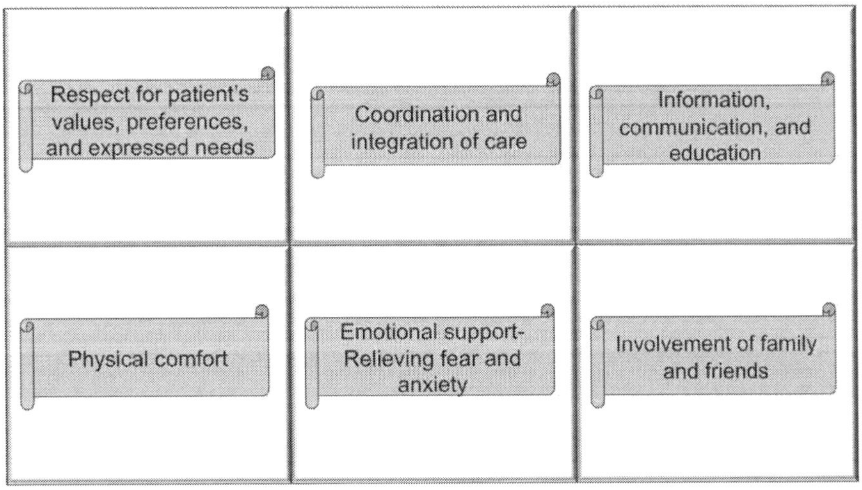

It is worth highlighting two of the elements, communication and coordination of care. Improved communication helps patients prevent disease, manage chronic conditions and understand steps they can take for better health, and allows network participants to turn the corner toward delivering higher-quality care. In the current health system, some patients feel uninformed and unsure of what is expected of them or what will come next in their treatment plan. As patients learn more about their medical conditions and health issues through the Internet, they close the knowledge gap that used to exist between patient and physician. In its place a partnership emerges that should reinforce trust in their physician. These partnerships result in *shared decision making*, whereby the physician's communication with patients and those closest to them forge stronger bonds that improve patient compliance with treatment plans resulting in better outcomes for the patient. Studies have also shown that patient-centered communications result in reduced numbers of diagnostic tests,

---

[119] Institute of Medicine, Patient-Centeredness. In: *Crossing the Quality Chasm: A New Health System for the 21st Century.* Washington, DC: National Academies Press, 2001: pp. 48–49.

referrals, and lower costs of care.[120] Thus, improved patient-physician communication, and involvement of family and friends not only improve the quality of care but also make it more affordable.

Coordination of care is one of the most difficult cultural changes for the current health system as it moves toward a patient-centric future. Effective coordination means knowing the resources available within a community and using those resources seamlessly available. This task is very difficult in the current system due to different technologies, different pricing structures, different insurance relationships, different ownerships and all the proprietary complexities that come with competing interests. Breaking through cultural barriers and making price transparency, quality outcomes, and personal preference the focal points of the care process will be necessary for ACOs to succeed over the long haul.

Technology Infrastructure and Information Services

To make the operations of any CIN or ACO effective and efficient the technology infrastructure must have certain essential elements. Health information technology is the driver of connectivity. These topics will be discussed in more detail in Chapter 6; a number of operational issues are addressed.

Health Information Technology

Health information technology is rapidly becoming the backbone of healthcare services. While electronic medical record implementations are in full swing across the nation, EMRs by themselves would be insufficient to manage a quality ACO or CIN. In fact, successful population health management has been done with little to no EMR technology at all. Instead, early adopters in this space have relied on paper-based registry systems in which relevant patient care information is entered into a common repository for quality reporting and proactive care management. Of course, as EMRs become more functional, manual

---

[120] Bertakis KD, Azari R. Patient-Centered Care is Associated with Decreased Health Care Utilization. *J Am Board Fam Med.* 2001 May-Jun;24(3):229-39.

entry will become less necessary and larger amounts of information will become available for more refined direct patient care and population health management.

CINs and ACOs also need to acquire the ability to analyze data and report on physician performance using scorecard capabilities. The ability to collect and use claims, laboratory, and pharmacy data are also important for programs to succeed. Claims data can either be collected directly from each physician or hospital management system, from payers, or more commonly, from regional clearinghouses. Laboratory data should include all relevant laboratory providers within the CIN market, including hospital and physician office-based laboratories. And finally, pharmacy data can come from e-prescribing directly or more commonly from pharmacy benefit managers within the market. Electronic medical records clinical data are currently not in a useful format. Their acquisition and use is a desirable long-range goal. Claims data are important as insurers and clearinghouses commonly use them to analyze total population health, stratify risk, and identify individual patients for interventions. Because of their long history and detailed nature, claims data are also the only way to obtain historical patient treatment data, therefore providing the basis for the Medicare ACO benchmark and shared savings analysis.

As systems mature they will invariably want to aggregate clinical information directly from medical records and combine it with the comprehensive view afforded by claims data. Start-up operations, however, will want to focus on such near term high-value investments as billed charges that can be instantly mined with many readily available applications. Many vendors are emerging in this space with data aggregation and reporting capabilities. In addition to aggregated repositories, population-based care management is largely dependent on ways to identify, intervene, and co-manage these patients. Cross-system cohort management capabilities, building links between clinical and claims databases as well as between disparate clinical medical records, are essential to helping ACOs effectively manage the populations they serve.

Helping physicians with implementation of EMRs should be considered in the start-up and ongoing operations of a CIN or ACO because of the need to access and mange patient \information from multiple points of care and to provide care management support and coordination. In addition, having a patients' portal with access to their clinical teams and self-management tools will become increasingly critical in a patient centered and value-based system, requiring improved outcomes for reimbursement.

In this age of the Internet and the technology revolution, health information for patients is now more important than ever. CINs and ACOs must introduce processes that strengthen patient engagement and self-management by ensuring patient-centeredness criteria are met.[121] Success in patient self-management requires the use of such enabling technologies as EMRs, personal health records, electronic communications, and remote monitoring. To support implementing these tools, CMS initiated the Meaningful Use of Electronic Health Records Program in 2009 and the ONC-HIT launched the Beacon Community initiatives. The benefits of the Meaningful Use program include setting up a structure and evaluation criteria to improve the interoperability of systems, strengthen quality, and improve safety. The Beacon Communities initiative is intended to establish best practices and models for health information technology advancement at the community level.

These new programs can also benefit the establishment of ACOs. Improving patient care is the central focus of each CIN and ACO. Over the last decade the patient population has been enabled in this technology driven era with iPads, smart phones, and laptops. The asymmetries of information that once existed between health professional and patient have changed in light of universal access to information via the Internet. CIN/ACOs and their participants can use these technologies to support patients, increase trust, and improve the accuracy of care delivered and health outcomes.

---

[121] Fed. Reg. Vol. 76, No. 67. April 7, 2011. II(B)(9)(b). Processes to Promote Patient Engagement and II(B)(10). Patient Centeredness Criteria. pp. 19547–19548.

Governance

Governance issues were introduced in the previous chapter. To launch a CIN or ACO requires a strong, agile, and multidisciplinary group of stakeholders engaged to do what is necessary to ensure the success and sustainability of the new organization. A passion for clinical and administrative transformation and a cultural transition from fee-for-service operations to a value-oriented way of delivering care will be essential. Consider the five potential ACO models illustrated in Chapter 3. Depending on the configuration and path chosen, the leadership structure of the organization will vary. The common characteristic is having a physician-led system with the necessary operational processes and infrastructure in place to work effectively toward improving patients' experience and clinical outcomes, and lowering cost while improving value.

Forming the board will likely involve detailed discussions about voting rights, initial and ongoing criteria for membership, incentive compensation formulas, and most importantly the quality care indicators and care management programs. Board committees of the board commonly include credentialing, quality or clinical performance, nominations, and contracting. Committees will vary in scope, type, and number depending on the ACO configuration, but they must address these fundamental issues and involve physicians so they understand their roles and responsibilities in making the network viable. An industry leader in CIN establishment is Advocate Physician Partners. In their 2011 Value Report their governance model employed in the seventh year of their clinical integration program is summarized below:[122]

---

[122] Advocate Physician Partners. 2011 Value Report. Benefits from Clinical Integration. Accessed online June 24, 2011, at http://www.advocatehealth.com/2009ValueReport.

Advocate Physician Partners- Clinical Integration Program Governance
"At any given time, over 100 Advocate Physician Partners member physicians hold governance positions on various boards and committees that guide the measure development process and monitor results. Advocate Physician Partners requires all board and committee members to participate in a comprehensive governance orientation program, an annual conference and business conduct programs to ensure they fully understand their duties and obligations. In addition, new leaders participate in a mentoring program in collaboration with an existing physician leader. Real physician representation in governance has facilitated a strong sense of group identity, enabled rapid expansion of the Program and fostered acceptance of ever more challenging performance goals and measures by the general physician membership."

The Advocate Physician Partners program includes more than 3,800 physicians. Over the years it has established programs that have achieved significant improvement in population health along with a positive economic impact in their communities. This excerpt from their report demonstrates the deep commitment and level of involvement from physicians in the strategic guidance of the program. Moreover, it shows the need to involve physicians in the development of performance goals against which they will be measured, and the importance of their acceptance of the changes needed to move from a procedure-based to a performance-based system.

Physician involvement and governance is even more critical for organizations interested in becoming a CIN, but not a full-risk ACO. This is because the antitrust enforcing agencies require physician involvement and collaboration from the beginning, to ensure every physician is committed to the goals of cost containment and quality improvement, and collective price negotiations are reasonably necessary and ancillary to achieve that goal. CIN formation is covered in more detail in Chapter 5.

Physician Relations

Identification, recruitment and retention of a panel of physicians and other providers capable of meeting needs in all areas of the CIN/ACO's patient population are essential for every ACO whether public or private payer. Physician relations are a dynamic field as the roles and responsibilities of physicians in today's healthcare environment and society are changing. Decades ago the physician's role involved autonomy, control, and prestige in both professional responsibilities and status in their communities. With the changes associated with healthcare reforms over the last two decades, the physician's position has shifted and the change is affecting the entire profession. Autonomy and control are giving way to an emphasis on collaboration, empowerment of others, and performance evaluation based on data-driven analysis and evidence. The "cottage industry" environment continues to shrink amid declining reimbursements and greater physician employment by integrated health systems and other provider organizations. In light of these issues, managing CIN/ACO physician relations will be increasingly vital. Clinical integration is growing across the industry, and will certainly intensify the need for stronger relations to retain the base of providers in each CIN/ACO to meet commitments to the patients served.

Important components of CIN/ACO physician relations include a strong physician network manager or director, and a physician relationship team. The network manager should be hired early by the CIN/ACO. Physicians are increasingly being asked to serve as leaders in addition to their patient care responsibilities. In these positions it is often helpful for the physicians to partner with healthcare administrators who can focus on overseeing the strategic and day-to-day operations of the provider organizations. Beyond the leadership team, every physician in the CIN/ACO will need a relationship that best promotes collaboration and the attainment of the goals set by the team. Having dedicated physician relationship team members that put a face and a name on the CIN or ACO is a way to bring to life the initiative on a personal level. Certainly physician-to-physician relations are key to success, but they should be supplemented by a relationship team that facilities bidirectional communication.

Regardless of how the relational functions are staffed or managed, ensuring physician engagement is maintained at all levels is paramount to the success of the new organization.

While physician recruitment does not take place officially until after the legal entity is formed and a physician participation agreement created, the recruitment process begins from the moment the first steering committee is convened. As CIN or ACO processes develop, a comprehensive communication and marketing plan will be essential to recruiting physicians. Value to physicians and setting expectations for network participants should be central to your communication plan.

A key component of the recruitment process is finding the so-called right docs. High-volume, high-quality, and low-cost providers are sought after. How to identify and access this level of information, particularly in markets in which the creating entity does not have an insurance product to rely upon for data intelligence, is not simple. Self-employed systems can look into their own data or third-party administrator information, and others may extrapolate from hospital-based data. In most cases insurers have the richest data source through their claims, and most have already identified physicians with the best outcomes. CINs and ACOs should consider partnering with insurers who are willing to share information and interested in collaborative relationships. Regardless of the process efforts should be undertaken early to assess this aspect of network formation.

In addition to "who gets on the bus," network recruitment will need to look at service coverage and make sure that the network is not violating antitrust rules. The legal aspects of this step are discussed elsewhere but must be considered in the recruitment process.

Clinical Quality and Outcomes

The ability to measure clinical quality and outcomes is critical to the efficiencies expected of CINs and ACOs. An old adage says you can't manage what you can't measure, and measuring physician performance is at the heart of CIN and ACO management and enhanced reimbursement.

Finding methods to provide accurate intelligence on clinical quality and outcomes to physicians and clinical teams is critical for CINs and ACOs. Quality initiatives include clinical quality improvement, administrative process improvement, organizational change management, educational programming for clinicians and physicians, and executive scorecard reporting on programs throughout the organization. Choosing and focusing on the most important clinical programs is an early task for the quality committees of CINs and ACOs. For organizations deciding to clinically integrate with independent physicians, the relationship must emphasize improved clinical outcomes and bringing enhanced value to the consumer. Moreover, if an integrated network wishes to function as a single contracting entity, antitrust laws require the network to prove that it can both monitor and deliver greater value to the consumer in the form of improved outcomes, or risk FTC legal challenges.

Clinicians are best suited to judge the available data and take the most appropriate courses of action for an individual patient. It takes expert systems and clinical decision support tools, however, to understand the entire breadth and depth of evidence-based guidelines, the latest medical findings, and up-to-date evidence-based medicine. Whether looking at such specific conditions as diabetes, asthma, or looking at such avoidable events as all cause hospital readmission, the network will need to develop quality programs informed by clinical decision support technologies that set care management and quality goals, identify care opportunities, notify clinicians, and measurably improve outcomes.

Development of such goals as benchmarks to measure quality and outcomes improvement is a critical step for the CIN or ACO. Several factors should be considered in the selection of these goals. Looking at disease prevalence, greatest opportunities for improvement, local expertise, and readiness to implement change are only a few of the considerations to be taken into account.

Claims analysis and clinical decision support tools can be used to analyze data, develop goals, and monitor progress.

Once the goals have been selected, the care management initiatives around those goals must be developed, communicated, and put into place. This process may include a team of such management staff as registered nurses or midlevel providers who assist physicians in caring for patients across practice types and locations. Here one begins to see the need for more advanced technologies for identification, stratification, intervention, and communication. In addition to monitoring patients and the care provided remotely, there needs to be coordination of efforts from all providers, including home care, post-acute care, hospital facilities and physician office settings.

Patient communication, including education, follow-up reminders, and other interventions, are important for patient self-management in improving the health of the managed population. Proactive engagement of patients, including persons without visible signs and symptoms who are at risk for serious illness, may be challenging for some physicians and their office staff. Having effective clinical decision support systems, an office communication strategy, and close relationships with patients has proven to be invaluable. Often the office staff members of the referral team and other clinician participants are best positioned to interact with patients and form the network that coordinates the patient experience.

Scorecards measuring physician performance at the individual patient and total population levels should guide the physicians so that they can see their progress and their relative status within the organization. Transparency of reporting, once agreed to by the clinician participants is a powerful motivator in helping moving the CIN/ACO to a higher level of performance, and is necessary to identify progress toward goals and enhanced reimbursements.

Budget and Finance

Financing compensation of physicians, care provider teams, and other ACO participants is a complex challenge that involves managing the revenue cycle, setting benchmarks and quality goals, regulatory/stakeholder reporting, ensuring accuracy of medical coding, and overseeing audit and risk management functions. Administering these functions under the Medicare ACO program is made more complicated by one-sided and two-sided risk models. Each risk model has a complex set of rules and calculations with benchmarks, quality scores, other factors regarding the ACO's beneficiary population, and their linkage to determining the share of financial incentives or losses by the ACO participants depending upon outcomes achieved.[123]

While complex and from an initial operations perspective, a simplified view of the starting point would be to look at how dollars flow into the CIN/ACO and how they flow out. Sources of network revenue may include third-party payers, self-insurance products, physicians, health systems and private investors. Physicians in some markets have personally contributed the startup capital to get the network off the ground. Such joint ventures can involve second and third capital calls depending on the status of the network. In other arenas, health systems have infused the startup capital to make such ventures operational. The Internal Revenue Service (IRS) has posted a special bulletin on the matter notifying nonprofit health systems that they may jeopardize their tax status if they participate in these ventures. To date the IRS has not provided adequate guidance and many nonprofits are awaiting further direction. As a result, the IRS has in some ways become a barrier to the creation of CINs. A common funding approach is for the proposed entity to approach third-party payers requesting creation of a shared risk pool based on mutually agreed-on goals. Ideally the network will select goals that will bring value to the patients and payers alike. One benefit of this approach is that a single set of goals is easier to implement than negotiating different goals with each payer. With negotiated contracts in

---

[123] Mulvany C. Medicare ACOs No Longer Mythical Creatures. *Healthc Financ Manage*. 2011 June. 65(6). Accessed online June 10, 2011 at http://www.hfma.org/Publications/hfm-Magazine/Archives/2011/June/Medicare-ACOs-No-Longer-Mythical-Creatures/.

hand, and funding of a shared risk pool in place, we now turn to the distribution of funds.

How do you manage a shared risk pool and distribute the funds equitably to physicians and other participants and ancillary providers? No single model will fit all situations; however, a few principles can be outlined. First, most observers would agree that the distribution model should have criteria for both individual and group performance. This feature offers physicians an incentive to cooperate to improve the overall performance of the CIN or ACO. Second, there may be bonus funds that individual physicians may be eligible to earn. Depending on membership status and attribution, there may be a desire to weight payments based on fully delegated or only partially delegated membership. Another consideration for bonus eligibility might be patient volume, such that a physician who manages a large volume of patients within a network receives greater consideration than one who manages a smaller number. For example, highly productive physicians might have greater eligibility than less productive physicians. This approach must be carefully designed, however, so as to avoid overutilization rather than rewarding higher quality and participation. Again, no one size fits all in analyzing these complex issues. The best way to begin is to look at what others have done and engage the leadership in creating a model that works in the specific situation at hand.

These issues must first be addressed at the board level within the CIN/ACO governance structure. Top-level executives will have a need for accurate information regarding the status of clinical operations performance and visibility to health outcomes in order to have an informed perspective on future performance against benchmarks and other quality measures. Once the performance goals are determined and communicated, the CIN/ACO can evaluate the effectiveness of its service delivery, change course as needed, and move toward improved quality and performance.

Payer Relations

CINs/ACOs are tasked with improving the quality of care for a targeted population while reducing costs, and participating in the resulting savings. Various healthcare stakeholders have similar goals for different segments of the American population. Medicare is of course the primary payer for those over 65 years of age and certain disabled persons while state Medicaid programs cover low-income, maternal, and pediatric subpopulations. Children's health insurance programs, some of which are also administered by Medicaid, serve low-income children not covered by Medicaid due to income ceilings. Such private payer organizations as employers and health insurance plans provide coverage for the largest segment of our nation's population. Each of these payer organizations is affected by health insurance reforms, and all must be taken into consideration in setting up a CIN/ACO.

Other forces at work make it imperative to interact with payers. The changing structure of regional markets is a major concern to payers as they see continued consolidation of health systems and physician groups (including primary and specialty care) that can shift the balance of power in contract negotiations.[124] The potential for hospitals and physician groups to concentrate market power and illegally leverage such power in negotiating prices for health services is one of the reasons for increased antitrust review by the FTC.[125] CINs and ACOs must carefully consider both how they establish their integration and the potential impact on the local market.

An important operational consideration for new CIN/ACO is engaging third-party payers and gauging their willingness to collaborate. Collaboration may take several forms, including funding of shared risk pools or other payment incentives to move from episodes of care to population- and quality-based payment methodologies. This variation means opening discussions with each payer and finding mutual opportunities to develop such relationships. Payers may not be

---

[124] Carroll J. FTC Antitrust Rules Offer Hope of Limiting ACO Market Power. *Managed Care*. May 2011. Accessed online June 11, 2011, at http://www.managedcaremag.com/archives/1105/1105.regulation.html.
[125] Fed. Reg. Vol. 76, No. 67. April 7, 2011. II(I)(4)(c). Competition, Price, and Access to Care. pp. 19630–19631.

able or willing to collaborate for a number of reasons. Increasingly, however, some payers are innovating and looking to enhance hospital and physician ability to provide the type and quality of care they do best while contributing the actuarial, underwriting, risk management, data mining, and clinical decision support services that payers do best.[126]

Administrative Operations

Administrative operational issues within an ACO/CIN include such program components as management, finance, human resources, budget, performance measurement, continuous quality improvement, internal communication and coordination, development schedules, and resource allocation. These issues also include managing inherent business risks and developing mitigation strategies. Finally they require developing the processes, policies, procedures, and workforce necessary to make the network successful.

One of the biggest issues facing new CINs and ACOs is underestimating the resources required for successful operations. Under sourcing will most certainly predetermine the new organization's demise. To make the kinds of sustainable change needed for a successful CIN/ACO means adequate resources and a change management initiative that touches every aspect of the organization in such a way that real change can occur and be maintained. A composite of good management skills, disciplined project management, and transparent dashboard reporting are required for adequate administration. In any case, managing operations takes adequate resources, a clear roadmap, and well-defined milestones. This book identifies elements of such a roadmap.

Strategic Planning

Executives of a CIN or ACO should have a core team that focuses on strategic and tactical planning initiatives. This function begins with the board as the entity

---

[126] One example of an innovative approach to collaboration is the Aetna Accountable Care Solution services. Accessed online August 14, 2011, at http://www.aetnaacs.com/accountable-care-solutions.html.

ultimately responsible for the organization, and assumes specific legal responsibilities for a CIN, Medicare ACO, or other public and private payer ACOs. As systems mature, staff members specializing in government affairs are essential to deal with the legal compliance and reporting requirements of federal and state insurance agencies and the changing requirements of public payers. There are many planning processes that organizations can draw upon and put to use in their strategic planning activities; however, there are some basic questions to answer at the inception of an organization's planning process:

- What is our mission?;
- Who are our customers?;
- What services do our customers need today, in the future, and what will they demand?;
- What resources (e.g. staff, technology, financial capital) do we have, and what other resources are needed to deliver these services?;
- What are the measurable and specific goals and objectives related to the organization's clinical operating efficiency, financial performance, quality, and safety to deliver these services?;
- Where are the gaps and how do we fill them?

The answers to these basic questions will vary for each organization. They ultimately set the tone and direction, however, of many activities across the spectrum of planning requirements for each CIN or ACO. Five key initiatives are provided as a framework for inclusion in each ACO's start-up planning and operational evolution.

Establish Mission and Vision. The mission and vision of a CIN/ACO should be communicated, understood, and embraced throughout the organization. They are developed and set by the governance team overseeing each CIN or ACO. To begin, each new organization should focus on its mission--to deliver and improve population health, which should also serve as its vision for the future.

Landscape Assessment. Understanding the environment in which the new

CIN/ACO and its stakeholders are operating is critical to its success. Physician executives and other healthcare leaders involved in the governance of CINs and ACOs need to assess the political, economic, societal, and industry issues that may affect their organization and the decisions they make. Any number of issues can be assessed; most assessments are tailored to the needs of the participating organizations. Some of the issues may include:

+ Market interest in new forms of care delivery.
+ The impact of regulatory changes on operations.
+ Availability of funding from public or private payers.
+ Identification of best practices and plans to adopt those practices.
+ Competitive assessments of regional provider and payer competitors.
+ Potential collaborations with other stakeholders, what those stakeholders bring to the relationship, and the legal structures of such collaborations.
+ Insights into the perceptions of customers, suppliers, and partners.

Having the right information at the right time helps improve the situational awareness of physicians, healthcare executives, and their team to ensure that their optimal decisions will improve their future prospects, and their ability to improve care of their patient population.

Weaknesses and Threats. Throughout the industry numerous strengths, weaknesses, opportunities, and threats (SWOT) analyses have been conducted. The most challenging aspect of this exercise is defining the organization's weaknesses and threats. Weaknesses and threats exist at both the individual and organizational level. Only through self-awareness and an ability to recognize and admit weaknesses can they be identified, discussed, and plans made to address and convert them into new strengths. Threats to any CIN or ACO can be both external and internal. External threats may come in the form of challenging contract issues with suppliers, competing regional health service providers, new legislation causing operational changes and unplanned expenditure of resources, or unforeseen events. Internal threats may include low morale, problems with staff retention, and attrition.

Intelligence Network. Real-time information from the field is critical but some valuable insights are readily available on the Internet. Physician executives and their peers can distill information and determine what is most pertinent to understand the environment and improve collaborative decision-making. In the area of government policies there is a complexity of hidden agendas and competing interests that must be factored into planning. State insurance commissioners and legislatures will largely influence not only by continued federal rule making, but Medicare ACO operations also. Each CIN/ACO should develop an intelligence network that focuses on state and federal government activities to identify the changes at each of these levels and the additional effects of grassroots initiatives, political posturing, and partisanship––each of which can influence future legislation that affects the ability of the CIN/ACO to continue operating.

Embrace Innovation. Healthcare organizations are faced with the need to reinvent much of what they have known as standard practice. Many industry-leading health systems have demonstrated a history of expanding operational boundaries and creating new and improved services with innovation in processes, technology, and workforce growth. Over the years many of these innovations have been tested and adopted by CMS and other health systems. With the passage of the Affordable Care Act, the CMS Innovation Center brings a national focus and platform to develop new models of health service delivery and payment reform. To thrive in the changing environment, healthcare organizations must welcome and embrace innovation. In his 2008 address to the World Economic Forum, Duke University's Chancellor for Health Affairs, Victor J. Dzau, noted an important framework for "determinants of innovation."[127] These determinants are development, ownership and diffusion. The realization of each determinant for any organization requires ideas, people and integrity. According to Dr. Dzau these determinants can foster innovations that will enable the growth of each CIN and ACO and its ability to establish a culture of open innovation with

---

[127] Dzau, VJ. *"Innovation in Healthcare in Emerging Economies."* Remarks to The World Economic Forum in Davos, Switzerland January 24, 2008. Accessed online June 24, 2009, at http://www.dukemedicine.org/Leadership/Chancellor/transforming_medicine/lectures_and_writings/3%20d.%20Innovation%20 Healthcare%20Davos%20Remarks%201-24-2008.pdf.

new pathways to deliver on our industry's obligation to improve patient care for generations to come.

Collectively and individually these strategic planning initiatives will enable the CIN/ACO, its leadership, caregivers, and other stakeholders to have greater confidence in the path they set for the future of their organization.

Legal and Regulatory Compliance

Contracting matters and compliance, are two significant issues faced by all healthcare provider organizations and physician practices. They take on added significance in a CIN/ACO context due to the additional applicable rules and regulations. Contracts with payer organizations will continue to be important for CINs and ACOs to generate revenue. Antitrust law has governed some of the relationships between providers and payers through rules established by the DOJ and FTC. The FTC is most concerned with the regional economic impact of organizations controlling the supply of services, especially if they focus on profit maximization instead of value of care delivery. Ensuring fair trade and preventing the development of monopolies is a major concern. Negotiation and contracting activities require the services of legal professionals as intermediaries and counsel to CIN, ACO, and managed care executives, especially given potential changes in antitrust regulations and waivers. Preventing market dominance while allowing for the growth of clinical integration programs that produce procompetitive benefits by improving the cost and quality of care is a goal of the FTC, and crucial to the success of CINs and ACOs.

Managing compliance involves a host of regulatory issues and is part of managing any contemporary healthcare organization. There are a myriad of issues ranging from patient safety, privacy and confidentiality, financial stewardship, and managing the legal medical record especially when you engage in continuity of care across care settings and among traditionally disparate care providers. To ensure these issues are covered appropriately, an internal auditing, compliance department or person is typically formed or hired to provide objective oversight and reporting. The Proposed Rule calls for five elements of a compliance plan to be in place for a Medicare ACO:[128]

- Assign a specific compliance official/officer who reports directly to the ACO's governing board.
- Put in place mechanisms that "identify and address compliance problems directly related to the ACO."
- Establish a method/system for employees or contractors of ACO participants to report compliance issues regarding the ACO's operations.
- Provide a compliance training program for all employees and contractors of the ACO.
- Have a requirement for employees and contractors of the ACO to report any "suspected violations of the law to appropriate law enforcement agencies."

Community Health Relations

An important part of any collaborative care arrangement that looks to drive efficiencies and value is finding and using resources already available in the community. The challenges of shrinking budgets and growth in uncompensated care have created socioeconomic challenges. To work toward remedying disease while improving quality and lowering costs, CIN and ACO leaders must seek out community and social service resources already available and build them into their operational plans by establishing a community engagement plan that builds strong ties with all services available, including those of managed care payers and social service providers.[129] Other organizations already providing services that should be part of the plan include area employers, school systems and clinics, economic development agencies, social service agencies, and safety net providers. Identifying the spectrum of stakeholders and nurturing the collective resources to optimize performance will not only benefit the new organization but also the entire community.

---

[128] Fed. Reg. Vol. 76, No. 67. April 7, 2011. II(B)(12)(a). Compliance Plans. p. 19552.
[129] Jarousse LA. Leadership in the Era of Reform. *H&HN Mag*. November 2010. Accessed online June 10, 2011, at http://www.hhnmag.com/hhnmag_app/jsp/articledisplay.jsp?dcrpath=HHNMAG/Article/data/11NOV2010/1110HHN_Fea_Gatef old&domain=HHNMAG.

Operating in this era of health reform requires a high degree of corporate citizenship. Accountability is vital, and is one of the three design principles noted in Chapter 1. A strong sense of empathy for the population is needed but will have to be balanced with fiduciary responsibilities to ensure that initiatives for aiding and improving the health of all population segments also helps the ACO grow stronger.

The United States is at a turning point in how we deliver care. The CIN and ACO focus on value rather than volume implies a greater focus on the community and improving total population health. Initiatives that emphasize wellness and preventative medicine are underlying themes of the Medicare ACO. Nevertheless, improving the health of a population involves complex challenges. To overcome these challenges and fulfill the dual missions of ensuring CIN and ACO operational soundness while improving the health of the community will require not only dealing with internal operations of the CIN and ACO but also creating an agile organization able to adjust course when needed based on the community needs and changes that inevitably occur as healthcare reform evolves.

Mapping the Operations

The path to effective operations of a network as described in this chapter is mapped below. Five functional streams have been identified to conceptually supplement the map in Chapter 1.

Figure 21. Roadmap 3: Operations of the Network

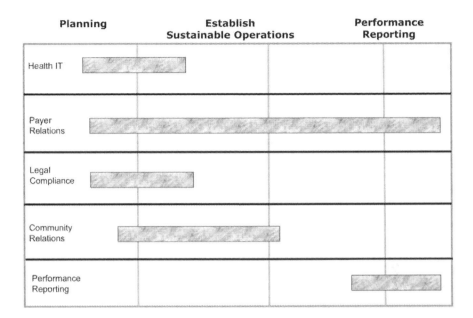

One of the first functional areas discussed is health information technology. The U.S. and global healthcare communities are in the midst of a technological revolution on many levels as technology solutions affects the processes, clinicians, and patients in every aspect of healthcare finance, administration, and delivery. In light of the cost of implementation, health information technology must be addressed early in the planning stages of an ACO or CIN initiative. Second is the issue of payer relations. As the CIN model in Chapter 3 indicates, establishment of a clinical integration program requires joint contracting with payers. As an organization moves toward the ACO model, providers and hospitals may assume more risk in the new organization as they accept more responsibility for quality and outcomes traditionally assumed by the payer. Transference and sharing of risk will be an ongoing process as the new care delivery models are put in place. The third functional area involves ensuring legal compliance to meet requirements of federal and state government agencies in antitrust and insurance domains along with IRS regulations on taxation of shared savings and distributions. Last is the area of quality and outcomes measurement and performance reporting. Monitoring, analyzing, and reporting to executives and team members on quality and outcomes allows transparency, course correction, and continuous improvements in clinical services. With new health information technologies, corrective actions can be taken and rewards given where positive economic and clinical impacts are demonstrated and verified.

INFOCUS: **Challenges Ahead**

In Chapter 3 we discussed the core elements of the CIN and five potential configurations of ACOs. Regardless of the model and path chosen by ACO stakeholders and participants, each of the elements described in this chapter must be addressed at various stages in the growth of the new organization. Ultimately the question must be asked, to whom are the operations of the CIN or ACO accountable? Our answer is to the patients, the communities in which they live, and to the taxpayers and consumers throughout the United States who pay for the health system and its services. The physician-patient relationship is sacred and the foundation of all activities in the healthcare industry, and without the patient there is no need for the technology, the facilities, or the staff to care for and support them.

So it is in this age of health reform that we are confronted with establishing new healthcare organizations. Networks of historically competing organizations are coming together to form accountable care organizations. We are reinventing a system that has evolved over the last two hundred years, a system that has been fragmented and appears broken, with an underlying dilemma of market competition combined with overregulation of the structure that has evolved.[130] The industry made significant changes through the managed care era but now we enter the period of accountable care. Operations may be physician led, but significant know-how must be obtained from other stakeholders with greater experience in improving quality and affordability.

---

[130] Porter E, Teisberg EO. Introduction. The Failure of Competition. In: *Redefining Healthcare. Creating Value-Based Competition on Results*. Boston, MA: Harvard Business School Press; 2006. p. 3.

Everyone agrees that the complexity of the current system must be managed better to reduce fragmentation, and make better use of technologies for patients' benefit. New coalitions and stronger partnerships are being formed among historically competing players throughout the industry in order to help CINs and ACOs work more effectively, embrace innovation, and focus on the Three Part Aim for the benefit of all consumers and stakeholders.

Table 14. Chapter 4 Challenges and Risks

Challenges	Risks
Securing an adequate physician and nursing professional workforce to meet patient demand for healthcare services.	Shortage of clinical professionals to care for a larger patient population and inability to meet new quality and productivity requirements.
Funding the determinants of innovation (development, ownership, diffusion) to maintain a pipeline of operational improvements.	Stalling the growth of the CIN or ACO and not being able to meet an ever increasingly greater demand for improvement in healthcare service quality.
Transitioning physician network operations from a traditional supplier focus to a partnership focus in relation to integrated delivery networks and physician-hospital organizations.	Continued and presence of barriers to collaboration and trust that affect movement toward the two-sided risk model.
Third-party payers may not wish to work with a developing CIN or ACO.	CIN/ACO administrative functions hampered due to lack of such expertise as underwriting and data mining in deriving population level health statistics.

Potential Mitigation Strategies
√ Engage the physicians early in the process and give them the resources to lead the process. Developing a formal communication plan with slide decks, collaterals, and other venues are worth the time and energy.
√ Clearly define the near term technologies needs and research vendors that can meet those narrowly defined needs. Avoid "world hunger" approaches to technology in the near term as you get your initiative underway.
√ Engage third party payers early enough to gauge their willingness to work with the CIN/ACO and to open dialog about clinical interventions that would bring the greatest value to your mutual patients.
√ Strive for an innovative approach and think "outside the box" to find novel arrangements that allow "win-win" situations for the stakeholders involved.

Chapter 5. Regulatory Matters and Antitrust Issues

There are no constraints on the human mind, no walls around the human spirit, no barriers to our progress except those we ourselves erect.

Ronald Reagan
40th President of the United States of America
(1911-2004)

Background

Regulatory issues for CINs and ACOs are extensive and complex. A wide range of regulations already covers all aspects of hospital and physician office operations, including state licensure, Medicare/Medicaid payments, taxes, human resources, certificates of need, occupational safety and health, professional liability, clinical laboratory, food and drug labeling and prescribing, anti-kickback laws, self-referral, health information privacy and security, human research subject protection, fraud prevention and detection, drug enforcement, and others. When a hospital or physician practice enters the realm of clinical integration or accountable care, however, another set of requirements looms large. These rules and regulations involve activities fundamental to ACO and CIN business models, such as joint agreements to negotiate prices and financial risk bearing. In addition to antitrust and state insurance laws, new provider organizations face additional regulatory requirements in such areas as tax exemption, licensing, antifraud, and other matters.

Many existing laws and regulations were established to govern the conduct of traditional hospitals and physicians, and are not designed for newer business models. In fact, some existing regulations actually prohibit or complicate the formation of such innovative provider configurations as CINs and ACOs.

Here we focus on some of the laws and regulations that are being relaxed or rewritten to accommodate the needs of CINs and ACOs. These include antitrust, anti-kickback, false claims, health information privacy and security, and tax laws and regulations.

This chapter is designed to be an overview to present some of the issues that can arise as providers implement CINs and ACOs. Because the following material is an overview and not meant to give legal advice, the reader is strongly encouraged to seek competent legal representation.

Antitrust Issues

Antitrust issues are discussed here first because of the large and growing body of law in this field, and because integration among and between hospitals and physicians, a fundamental activity of CIN and ACO, raises major antitrust issues. Over the last several decades antitrust laws and regulations applied to health care settings have evolved, especially in such areas as price fixing, market concentration in specific geographic areas, and non-price competition.[131]

The basic antitrust rule is that any activities between competitors, such as physicians who practice separately in the same market, that involve setting or "fixing" prices restrain trade in violation of antitrust laws and are by definition ("per se") illegal.[132] There are, however, instances in which joint arrangements between otherwise competing physicians can improve efficiencies, bring economies of scale, and increase competition. In fact, the HMO Act of 1973 recognized this potential and encouraged collective activity by physicians, causing a conflict with the fundamental antitrust prohibition against collective actions by otherwise competing sellers of services. As a result, the federal government has worked to define situations in which joint activities do improve competition and will not be deemed per se illegal. Here we look at some of the ways the federal government has defined allowable joint activities.

---

[131] Jacobs P, Rapoport J. Regulation and antitrust policy in health care. In: *The Economics of Health and Medical Care*. 5th ed. Sudbury, MA: Jones and Bartlett Publishers; 2004,: Chapter 16.
[132] *Arizona v Maricopa County Medical Society*, 457 U.S. 332 (1982).

Collective activity by physicians and hospitals that might otherwise be per se illegal will be allowed if procompetitive results of the activity can be found, such as improvement in quality or lowered costs. A balancing test called the "rule of reason" analysis, which compares the procompetitive effects of the activities against their anticompetitive effects, is generally used by the FTC to determine whether an activity is illegal. Both case law and statements by the federal government indicate that the FTC will scrutinize whether the joint activities by providers create a product or service new and different from what existed previously; whether the persons participating in the venture share substantial financial risk; and whether care delivery has been integrated in such a way that procompetitive results justify joint price negotiation.[133] Fundamental to rule of reason analysis is a review of the facts behind the joint venture pricing arrangements. To avoid per se treatment, agreements to set and negotiate prices must be "reasonably necessary" or "ancillary" to achievement of procompetitive efficiencies.

Although the American Medical Association and others have argued that antitrust laws should not apply to the "learned professions," such as physicians, engineers, and lawyers, the Supreme Court overturned the learned professions exception to the Sherman Act in the 1975 decision *Goldfarb v. Virginia State Bar*.[134] Since that decision, FTC scrutiny of physicians and hospital collaborations began in earnest and has continued to this day. A 2007 article in a journal of health law noted:

> . . . as early as 1976, the FTC was challenging physician attempts to thwart competition by denying reimbursement to physicians providing services to HMOs, penalizing physicians who accepted salaries or payment on other than a fee-for- service basis or limiting price competition by other means.[135]

---

[133] Statements of Antitrust Enforcement Policy in Health Care, Statement 8.A.4 (1996); see also Arizona v Maricopa County Medical Society, 457 U.S. 332 (1982)

[134] See *Goldfarb vs. Virginia State Bar*, 421 U.S. 773 (1975)

[135] Greaney T. Thirty years of solicitude: antitrust law and physician cartels. *Houston Journal of Health Law and Policy*. 2007;72:189-226. Accessed online July 24, 2011, at http://www.law.uh.edu/hjhlp/Issues/Vol_72/Greaney.pdf.

Antitrust Laws

Antitrust laws are enforced by the Antitrust Division of the DOJ, FTC, state attorneys general, and by private suits brought by plaintiffs. The FTC is chartered with "both consumer protection and competition jurisdiction in broad sectors of the economy."[136] In the healthcare industry the FTC ensures fair pricing of health services and products within and across geographic markets and enforces laws that prohibit any activity that restrains trade. Congress has passed a body of antitrust laws that the DOJ and FTC use to enforce fair trade in the Unites States and global marketplace. Three laws form the framework for antitrust enforcement: the Sherman Act of 1890, the Federal Trade Commission Act of 1914, and the Clayton Act of 1914. The Sherman Act, the first United States antitrust law, prohibits unreasonable restraint of trade, including "every contract, combination, or conspiracy in restraint of trade and any monopolization, attempted monopolization, or conspiracy or combination to monopolize."

Figure 22. Framework of Antitrust Laws

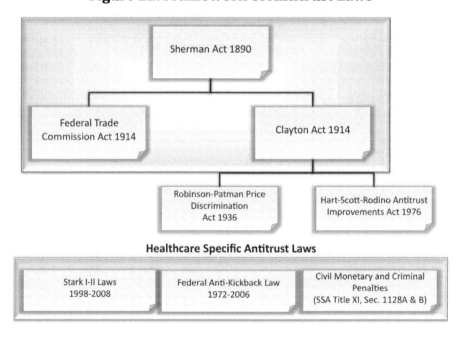

[136] Federal Trade Commission. About the Federal Trade Commission. Accessed online July 12, 2011, at http://www.ftc.gov/ftc/about.shtm.

The Federal Trade Commission Act created the FTC; it bans "unfair methods of competition and unfair or deceptive acts or practices." The Clayton Act "prohibits mergers and acquisitions where the effect may be substantially to lessen competition, or to tend to create a monopoly." The Clayton Act has been amended over the years: notably, by the Robinson-Patman Act of 1936 banning "discriminatory pricing and allowances in dealings between merchants"; and the Hart-Scott-Rodino Act of 1976 requiring advance notice of large planned mergers to the FTC. [137]

Antitrust Issues Facing CINs and ACOs

CINs and ACOs require collaboration among and between hospitals and physicians to obtain the economies of scale necessary to reduce cost and improve quality. One way to collaborate for greater efficiency is through a joint venture or agreement whereby providers band together to achieve greater efficiency and collectively negotiate their fees with payers. Such collective negotiation with single signature authority for hospital and physician contracting is generally considered anticompetitive and hence problematic. Competitive pressures and government reform efforts, however, are resulting in unprecedented mergers, acquisitions, and the formation of new alliances. Many of the new structures have economies of scale that are procompetitive and bring down the cost of care while increasing quality and accessibility. Because these efficiencies are sought by all stakeholders, exceptions to the antitrust rules have been created for certain kinds of organizations and the government is looking at new waivers for other categories of joint arrangements. The antitrust laws, regulations, and exceptions are important for any hospital or physician collaboration.

In 1996 the FTC and DOJ issued their Statements of Antitrust Enforcement Policy in Health Care in 1996 (hereinafter referred to as the Joint Statements). The Joint Statements provide basic guidance to the healthcare industry on collaborative arrangements that comply with antitrust laws, introduced the clinical integration concept and create "safety zones." Since the Joint Statements

---

[137] Federal Trade Commission. FTC guide to the antitrust laws. Accessed online July 24, 2011, at http://www.ftc.gov/bc/antitrust/antitrust_laws.shtm.

were released the FTC has set forth numerous rulings and pursued many lawsuits against physician and hospital organizations for collective activity, many of which have been pronounced illegal as they have not found significant, procompetitive improvements in quality of care and reductions in costs necessary to outweigh potentially anticompetitive effects.

Medicare Shared Savings Program ACO

The creation of Medicare ACOs in the Affordable Care Act and private sector arrangements developing around the country have made CMS, the FTC, and the DOJ realize the importance of providing guidance for payment reform and health system transformation. Recognizing that collaboration among competing providers to improve efficiency is a desirable endpoint, FTC chair Jon Leibowitz commented at an October 2010 ACO workshop:

> From an antitrust perspective, we want to explore how to develop safe harbors so doctors, hospitals and other medical professionals know when they can collaborate and when they cannot. And we're also considering whether we can put in place an expedited review process for those ACOs that fall outside of safe harbors as some may. And let me assure you, if we can do this we will.[138]

Since the time of this workshop, work has continued with a significant interagency effort among CMS, DHHS Office of the Inspector General, FTC, DOJ, and the Internal Revenue Service (IRS). In the Proposed Rule are three specific waivers for organizations participating in the Medicare ACO program. The three waivers are:

- **CMS/DHHS Office of the Inspector General**- Proposed waiver of CMPL, federal Anti-Kickback Statutes, and Stark Laws I and II for Medicare ACO and CMS Innovation Center initiatives.

---

[138] Leibowitz J. Accountable care organizations and implications regarding antitrust, physician self-referral, anti-kickback, and civil monetary penalty laws. Remarks made at the Centers for Medicare and Medicaid Services workshop; October 5, 2010. p. 11. Transcript available at: http://www.cms.gov/PhysicianFeeSched/downloads/10-5-10ACO-WorkshopAMSessionTranscript.pdf .

- **IRS**- Proposed waiver on unrelated business income for tax-exempt organizations involved in the Medicare ACO Program.

- **DOJ/FTC**- Establishment of antitrust "safety zones" for Medicare ACOs based on participant's percentage share of common services within their designated primary service areas.[139] (NOTE: these safety zones are in addition to the original safety zones outlined in the FTC's enforcement policy on physician network joint ventures).[140]

These waivers are designed to provide added flexibility for industry participants and help reduce potential regulatory barriers to Medicare ACO formation. The waivers are specifically designed around the formation of clinically integrated networks and also apply to ACOs. The new rules and waivers bring the potential to expedite creation of ACOs and CINs, and help develop innovations at an accelerated pace.

The remainder of this chapter deals with insights on these laws, waivers and other important laws and regulations that affect the creation and operation of ACOs and CINs.

The Joint Statements

The FTC and DOJ Joint Statements form the current framework for guidance on collaborative arrangements between and among hospitals and physicians.[141] Of particular importance to ACOs and CINs are Statements #8 (physician network joint ventures) and #9 (multiprovider network joint ventures). These two statements provide a framework of rules applied by the FTC in its rule of reason analysis to determine whether joint ventures are legitimate networks producing procompetitive efficiencies that outweigh their anticompetitive effects.

---

[139] Fed. Reg. Vol. 76, No. 67. April 7, 2011. I. Coordination With Other Agencies. p. 19628.
[140] Department of Justice and Federal Trade Commission. Enforcement policy on physician network joint ventures. Statement #8, Section 8A. Accessed online July 26, 2011, at http://www.ftc.gov/bc/healthcare/industryguide/policy/statement8.htm
[141] Department of Justice and Federal Trade Commission statements of antitrust enforcement policy in health care. Accessed online July 26, 2011, at: http://www.ftc.gov/bc/healthcare/industryguide/policy/.

If competitors are economically integrated and share substantial financial risk, arrangements that set prices and are ancillary to the procompetitive benefits achieved either fall under a safety zone, or may be reviewed under rule of reason analysis. When providers agree to share financial risk of overutilization of resources, they have an incentive to reduce costs and it becomes necessary for them to agree on the prices charged for services to manage the financial risk. The Joint Statements describe several financial risk sharing arrangements, including capitation, percent of premium, withholds, shared savings, global fee, and all-inclusive case rates. ACOs, by definition are a risk sharing or bearing entity; still need to document how financial risk is shared.

For clinically integrated networks who don't share substantial financial risk or meet safety zone requirements, but wish to collaborate to negotiate prices, the analysis is more detailed and depends on the facts of the situation. Statement #8 defines a clinically integrated network as:

> ...implementing an active and ongoing program to evaluate and modify practice patterns by the network's physician participants and create a high degree of interdependence and cooperation among the physicians to control costs and ensure quality. This program may include:
>
> (1) Establishing mechanisms to monitor and control utilization of health care services that are designed to control costs and assure quality of care;
>
> (2) Selectively choosing network physicians who are likely to further these efficiency objectives; and
>
> (3) The significant investment of capital, both monetary and human, in the necessary infrastructure and capability to realize the claimed efficiencies.[142]

A joint arrangement between or among hospitals or physicians must meet the requirements discussed above to avoid being labeled per se illegal, and instead be reviewed by the FTC under the rule of reason analysis. Rule of reason analysis

---

[142] Department of Justice and Federal Trade Commission statement on policy enforcement on physician network joint ventures, §8B(1). Accessed online July 26, 2011, at: http://www.ftc.gov/bc/healthcare/industryguide/policy/statement8.htm.

will determine whether economic actions collectively taken by the participants are highly likely to create procompetitive benefits for consumers and whether any pricing or market allocation arrangements are reasonably necessary to achieve the procompetitive efficiencies.

To assist with legitimate healthcare integration, the DOJ and FTC jointly issued a healthcare industry report in 2004 that identified four primary indicators of clinical integration. Additional indicia of clinical integration are listed in Statements #8 and #9.

Figure 23. FTC Identified Indicia of Clinical Integration[143]

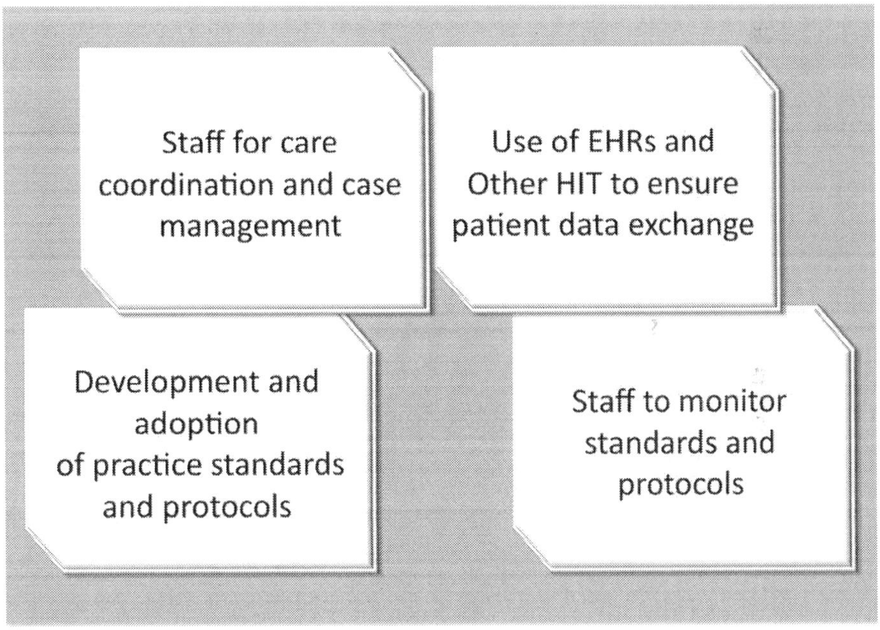

Implementation of these elements of clinical integration requires proper planning and the right people, processes and technology. To begin, recruiting and retaining the clinical and administrative staff necessary to meet all the indicators of clinical integration is critical. Administration and management personnel are needed to help develop, measure, and maintain practice standards and protocols.

---

[143] Department of Justice and Federal Trade Commission. Improving health care: a dose of competition, July 2004. Accessed online August 30, 2011, at: http://www.justice.gov/atr/public/health_care/204694/chapter2.htm#4b3. Federal Trade Commission. Statement #8. Paragraph 8(C)1: Examples of clinical integration. Accessed online August 30, 2011, at: http://www.ftc.gov/bc/healthcare/industryguide/policy/statement8.htm.

Appropriate staff members are needed to monitor standards and protocols, enabling implementation of an "ongoing program to evaluate and modify practice patterns." This process requires development of benchmarks and report cards so that everyone knows how they are doing and that clinical quality improvements are achieved. Staffing for care coordination, including physicians and other clinicians as nursing care managers and other ancillary personnel is are usually needed to ensure appropriate care continues between office visits. Care coordination requires both primary and specialty care participation, and appropriate transitions between physicians, which may be facilitated by clinicians or non-clinicians. Health information technology staff and management are also needed to meet these requirements.

Processes and the policies and procedures to implement them are necessary to meet the legal requirements of clinical integration and accountable care. Practice standards and protocols are focused on creation of clinical protocols from evidence-based guidelines and other medical and scientific findings to create benchmarks against which clinicians may be measured and practice patterns modified for clinical improvement. Measurable outcomes are critical for the program to succeed.

Many organizations develop and adopt practice standards and protocols through committees of physicians and clinicians. It is important for the physicians to be involved in both development and adoption of the protocols, as they will be called upon to follow them and demonstrate their commitment to the goals of improved quality and cost reduction. The protocols may also use clinical, safety, and other quality metrics developed by external regulatory agencies and such industry-developed guidelines as the National Quality Forum, Joint Commission standards, CMS Hospital Quality Initiative metrics, and Agency for Healthcare Research and Quality guidelines. Moreover, clinical and business process redesign is crucial to ensuring an "active and ongoing program" is implemented and adopted by physicians and clinicians.

Finally, implementing electronic health records, health information exchanges, information-sharing tools, and other clinical information systems across integrated delivery networks, affiliated and unaffiliated physician practices, and payer organizations is necessary to achieve the "interdependence and cooperation" required "to control costs and ensure quality."

Case Studies: GRIPA

The FTC's willingness to redefine safe harbors resulted from a number of cases and opinions. Three FTC rulings are provided here as examples of clinical integration. First is the ruling by the FTC in 2007 regarding the Greater Rochester Independent Practice Association (GRIPA) in their evaluation of that entity's clinically integrated program. A 2010 Robert Wood Johnson Foundation policy paper summarized the FTC's opinion:

> GRIPA offers an example of a clinically integrated physician arrangement that successfully met the FTC's standard as set forth in the revised 1996 Statements. GRIPA positioned its venture as one offering a new health care product that would combine clinical practice with an integrated clinical improvement program designed to improve the quality of care and create efficiencies in the practice of medicine. GRIPA claimed that this new product would be "intertwined" with its proposed joint contracting practices with payers (health insurance companies) on behalf of its 500 independent and hospital-affiliated primary care physicians and specialists in practice across 40 separate areas. The FTC agreed that collective bargaining was reasonably necessary to achieve the program's likely efficiencies.[144]

In the FTC's GRIPA opinion the agency provided in-depth analysis of each element of clinical integration and validated that GRIPA's proposed clinical improvement services program showed evidence that the program was likely to

---

[144] Burke T, Rosenbaum S. Accountable care organizations: implications for antitrust policy. Robert Wood Johnson policy analysis paper, March 2010. Accessed online July 27, 2011, at http://www.rwjf.org/files/research/57509.pdf; Federal Trade Commission. Advisory opinion, September 17, 2009. Accessed online July 27, 2011, at http://www.ftc.gov/bc/healthcare/industryguide/advisory.htm.

produce substantial cooperation among participating physicians.[145] On the subject of physician collaboration, the FTC's opinion indicated that GRIPA presented appropriate clinician responsibility and interdependence in a number of collaborative initiatives with its physicians that planned to implement or build "from its risk-sharing program as evidencing the physicians clinical integration through the proposed program."

Table 15. Summary of GRIPA's Collaborative Physician Activities[146]

Topic	Description of Activity
1. Coordination of care	Develop a collaborative, independent network of primary care and specialty care physicians to provide medical care services in a seamless and coordinated manner.
2. Evidence-based practices and performance measurement	Promote physician collaboration in: a) Design, implementation and application of evidence-based practice guidelines or protocols and quality benchmarks; b) Monitoring one another's individual and GRIPA's aggregate performance in applying the guidelines in achieving the network's benchmarks.
3. Use of integrated CIS	Integrate its physicians and ancillary services through a Web-based electronic clinical information system (CIS) that ensures sharing of clinical information.
4. Decrease burdens	Decrease overall administrative/regulatory burden of participating physicians by reducing paperwork and time to process treatment information.

The FTC's plan also included expanding the scope of diseases that GRIPA covered in its disease management services; ensured nonexclusivity options for contracting; and established a clinical integration committee comprising 12 physicians.[147] The FTC recommended in its conclusion that the Commission not challenge GRIPA's clinical integration program as its joint negotiation of contracts was "reasonably related to" GRIPA's ability to achieve potential

---

[145] Federal Trade Commission. GRIPA advisory opinion, September 17, 2007. Detailed analysis of FTC review of GRIPA evidence for meeting the indicia of clinical integration. Accessed online July 27, 2011, at: http://www.ftc.gov/bc/adops/gripa.pdf, 11-16.

[146] Federal Trade Commission. GRIPA advisory opinion, September 17, 2007, 5. Accessed online July 27, 2011, at http://www.ftc.gov/bc/adops/gripa.pdf.

[147] Federal Trade Commission. GRIPA advisory opinion, September 17, 2007, 6. Accessed online July 27, 2011, at http://www.ftc.gov/bc/adops/gripa.pdf.

efficiencies and in view of the "pro-competitive potential of GRIPA's proposed program."[148]

Case Studies: TriState Health Partners

A second opinion rendered by the FTC was the TriState Health Partners, Inc. (TriState) in April 2009.[149] TriState was a physician-hospital organization located in Maryland with over 200 physicians engaged in a multiprovider network joint venture. In this case TriState proposed a clinical integration program that would require a joining fee of $2,500 per physician with no additional investment required (which met the financial risk requirement). TriState also proposed joint contracting among all member physicians to maximize the number of patients in the program and the engagement of physicians to maximize the integration of care services within the network. TriState met a similar but slightly more extensive set of clinical integration requirements than GRIPA. Its collaborative physician activities are aligned with the four primary indicators noted above.

Table 16. Summary of TriState's Collaborative Physician Activities[150]

Topic	Description of Activity
Physician engagement	Requires extensive participation by clinical integration program's physicians in program development, implementation, and operations.
Coordination of care	Maintains continuity and care coordination through a within-network referral policy.
Evidence-based practices	Establishes a mostly closed panel of providers committed to practices consistently with evidence-based standards and clinical guidelines created or tailored by the clinical integration program's participants.
Performance measurement	Sets up mechanisms to collect and evaluate clinical treatment and performance measurement data, with appropriate feedback and action, including information on appropriate use of clinical resources.

---

[148] Federal Trade Commission. GRIPA advisory opinion, September 17, 2007, 29. Accessed online July 27, 2011, at http://www.ftc.gov/bc/adops/gripa.pdf.

[149] Federal Trade Commission. Tristate advisory opinion, April 2009. Accessed online July 27, 2011, at www.ftc.gov/os/closings/staff/090413tristateaoletter.pdf.

[150] Federal Trade Commission. Tristate advisory opinion, April 2009, Part B, 3) Infrastructure and program capability for integrating the provision of care and achieving efficiencies, 19-20. Accessed online July 27, 2011, at www.ftc.gov/os/closings/staff/090413tristateaoletter.pdf.

Table 16. Summary of TriState's Collaborative Physician Activities, cont.

Topic	Description of Activity
Use of health information technology	Requires the use of health information technology, including electronic health records to coordinate care, clinical decision support, communicate effectively communications with network physicians, collect performance improvement information, and mitigate occurrence of duplicate tests.
Governance and peer review	Establishes procedures and mechanisms, including committees of physicians providing feedback and action on individual and group performance; addressing deficiencies in performance within the network; and when necessary, imposing sanctions on physicians whose "performance is chronically deficient regarding program requirements and standards."

TriState went further in demonstrating clinical integration program through their physician engagement, governance, and peer review. These elements indicate deeper commitment by physicians in the network to ensure an emphasis on quality improvement in patient care and controlling costs.

Case Studies: Advocate Physician Partners

A third opinion to note is that of Advocate Physician Partners (Advocate) and their clinical integration program. Advocate's president, Lee B. Sacks, indicated in a May 2008 presentation that the goal of its program is "to drive targeted improvements in health care quality and efficiency through our relationship with every major insurance plan offered in the Chicago metropolitan area, thus uniting payer, employer, patients, and physicians in a single program to improve outcomes."[151]

The Advocate Clinical Integration Program (CIP) was launched on January 1, 2004. It was initially controversial as some stakeholders thought that collective activities by independent physicians to jointly negotiate contracts with fee-for-service health plans were illegal. The activities of Advocate drew FTC scrutiny and a lawsuit by a major national health plan. After years of investigation, the

---

[151] Sacks LB. Presentation at Federal Trade Commission clinical integration workshop; May 2008,; Washington, DC. Accessed online July 27, 2011, at http://www.ftc.gov/bc/healthcare/checkup/pdf/Sacks%20Presentation%20-%20Clinical%20Integration%20Workshop.pdf.

FTC issued a consent decree in 2006 specifically allowing Advocate's CIP to proceed, including the contracting practices. The consent decree was the first time the FTC granted such permission, but the commission also commented that it would continue to monitor the CIP.[152] We can see from the Advocate Physician Partners' 2011 Value Report on Clinical Integration that a number of benefits were derived from the program.

Table 17. Highlights from AHP 2011 Value Report[153]

Clinical Area	Value Generated
Comprehensive asthma outcomes initiative	This initiative produced direct and indirect medical cost savings of $13M and an asthma control rate of 38 percent above the national average. The program also resulted in saving an "additional 58,436 days saved from absenteeism and lost productivity."
Generic prescribing initiative	The initiative resulted in prescribing rates of 4 to 6 percentage points higher than those of two large Chicago-area insurers. The initiative generated savings of "$26.5M annually to Chicago-area payers, employers and patients above community performance."
Diabetic care outcomes initiative	This initiative resulted in an additional 16,430 years of life saved, 26,288 years of eyesight preserved and 19,716 years free from kidney disease. Additionally, improvement in poor Hemoglobin A1c levels resulted in nearly $1.6M annual savings above national averages.
Postpartum depression screening	Screening of 93 percent of new mothers that exceeded the national average of 50 percent. Resulted in saving of almost $600K annually and in excess of 1,638 workdays per year.

Advocate's efforts demonstrate the economic impact on its community and improvements in population health in the market it serves. Proving measurable benefits to the community, consumers, and patients is crucial to a successful

---

[152] Federal Trade Commission. Analysis of agreement containing consent order to aid public comment in the matter of Advocate Health Partners, et al., file No. 031 0021. Accessed online July 27, 2011, at http://www.ftc.gov/os/caselist/0310021/061229ana0310021.pdf; Federal Trade Commission. Press release, December 29, 2006. FTC charges Chicago-area doctor groups with price fixing. Accessed online July 27, 2011, at http://www.ftc.gov/opa/2006/12/ahp.shtm.

[153] Advocate Health Partners. The 2011 value report: benefits from clinical integration. Accessed online July 27, 2011, at http://www.advocatehealth.com/documents/app/Full%20Value%20Report%20-%20Final.pdf.

clinical integration program and compliance with existing FTC rulings and regulations.

The foregoing cases are examples of FTC approval of clinical integration programs; however, there are other cases in which the commission did not approve joint activities by physicians and hospitals. Cases of interest include *Arizona v. Maricopa County Medical Society*;[154] Evanston Northwestern Health System;[155] and North Texas Specialty Physicians.[156] Each case or administrative opinion has its unique circumstances, but ultimately each comes down to the rule of reason balancing of anticompetitive actions versus procompetitive effects, including improvements in quality and reductions in cost of healthcare services in each geographic market.

As health systems strengthen their relationships with physician practices and develop both ACOs and clinically integrated networks, one compelling truth appears: the primary reason for these participants to come together must be improving quality and value in healthcare services. Discussions and negotiations must focus on both economic incentives (such as joint contracting) and improvements in quality and value of services. Otherwise the initiative will violate legal, regulatory, and antitrust requirements from the outset.

Antitrust Safety Zones

One of the most important steps taken by the DOJ and FTC in the Joint Statements is the creation of antitrust safety zones.[157] Safety zones are requirements that reduce the likelihood of raising substantial competitive concerns, and make a joint venture unlikely to be challenged by the Antitrust Agencies. Safety zone treatment differs for exclusive and nonexclusive physician network joint

---

[154] *Arizona v. Maricopa County Medical Soc.*, 457 U.S. 332 (1982). Accessed online July 20, 2011, at http://biotech.law.lsu.edu/cases/antitrust/maricopa.htm.

[155] Federal Trade Commission, Press release, August 7, 2007. Commission rules that Evanston Northwestern Healthcare Corp.'s acquisition of Highland Park hospital was anticompetitive. Accessed online July 20, 2011, at http://www.ftc.gov/opa/2007/08/evanston.shtm.

[156] *North Texas Specialty Physicians v. FTC*, 528 F.3d 346 (5th Cir. 2008). Federal Trade Commission, Press release, September 12, 2008. FTC issues final order on remand in case of North Texas Specialty Physicians. Accessed online July 20, 2011, at http://www.ftc.gov/opa/2008/09/ntsp.shtm.

[157] Department of Justice and Federal Trade Commission. Enforcement policy on physician network joint ventures. Statement #8, Section 8A. Accessed online July 22, 2011, at http://www.ftc.gov/bc/healthcare/industryguide/policy/statement8.htm.

ventures. The multiprovider network structure, which involves a combination of different kinds of providers, will be addressed later. Figure 24 illustrates the decision tree for determining whether the physician network qualifies for an antitrust safety zones (and what happens if it does not qualify).

Figure 24. Antitrust Safety Zones

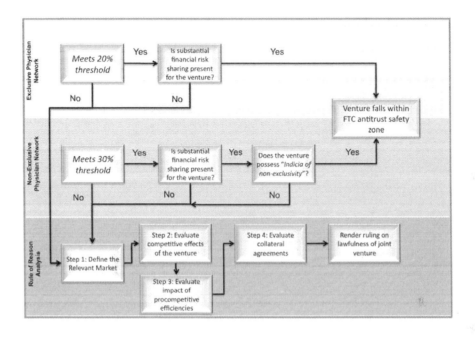

The figure shows two pathways for determining a joint venture's ability to meet the FTC's criteria for an antitrust safety zone. Rule of reason analysis provides the mechanism to evaluate relationships that do not meet the criteria for antitrust safety zones.

Two key factors are evaluated for both types of network arrangements: market share and sharing of substantial financial risk. The exclusive antitrust safety zone has the following market share requirements:

1. Network has 20% or fewer of its physicians with active hospital staff privileges in each specialty area within a given geographic market.

2. In a market having fewer than five physicians in any specific specialty area, "an exclusive network otherwise qualifying for the antitrust safety zone may

include one physician from that specialty, on a nonexclusive basis, even though the inclusion of that physician results in the venture consisting of more than 20 percent of the physicians in that specialty."

If an entity does not meet the criteria for an exclusive network, it is considered for evaluation as a nonexclusive physician network. Nonexclusive antitrust safety zone market share requirements are:

1. Network having 30% or less "of the physicians in each physician specialty with active hospital staff privileges who practice in the relevant geographic market."

2. In markets having fewer than four physicians in any specific specialty area, "a non-exclusive physician network joint venture otherwise qualifying for the antitrust safety zone may include one physician from that specialty, even though the inclusion of that physician results in the venture consisting of more than 30 percent of the physicians in that specialty."

The elements required by the FTC for an entity to qualify as nonexclusive are provided in Table 18 below. It is important for physicians to understand these characteristics to ensure that if an organization claims to be a nonexclusive network, it is properly structured and has appropriate contractual relationships with insurance payers and physicians engaged in the network.

Table 18. Nonexclusive Physicians' Activities: Indicia of Nonexclusivity[158]

No.	Indicia
1	Viable competing networks or managed care plans with adequate physician participation currently exist in the market;
2	Physicians in the network individually participate in or contract with other networks or managed care plans; or there is other evidence of their willingness and incentive to do so;
3	Physicians in the network earn substantial revenue from other networks or through individual contracts with managed care plans;
4	The absence of any indications of significant de-participation from other networks or managed care plans in the market;
5	The absence of any indications of coordination among the physicians in the network regarding price or other competitively significant terms of participation in other networks or managed care plans.

Nonexclusive networks give providers flexibility in contractual relationships with payers and keep the geographic market open to competition. In April 2011, at the same time the Proposed Rule was published, the FTC and DOJ's Antitrust Division (Antitrust Agencies) issued a Proposed Statement of Antitrust Enforcement Policy Regarding Accountable Care Organizations Participating in the Medicare Shared Savings Program (Proposed Policy Statement) that provided additional guidance for Medicare ACOs and their participant organizations.[159] Within this statement the Antitrust Agencies clarified that "Any hospital or ambulatory surgery center ("ASC") participating in [a Medicare] ACO must be non-exclusive to the ACO. . . ."[160] This requirement ensures that providers retain flexibility in their ability to contract with multiple entities, including other ACOs, private payers, and the public payers.

---

[158] Department of Justice and Federal Trade Commission. Enforcement policy on physician network joint ventures. Statement #8. Paragraph 8(A)3: Examples of clinical integration. Accessed online July 20, 2011, at http://www.ftc.gov/bc/healthcare/industryguide/policy/statement8.htm.
[159] Fed. Reg. Vol. 76, No. 75, April 19, 2011. Federal Trade Commission and Department of Justice. Proposed Statement of Antitrust Enforcement Policy Regarding Accountable Care Organizations Participating in the Medicare Shared Savings Program. pp. 21894–21902.
[160] Fed. Reg. Vol. 76, No. 75, April 19, 2011. IV(A). The Antitrust Safety Zone for ACOs in the Shared Savings Program. p. 21897.

Once market share and exclusivity issues are determined, the issue of evaluating substantial financial risk in the joint venture arrangement is next. When physicians assume financial risk, they have a greater interest in clinical and financial outcomes, and the joint venture is more likely to produce intended efficiencies, including improved quality of care and reduced costs for the patient population and geographic market served. A number of financial risk arrangements for physician joint ventures (either exclusive or nonexclusive) are identified by the FTC.

Table 19. Arrangements for Substantial Financial Risk for Physician Network Joint Ventures[161]

No.	Arrangement Description
1	Agreement by participants to provide services at a capitated rate.
2	Agreement by participants to provide designated services or classes of services to a health plan for a predetermined percentage of premium or revenue from the plan.
3	Participants' use of significant financial incentives for its physician participants as a group to achieve specified cost-containment goals. Two methods that the venture can use to accomplish these goals include: (a) Withhold from all physician participants in the network a substantial amount of the compensation due to them, with distribution of that amount to the physician participants based on group performance in meeting the cost-containment goals of the network as a whole; or (b) Establish overall cost or utilization targets for network physicians in whole, with the network's physician participants subject to subsequent substantial financial rewards or penalties based on group performance in meeting the targets
4	Agreement by participants to provide a complex or extended course of treatment requiring the substantial coordination of care by physicians in different specialties offering a complementary mix of services, for a fixed, predetermined payment, where the costs of that course of treatment for any individual patient can vary greatly due to the individual patient's condition, the choice, complexity, or length of treatment, or other factors.

[161] Department of Justice and Federal Trade Commission. Enforcement policy on multiprovider networks. Statement #8. Paragraph 8(A)4. Accessed online July 20, 2011, at http://www.ftc.gov/bc/healthcare/industryguide/policy/statement8.htm.

If it is determined that substantial financial risk has been undertaken and the entity meets the requirements for one of the two safety zones, the FTC's analysis is complete and the entity qualifies for safety zone treatment. If it does not qualify, then the rule of reason analysis is initiated to determine whether it will be challenged.

Additional guidance is provided within the Proposed Rule.[162] While these proposals may be changed in a final rule, some key points may be noted here. First is the establishment of a process for Medicare ACOs and their suppliers/providers to determine whether their arrangement would require review by the Antitrust Agencies, based on their Primary Service Area (PSA) market share.

Table 20. ACO Service Market Share and Review Process[163]

"ACO PSA Share	Review Process"
< 30% (with a rural exception)	"*Safety Zone-* No antitrust review necessary by the Antitrust Agencies."
> 30% and < 50%	"*Expedited review-* Compliance with list of conduct restrictions, or proceed without antitrust assurances- ACOs may: 1. Request expedited review by Antitrust Agencies by submitting a letter from the reviewing Antitrust Agency confirming that it has no present intent to challenge or recommend challenging the ACO. 2. Begin to operate and abide by a list of conduct restrictions, reducing significantly the likelihood of an antitrust investigation, or 3. Begin to operate and remain subject to antitrust investigation if it presents competitive concerns."
>50%	"*Required expedited review-* ACO must seek review by the Antitrust Agencies to assess likelihood of procompetitive and anticompetitive effects. ACO eligibility to participate in the Shared Savings Program is contingent on the ACO's submission of a letter from the reviewing Antitrust Agency confirming that it has no present intent to challenge or recommend challenging the proposed ACO."

---

[162] Fed. Reg. Vol. 76, No. 75, April 19, 2011,. Federal Trade Commission and Department of Justice. Proposed Statement of Antitrust Enforcement Policy Regarding Accountable Care Organizations Participating in the Medicare Shared Savings Program.
[163] Fed. Reg. Vol. 76, No. 67. April 7, 2011. I.(3). Antitrust Policy Statement. pp. 19628–19629.

The wording of the Proposed Policy Statement provides an extension of the previous safety zone language and framework applicable to CIN physician joint ventures involving hospitals and physician practice collaborations. It takes into account the new ACO entity's market share, involvement of critical access hospitals and sole community hospitals, prior review by the Antitrust Agencies, and the competitive effects of the clinical integration program implemented between providers and hospitals. The involvement of rural hospitals is specifically covered by the Rural Exception[164] that notes a Medicare "ACO may include one physician per specialty in each rural county on a non-exclusive basis and may include a rural hospital also on a non-exclusive basis." An additional issue discussed by the Antitrust Agencies is the conduct that ACO participants should avoid to reduce the likelihood of antitrust investigation.

Table 21. Conduct to Avoid to Reduce Likelihood of Antitrust Investigation

No.	Type of Conduct to Avoid[165]
1	Taking actions to keep commercial payers from directing or incentivizing patients to choose certain providers.
2	Implicit or explicit linkage of sales (through pricing policy) of ACO services to commercial payers' purchase of other services from providers outside the ACO including providers affiliated with an ACO participant.
3	Except for primary care physicians, "contracting with other ACO physician specialists, hospitals, ambulatory service centers, or other providers on an exclusive basis, thus preventing or discouraging them from contracting outside the ACO, either individually or through other ACOs or provider networks."
4	"Restricting a commercial payer's ability to make available to its health plan enrollees cost, quality, efficiency, and performance information to aid enrollees in evaluating and selecting providers in the health plan..."
5	"Sharing among the ACO's provider participants competitively sensitive pricing or other data that they could use to set prices or other terms for services they provide outside the ACO."

---

[164] Fed. Reg. Vol. 76, No. 75, April 19, 2011. IV(A). The Antitrust Safety Zone for ACOs in the Shared Savings Program (Rural Exception Statement). p. 21897.
[165] Fed. Reg. Vol. 76 No. 75, April 19, 2011. IV(C). ACOs Below the 50 Percent Mandatory Review threshold and Outside the Safety Zone. p. 21898.

The Antitrust Agencies go on to note that the first four types of questionable conduct are intended to ensure that payers maintain flexibility in product offerings to local market providers. The last type of conduct is an action that would create collusion in the market if practiced by ACO participants. Avoiding this type of conduct demonstrates an effort to avoid illegal collusion and helps ensure that procompetitive market activity is reinforced.

The CIN/ACO and Disruptive Innovation

ACOs as clinically integrated entities have the potential to produce disruptive innovation in care delivery, payment models, quality, and performance measurement as part of new value networks. Clayton Christensen, a Harvard professor and noted author on innovation, defined disruptive innovation:

> A process by which a product or service takes root initially in simple applications at the bottom of a market and then relentlessly moves 'up market,' eventually displacing established competitors.[166]

Christensen noted that some organizations, such as Kaiser Permanente, Intermountain Healthcare, Geisinger Health System, and the Veterans Health Administration all have the "scope within themselves to create disruptive value networks."[167] Moreover, as noted in Chapters 2 and 3, these organizations have achieved advanced levels of integration and operate under many of the same principles of accountable care. The next figure, adapted from Christensen's book *The Innovator's Prescription* (2009), illustrates the concept of disruptive innovation and the theoretical shift that can occur as new models of care delivery enter the market place.

According to this theory, the current market (Plane of Competition 1) for healthcare services was created by managed care and fee-for-service payment systems in the 1980s and 1990s. As of 2011 the industry is moving in the

---

[166] Christensen C, Grossman J, Hwang J. *The Innovator's Prescription: A Disruptive Solution for Healthcare*. New York, NY: McGraw Hill; 2009. Introduction, xxix, Figure I.2 Existing and disruptive value networks in healthcare; Chapter 1, 3–8, Figure 1.1 Model of disruptive innovation; definition of disruptive innovation. Accessed July 20, 2011, at http://claytonchristensen.com/disruptive_innovation.html.
[167] Christensen C,. *The Innovator's Prescription: A Disruptive Solution for Healthcare*. 2009. Introduction, xxix, Figure I.2 Existing and disruptive value networks in healthcare; Chapter 6, 198–207, Figure 6.3 Assessment of candidate entities for managing our healthcare. Accessed July 20, 2011, at http://claytonchristensen.com/disruptive_innovation.html.

direction of more pay-for-performance and value-based compensation and reimbursement systems. The Antitrust Agencies and their Proposed Policy Statement help to maintain a fair and procompetitive balance among healthcare market participants in this new era while encouraging such procompetitive programs as clinical integration.

CINs can be part of the foundation of ACOs and have evolved over the last two decades (e.g. GRIPA, TriState, and Advocate) as viable business models. This evolution has created an environment ripe for public and private ACOs to create a future market (Plane of Competition 2) serve as a vehicle for innovative care delivery and disruptive innovation.

Figure 25. ACOs and CINs: Changing the Game

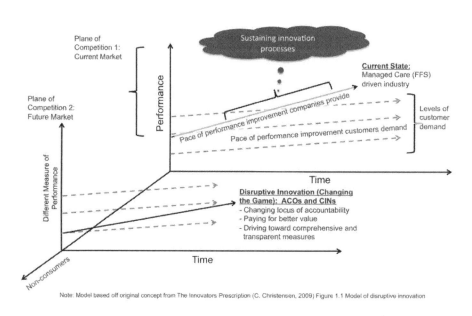

Note: Model based off original concept from The Innovators Prescription (C. Christensen, 2009) Figure 1.1 Model of disruptive innovation

Consumer expectations, the need to improve quality and reduce the cost of care, and health reform will continue to fuel disruptive transformation and drive changes in the market. Within the Proposed Rule, CMS and the Antitrust Agencies noted that "competition fosters improvements" and motivates market participants to bring new innovations to the market.[168] CINs have demonstrated the ability to foster improvements, and early demonstrations of ACOs are designed to continue these innovations. Other potential improvements noted included:

♦ Increasing utilization of evidence-based best practices in markets;

♦ Raising the probability of ensuring that alternative health service solutions exist for consumers in the market;

♦ Strengthening the validity and applicability of benchmarks for evaluating and comparing gains in financial and clinical effectiveness and efficiency.

As ACOs and CINs become more widespread and move from pilots and demonstrations to mainstream models of care delivery, the nation's framework of antitrust laws will evolve, hopefully maintaining the flexibility needed to foster innovation and improvements in care. The vision of policy makers is a future state in which medical errors are reduced, quality of care improved, collaboration and new health information technology used to improve care coordination, and market competition allowed for these improvements without creating anticompetitive side effects.

Other Critical Laws: Implications for ACOs

Stark Laws I and II

The Stark Law (Section 1877 of the Social Security Act) is also known as the physician self-referral law. The law has been defined in three phases since 1998; its general provisions are as follows:

1. Prohibits a physician from making referrals for certain designated health services payable by Medicare to an entity with which he or she (or an immediate family member) has a financial relationship (ownership, investment, or compensation), unless an exception applies.

2. Prohibits the entity from presenting or causing to be presented claims to

---

[168] Fed. Reg. Vol. 76, No. 67, April 7, 2011. I(4)(b). Competition and Quality of Care, p. 19630.

Medicare (or billing another individual, entity, or third-party payer) for those referred services.

3. Establishes a number of specific exceptions and grants the Secretary the authority to create regulatory exceptions for financial relationships that do not pose a risk of program or patient abuse.[169]

The Stark Laws and regulations generally prohibit a physician from referring a Medicare patient to him- or herself for additional services that would increase utilization and the costs of care inappropriately or unnecessarily. As the federal law governing physician self-referral activities, the Stark Law has a significant impact on business relationships in the practice of medicine. The Stark Law must be considered in ACO and CIN implementations because of the involvement of physicians, hospitals, and ancillary service providers. CMS has issued two primary rules (Stark I and II), with two separate phases for Stark II.

---

[169] Centers for Medicare and Medicaid Services. Overview of physician self-referral laws. Accessed online July 27, 2011, at: http://www.cms.gov/PhysicianSelfReferral/.

Figure 26. Stark I-II Summary[170]

Stark I- Phase I	Stark II- Phases II-III
• Chronology- Proposed rule 1998; finalized Jan. 2001. • Applies only to physicians that refer CMS patients for designated health services to organizations they (or an immediate family member) have a financial relationship. • 20 exceptions are defined. • Covers 10 designated health services. • Exceptions apply only to group practices (2 or more physicians). • Violations are punishable by up to $15,000 in civil monetary penalties.	• Chronology- Phase II proposed March 2004; finalized July 2004. Phase III proposed rule Sept. 2007; final rule Sept. 2008 (with noted proposed revisions) • (Sept 2007) Phase III- "Stand in Shoes" provision introduced but not finalized. (updated Nov. 2009) noting that physician "titular" ownership does not require the physician to stand in the shoes of the physician organization. • This provision impacts the physician's compensation arrangement analysis for determining if one receives direct or indirect compensation in regards to the exception established on this issue. • (Sept 2008) Phase III- Finalized prohibition of unit of service ("per click") payments in lease agreements. • (Mar 2004) Phase II- "safe harbor" added for referring physician that spends at least 20% of their professional time or 8 hours per week providing academic services or clinical teaching services.

Stark I–Phase I allowed 20 exceptions to the self-referral prohibition, including physicians in the same group practice, in-office ancillary services, rental of office space or equipment, prepaid plans (HMOs or Medicare/Medicaid plans), and compensation received in physician recruitment.[171] Stark I–Phase I also specified ten designated health services that include the following:

♦ Clinical laboratory services;

♦ Physical therapy, occupational therapy, and speech-language pathology services;

♦ Radiology and certain other imaging services;

♦ Radiation therapy services and supplies;

---

[170] Centers for Medicare and Medicaid Services. Physician self-referral laws: statutory history. Accessed online July 27, 2011, at: https://www.cms.gov/PhysicianSelfReferral/90_statutory_history.asp#TopOfPage; Gosfield AG. The stark truth about the Stark law. Part I. *Fam Pract Manag.* 2003;10(10):27-33. Accessed online July 27, 2011, at: http://www.aafp.org/fpm/2003/1100/p27.pdf; Katayama AC, Coyne SE, Moskol KL. Another round of Stark law changes coming your way as early as October 1, 2008. *WMJ* 2008;107(6):305-306. Accessed online July 27, 2011, at: http://www.wisconsinmedicalsociety.org/_WMS/publications/wmj/issues/wmj_v107n6/107no6_katayama.pdf.
[171] Social Security Act §1877, Limitation on certain physician referrals. [42 U.S.C. 1395]. Accessed online July 27, 2011, at http://www.socialsecurity.gov/OP_Home/ssact/title18/1877.htm.

- Durable medical equipment and supplies;

- Parenteral and enteral nutrients, equipment, and supplies;

- Prosthetics, orthotics, and prosthetic devices and supplies;

- Home health services;

- Outpatient prescription drugs;

- Inpatient and outpatient hospital services.[172]

Stark II consisted of two phases with numerous proposed rules and final versions, the last being Phase III, made final in September 2008[173]; however, several issues remain open for revision based on the needs of health reform legislation and future statutory changes. Figure 26 gives highlights from the Stark Law. The Stark rules are complex and should be examined to ensure compliance and avoid sanctions. Sanctions can include civil monetary penalties and criminal penalties for arrangements established with the intent to assure referrals.

Concurrent with release of the Proposed Rule, CMS and the DHHS Office of the Inspector General issued a waiver that covered Stark Laws I and II, CMPL, and the Federal Anti-Kickback Statute.[174] The waiver grants a Medicare ACO permission to avoid Stark Law restrictions on distributions of Medicare ACO shared savings based on two requirements. First, that the distributions are made to ACO participants; second, that the distribution is directly related to "activities" required for the ACO's participation in the Medicare Shared Savings Program.[175] Potential issues or pitfalls that the waiver did not address include: 1) development and operating costs; 2) downside risk under the "two-sided model"; and 3) private payer ACO shared savings distributions and quality

---

[172] Health Care Financing Administration, 42 CFR Parts 411 and 424. *Federal Register*, January 4, 2001. Physician self-referral, final rule (Stark I- Phase I), Vol. 66, No. 3. 856—904.

[173] Physician Self Referral-Final Rule (Stark II- Phase III). *Federal Register*. August 19, 2008. Vol. 73, No. 161, 48688—48732.

[174] Fed. Reg. Vol. 76, No. 67, April 7, 2011. Center for Medicare and Medicaid Services and DHHS Office of the Inspector General. Medicare Program; Waiver Designs in Connection With the Medicare Shared Savings Program and the Innovation Center. II(B). Scope of the Proposed Waivers, p. 19657.

[175] Charrow RP, Taylor NE. Accountable Care Organization ("ACO") —- The Real Journey Begins. *National Law Review*, April 11, 2011. Accessed online May 27, 2011, at http://www.natlawreview.com/article/accountable-care-organization-aco-real-journey-begins.

performance incentive payments.[176] The waiver should be evaluated for impact on each ACO participant and to ensure that risk mitigation plans are in place to deal with pitfalls that may arise as the ACO becomes operational.

Federal Anti-Kickback Statute and Safe Harbors

The federal Anti-Kickback Statute was issued in 1972; it provides protection for patients and federal healthcare programs from fraud and abuse that occurs due to illegal kickbacks that attempt to capitalize on healthcare decisions. The law states:

> ... anyone who knowingly and willfully receives or pays anything of value to influence the referral of federal health care program business, including Medicare and Medicaid, can be held accountable for a felony. Violations of the law are punishable by up to five years in prison, criminal fines up to $25,000, administrative civil money penalties up to $50,000, and exclusion from participation in federal health care programs.[177]

Cases involving Medicare and Medicaid fraud[178] are prosecuted regularly. The anti-kickback laws are enforced by the DOJ and are designed to protect the practice of medicine. In this context two examples of violations of the Anti-Kickback Statute are provided. First is the landmark case of *U.S. v. Greber,* 760 F.2d 68 (3d Cir. Pa. 1985).[179] The defendant, president of Cardio-Med, Inc., argued that payments made to his company for professional services related to tests performed by a laboratory do not constitute Medicare fraud. In the original trial and decision, upheld on appeal, the defendant was convicted on twenty of 23 counts for violations of mail fraud, Medicare fraud, and false statement statutes.

---

[176] Melvin DH, Millsaps W. The Proposed Waivers of the Fraud & Abuse Laws for ACOs: Have OIG and CMS Gone Far Enough? *National Law Review*, April 28, 2011. Accessed online July 11, 2011, at
http://www.natlawreview.com/article/proposed-waivers-fraud-abuse-laws-acos-have-oig-and-cms-gone-far-enough.
[177] Office of Inspector General, fact sheet, November 1999. Federal anti-kickback law and regulatory safe harbors. Accessed online July 28, 2011, at http://oig.DHHS.gov/fraud/docs/safeharborregulations/safefs.htm.
[178] Department of Justice, press release, June 26, 2003. Largest health fraud case in U.S. history settled. Accessed online July 28, 2011, at http://www.justice.gov/opa/pr/2003/June/03_civ_386.htm; Commons J. DOJ indicts 73 in massive Medicare fraud case. *Modern Healthcare*, October 14, 2010. Accessed online July 27, 2011, at http://www.healthleadersmedia.com/page-1/FIN-257713/DOJ-Indicts-73-in-Massive-Medicare-Fraud-Case; Clark C. Physician to settle Medicare fraud case for $20M. *HealthLeaders Media*, October 1, 2010. Accessed online July 26, 2011, at http://www.healthleadersmedia.com/content/PHY-257184/Physician-to-Settle-Medicare-Fraud-Case-for-20M.html.
[179] *U.S. v. Greber,* 760 F.2d 68 (3d Cir. Pa. 1985). Accessed online July 26, 2011, at
http://biotech.law.lsu.edu/cases/FCA/greber.htm.

The second case is *U.S. v. LaHue*, 261 F.3d 993 (10th Cir. (Kan.) (Aug 17, 2001). In this case the defendants, two principals (physicians) of a specialized medical practice and a chief executive officer of a hospital, had each benefited from fraudulent kickback activities. The principals of the medical practice received over $1.8M from a medical center, and the medical center received over $39.5M from Medicare for services rendered to the practice's patients as a result of contracts with the specialized medical practice.[180] On appeal, the Tenth Circuit Court affirmed the original decision, resulting in prison time and monetary penalties for all three defendants. The court was able to adopt the "one purpose test" (which originated in *Greber*), in which the Anti-Kickback Statute is violated if only one purpose of a payment in question was to induce future referrals.

In light of the serious impact these issues have on the nation's financing of healthcare, members of the Government Accountability Office testified before Congress on March 9, 2011, addressing the issues of Medicare and Medicaid fraud, waste, and abuse and summarized a number of key strategies used to attack this problem.[181]

Table 22. Approaches to Address Fraud, Waste, and Abuse in Medicare and Medicaid

Number	Key Strategies
1	Strengthening provider enrollment standards and procedures.
2	Improving prepayment review of claims.
3	Focusing post payment claims review on most vulnerable areas.
4	Improving oversight of contractors.
5	Developing a robust process for addressing identified vulnerabilities.

Physicians and healthcare executives involved in establishing ACOs and CINs should be aware of these strategies as they set up their financial and health information operations. In the case of Medicare ACOs, in which enrollment and

---

[180] *U.S. v. LaHue*, 261 F.3d 993 (10th Cir. (Kan.) Aug 17, 2001). Para. 45, note on the financial benefits received by defendants. Accessed online July 26, 2011, at http://biotech.law.lsu.edu/cases/FCA/US_v_LaHueII.htm.
[181] U.S. Government Accountability Office. Testimony of Kathleen King and Kay Daly before U.S. Senate Subcommittee on Federal Financial Management, Government Information, Federal Services, Effective Implementation of Recent Laws and Agency Actions Could Help Reduce Improper Payments,. March 9, 2011. Accessed online July 14, 2011, at http://www.gao.gov/new.items/d11409t.pdf.

maintaining sufficient beneficiary volumes is important, it will be critical to understand any changes in enrollment standards and procedures (Strategy #1). ACO and CIN financial staff should monitor developments on these issues for impact to the financial and administrative operations.

Considering the seriousness of penalties resulting from violations of the Anti-Kickback Statute, safe harbors are important to understand as they reduce or eliminate legal liability, provided that actions are made in good faith. Exceptions to the Anti-Kickback Statute provide flexibility for lawful activities. There were ten original safe harbors for the Anti-Kickback Statute in 1991 listed in Table 23:[182]

Table 23. Original Anti-Kickback Law Safe Harbors (1991)

Types of Safe Harbors				
Investment interests	Space Rental	Equipment rental	Personal services and management contracts	Sale of practice
Referral services	Warranties	Discounts	Employees	Group purchasing organizations

While these safe harbors established a baseline of exemptions to the law, more safe harbors were needed as the health system, policies, and practices evolved during the 1990s. In view of the transformation occurring throughout the industry during the managed care era, another set of safe harbors was proposed by the DHHS's Office of the Inspector General in 1999 covering joint ventures, sales of practices, investments, malpractice insurance subsidies, and other key topics.

---

[182] U.S. Department of Health and Human Services, Office of Inspector General. Medicare and state health care programs: fraud and abuse; Office of Inspector General anti-kickback provisions, final rule. 42 CFR, Part 1001,. July 29, 1991 (56 FR 35952). Accessed online July 27, 2011, at http://complianceland.com/aks/fedreg-7-29-91.html.

Table 24. Additional Anti-Kickback Safe Harbors (1999)

Types of Safe Harbors			
Investments in ambulatory surgical centers	Joint ventures in underserved areas	Practitioner recruitment in underserved areas	Sales of physician practices to hospitals in underserved areas
Subsidies for obstetrical malpractice insurance in underserved areas	Investments in group practices	Specialty referral arrangements between providers	Cooperative hospital service organizations

A number of other safe harbors have been created since 1999; however, one rule that is particularly important to ACOs and CINs is the August 6, 2008, final rule on safe harbors for "Certain Electronic Prescribing and Electronic Health Records Arrangements Under the Anti-Kickback Statute; Final Rule."[183] This rule provides a much-needed set of safe harbors for protection of lawful transactions between hospitals and physician practices designed to accelerate the adoption of health information technologies and electronic prescribing systems.

The primary tenets of the electronic health record safe harbors are included in Table 25. One of the key elements of clinical integration discussed earlier is the use of electronic health records to enhance the ability of physicians, healthcare organizations, and others involved in clinical integration programs to exchange patient data. This is a critical function to ensure the efficient flow of information and improve care coordination and quality. Thus the electronic health records safe harbors support industry-wide initiatives to adopt electronic health record technologies as required by the CMS meaningful use rules.

---

[183] 42 CFR Part 1001 Medicare and state health care programs: fraud and abuse; safe harbors for certain electronic prescribing and electronic health records arrangements under the anti-kickback statute; final rule. *Federal Register*, August 8, 2006. Accessed online September 15, 2011, at http://oig.hhs.gov/authorities/docs/06/OIG%20E-Prescribing%20Final%20Rule%20080806.pdf.

Table 25. EMR Safe Harbor Tenets (August 6, 2008)[184]

Topic	Explanation
Covered technology	Software used predominantly to create, maintain, transmit, or receive electronic health records. Software must include an electronic prescribing component. Software packages may also include functions related to patient administration; for example, scheduling, billing, and clinical support. Information technology and training services, which could include Internet connectivity and help desk support services. Does not include hardware.
Compliance standards with donated technology	Electronic health records software that is interoperable. Certified software may be deemed interoperable under certain circumstances. Electronic prescribing capability must comply with final standards for electronic prescribing adopted by the Secretary.
Donors and recipients	Protected donors are (i) individuals and entities that provide covered services and submit claims or requests for payment, either directly or through reassignment, to any federal health care program; and (ii) health plans. Protected recipients are individuals and entities engaged in the delivery of health care.
Selection of recipients	Donors may not select recipients using any method that takes into account directly the volume or value of referrals from the recipient or other business generated between the parties.
Value of protected technology	Recipients must pay 15% of the donor's cost for the donated technology. The donor or any affiliate must not finance the recipient's payment or loan funds to the recipient for use by the recipient to pay for the technology.
Expiration of safe harbor	Safe harbor sunsets December 31, 2013.

[184] 42 CFR Part 1001 Medicare and state health care programs: fraud and abuse; safe harbors for certain electronic prescribing and electronic health records arrangements under the anti-kickback statute; final rule. *Federal Register*, August 8, 2006. Accessed online September 15, 2011, at http://oig.hhs.gov/authorities/docs/06/OIG%20E-Prescribing%20Final%20Rule%20080806.pdf.

On April 7, 2011, the federal government published Waiver Designs in Connection with the Medicare Shared Savings Program and the CMS Innovation Center. CMS and the Antitrust Agencies proposed in that document that permission would be granted for waiver of the Anti-Kickback Statute under two scenarios:

1. Distributions of shared savings that go to an ACO's participants, suppliers, or providers in the year that the savings were earned; and for activities directly tied to involvement in the Medicare shared savings Program.

2. Financial relationships involving the ACO participants, suppliers, or providers "necessary for and directly related to the ACO's involvement in the Medicare shared savings program" that implicates the Stark Law and complies with one of its exceptions.[185]

Part of the intent of these waivers is to minimize regulatory burdens and increase ACO abilities to implement new models of health services delivery. It is recommended to enlist legal counsel to ensure ACO and CIN relationships are legal and take advantage of appropriate safe harbors.

False Claims Act

The Affordable Care Act granted DHHS waiver authority on sections 1128A, 1128B, and Title XVIII of the Social Security Act "as may be necessary to carry out the provisions of this section."[186] Section 1128A [42 U.S.C. 1320a–7a] pertains to civil monetary penalties when any person that knowingly presents a claim for medical services or items that they know or should know to be false or fraudulent.[66] Section 1128B [42 U.S.C. 1320a–7b] pertains to criminal acts involving federal healthcare programs in which someone knowingly and willfully makes false statements or misrepresentations to request receipt of any benefit or payment from a federal healthcare program, determine rights to such benefit or

---

[185] Fed. Reg. Vol. 76, No. 67, April 7, 2011. Center for Medicare and Medicaid Services and DHHS Office of the Inspector General. Medicare Program; Waiver Designs in Connection With the Medicare Shared Savings Program and the Innovation Center. II(B)(2). The Anti-Kickback Statute (Sections 1128B(b)(1) and (2) of the Act, p. 19658.
[186] H.R. 3590, Patient Protection and Affordable Care Act, §3022(b)(2)(G). Section 1128A pertains to civil monetary penalties; available at: http://www.socialsecurity.gov/OP_Home/ssact/title11/1128A.htm. Section 1128B pertains to criminal penalties for acts involving federal health care programs. Accessed online July 26, 2011, at http://www.socialsecurity.gov/OP_Home/ssact/title11/1128B.htm.

payment, and presents a claim, or causes to be presented for a physician's service when they know the individual who provided the service was not a licensed physician.[66]

This waiver authority provides DHHS with additional flexibility in reducing regulatory barriers to the development of CINs and ACOs. Added flexibility may improve the ability of physicians and hospitals to integrate clinically and financially; spur development of ACOs; and increase their ability to implement and test innovations in healthcare finance and delivery.

Health Insurance Portability and Accountability Act Implications for ACOs

The Health Insurance Portability and Accountability Act of 1996 (HIPAA) privacy and security rules govern the use and management of protected health information. Industry adoption of EHRs, increased focus on care coordination, and the move toward state and national interoperability has led to additional rule making to deal with the increased amount and availability of health information. DHHS is currently working toward several changes to HIPAA through the rule making process. On July 14, 2010, a proposed rule was issued,[187] which when final will increase regulatory requirements for both "business associates" and "covered entities."

Health information privacy and security issues are complex and the new rules are still in the regulatory deliberation process. The 2010 proposed rule affected Chapter 45 in the Code of Federal Regulations, Parts 160 and 164. It involved major changes to the definition of a business associate; broadened the application of civil monetary penalties (amending the definition of reasonable cause); and added new provisions for the "permitted and required uses and disclosures of protected health information by business associates." The proposed rule identifies new requirements for covered entities (applicable to ACOs and CINs) that include being responsible for retaining and protecting the

---

[187] 45 CFR Parts 160 and 164. Modifications to the HIPAA privacy, security, and enforcement rules under the Health Information Technology for Economic and Clinical Health Act; proposed rule. *Federal Register*. July 14, 2010. Accessed online July 27, 2011, at http://edocket.access.gpo.gov/2010/pdf/2010-16718.pdf.

personal health information of deceased patients for 50 years after death rather than protecting it in perpetuity. Challenges regarding implementation requirements and deadlines along with the need for more detailed descriptions of disclosures resulted in the issuance of the new proposed rule on May 31, 2011, for Part 164 in Chapter 45 of the Code of Federal Regulations.[188] Key issues in the proposed rule include:

PURPOSE: "Revise §164.528 of the Privacy Rule by dividing it into two separate rights for individuals: paragraph (a) would set forth an individual's right to an accounting of disclosures and paragraph (b) would set forth an individual's right to an access report (which would include electronic access by both workforce members and persons outside the covered entity)."

EFFICIENCY FOCUS: Transition the accounting provision for disclosures from a manual to automated process.

CHANGE IN TIME PERIOD: Propose changing the time period for accounting of disclosures by covered entities and business associates from six years to three years.

DEADLINES: "Covered entities and business associates provide individuals with a right to an access report beginning January 1, 2013, for electronic designated record set systems acquired after January 1, 2009, and beginning January 1, 2014, for electronic designated record set systems acquired as of January 1, 2009."

ACO and CIN participant organizations should monitor the development of these rules, as they affect policies and procedures regarding privacy and security of protected health information.

---

[188] Fed. Reg., Vol. 76, No. 104, May 31, 2011. 45 CFR Part 164. HIPAA Privacy Rule Accounting of Disclosures Under the Health Information Technology for Economic and Clinical Health Act. Accessed online July 14, 2011, at http://www.gpo.gov/fdsys/pkg/FR-2011-05-31/pdf/2011-13297.pdf.

Internal Revenue Service Implications

Two federal tax issues of concern to ACOs are nonprofit status and taxability of unrelated business income. These issues affect physicians, hospitals, integrated delivery networks, and CINs as new business relationships are created in forming ACOs. It is important to understand whether clinical and financial integration initiatives affect tax status and whether nonprofit organizations are an asset to a newly formed ACO.

The IRS issued a notice regarding involvement of tax-exempt hospitals or other healthcare organizations (i.e. § 501(c)(3) organizations) in the Medicare ACO concurrently with release of the Proposed Rule on March 31, 2011. One of the primary concerns for the IRS is to ensure that involvement of a tax-exempt entity is "not to result in its net earnings inuring to the benefit of its insiders or in its being operated for the benefit of private parties participating in the ACO."[189] Tax-exempt healthcare organizations and hospitals must meet specific regulations for conducting business as charitable entities per the IRS Code and U.S. Treasury Department regulations.[190] The following requirements should be considered for tax-exempt organizations that pursue involvement in a Medicare ACO.

---

[189] IRS Notice 2011–20, p. 7. Accessed online July 9, 2011, at http://www.irs.gov/pub/irs-drop/n-11-20.pdf.
[190] IRS Code §501(c)(3); U.S. Treas. Reg. § 1.501(c)(3)-1(c)(1); U.S. Treas. Reg. § 1.501(c)(3)-1(c)(2); U.S. Treas. Reg. § 1.501(c)(3)-1(d)(1)(ii).

IRS Proposed Waiver: Participant Requirements

The IRS anticipates that "...it will not consider a tax-exempt organization's participation in the MSSP through an ACO to result in inurement or impermissible private benefit to the private party ACO participants where:

- The terms of the tax-exempt organization's participation in the MSSP through the ACO (including its share of MSSP payments or losses and expenses) are set forth in advance in a written agreement negotiated at arm's length.
- CMS has accepted the ACO into, and has not terminated the ACO from the MSSP.
- The tax-exempt organization's share of economic benefits derived from the ACO (including its share of MSSP payments) is proportional to the benefits or contributions the tax-exempt organization provides to the ACO. If the tax-exempt organization receives an ownership interest in the ACO, the ownership interest received is proportional and equal in value to its capital contributions to the ACO and all ACO returns of capital, allocations and distributions are made in proportion to ownership interests.
- The tax-exempt organization's share of the ACO's losses (including its share of MSSP losses) does not exceed the share of ACO economic benefits to which the tax-exempt organization is entitled.
- All contracts and transactions entered into by the tax-exempt organization with the ACO and the ACO's participants, and by the ACO with the ACO's participants and any other parties are at fair market value."[191]

Organizations will have different levels of involvement in a Medicare ACO based on contractual arrangements and their specific role in the new organization. Understanding the flow of funds, capital contributions, and economic benefits to all parties are key to managing these new care delivery models, and help ensure tax laws are followed.

Another issue raised in the IRS notice is taxability of unrelated business income. Tax-exempt hospitals and healthcare organizations offer multiple service lines, especially considering the diverse range of private and public payers, and the needs and demographics of the patient population they serve. It is not uncommon for these organizations to expand into a new service; however, this move can have adverse consequences for their tax-exempt status if the service has no relation to the charitable purposes for which the organization was established. The key to this issue is understanding whether the "activities generating the Medicare shared savings program payments are substantially

---

[191] IRS Notice 2011-20. pp. 7-8. Accessed online July 9, 2011 at http://www.irs.gov/pub/irs-drop/n-11-20.pdf.

related to the exercise or performance of the tax-exempt organization's charitable purposes constituting the basis for its exemption under §501."[192]

Changes to these proposed rules should be expected as public comments are reviewed and the proposed rule made final. Organizations should monitor IRS proceedings as the rules evolve and change.

State Laws and Regulations

State governments have antitrust and other laws that impact healthcare organization activities. State authorities have responsibilities for regulating health insurance payers, administering state Medicaid programs, and even health reform initiatives within their state boundaries. Responsibility for maintaining fair and open competition in each state's geographic market is shared by federal and state authorities.[193]

Certificate of need (CON) programs are used by states to help ensure fair competition. CON laws regulate health facility volume and capacity to ensure affordability and availability of health services. These programs exist in 36 states as of 2011.[194] As part of the early design phase and as ACOs grow and expand into states with CON laws, they should check with state agencies to determine whether they might be affected by any planned CON activities.

Vermont is one example of state involvement in health reform. As we noted earlier in Chapter 1, Vermont has taken a very aggressive approach to adoption of medical homes and ACOs. The Vermont state legislature began in 2003 to develop a health reform initiative covering all Vermont citizens. In addition to a statewide medical home program involving community health teams, Vermont has used Medicaid laws and the Affordable Care Act to include public payers in their reform initiatives. In 2010 the state established a task force to analyze the

---

[192] IRS Notice 2011–20, p. 8. Accessed online July 9, 2011, at http://www.irs.gov/pub/irs-drop/n-11-20.pdf.

[193] Hellinger FJ. Antitrust enforcement in the healthcare industry: the expanding scope of state activity. *Health Serv Res.* 1998;33 (5 Pt 2): 1477–1494. Accessed online July 27, 2011, at http://www.ncbi.nlm.nih.gov/pmc/articles/PMC1070330/pdf/hsresearch00031-0086.pdf.

[194] National Conference of State Legislatures. Certificate of need: state health laws and programs. Accessed online July 27, 2011, at http://www.ncsl.org/IssuesResearch/Health/CONCertificateofNeedStateLaws/tabid/14373/Default.aspx.

impact of the Affordable Care Act on Vermont's ongoing health reform program.[195] This task force made specific recommendations in a report issued on October 13, 2010. Recommendations related to supporting the evolution of ACO models include:

◆ Continue pursuit of initiatives already underway by the Department of Vermont Health Access by including publicly funded insurance programs related to the Affordable Care Act;

◆ Continue pursuit of initiatives by the Vermont Information Technology Leaders focused on supporting CMS meaningful use compliance, electronic prescribing, and health information exchange;

◆ The Vermont Banking, Insurance, Securities and Health Care Administration should identify legal barriers and any opportunities for state assistance, such as working toward antitrust exemptions.

State Medicaid agencies are responsible for administration of state Medicaid programs. Medicaid Fraud and Abuse offices[196] monitor and enforce laws preventing fraudulent activities. Enforcement of federal civil monetary and criminal penalties is an important component of state antifraud and abuse activities. As Medicaid-focused ACOs develop, state Medicaid offices will be engaged at some level to ensure that new healthcare organizations meet legal requirements.

Future Legislative Impact

As this chapter illustrates, federal and state laws have a significant impact on the planning and formation of new healthcare organizations. The impact of ACOs (public and private) and CINs will change the landscape of how healthcare

[195] Report of the Health Care Reform Readiness Taskforce, October 13, 2010. Accessed online July 27, 2011, at http://www.vtmd.org/HCRR%20TF%20Report%2010-13-10.pdf; Vermont House of Representatives. An act relating to containing health care costs by decreasing variability in health care spending and utilization. S. 129, 2009. Accessed online July 27, 2011, at http://www.leg.state.vt.us/docs/2010/bills/House/S-129.pdf.
[196] Florida Agency for Health Care Administration, Bureau of Medicaid Program Integrity. Accessed online July 27, 2011, at http://ahca.myflorida.com/Executive/Inspector_General/medicaid.shtml; State of California, Department of Justice, Bureau of Medi-Cal Fraud and Elder Abuse. Accessed online July 27, 2011, at http://ag.ca.gov/bmfea/index.php; Attorney General of Virginia, Medicaid Fraud Control Unit (MFCU). Accessed online July 27, 2011, at http://www.oag.state.va.us/Programs%20and%20Resources/Medicaid_Fraud/index.html.

services are financed and delivered. As the Medicare ACO program is implemented, lessons will be learned and regulations will continue to change. This process will coincide with such complementary programs as the CMS meaningful use program, Electronic Prescribing Initiative, Hospital Quality Initiative, and Physician Quality Reporting System. New CINs and ACOs should ensure that government affairs regulatory activities closely cover state government agencies as they have the ability to issue new rules and regulations that affect the operations of these new care delivery organizations. Ensuring resources are in place to monitor government policies and rule-making processes at both federal and state levels will allow CIN and ACO leaders to mitigate risk, deal with changes, and adjust operating or financial plans accordingly.

Innovations that emerge throughout the industry will result in new modes of operation for healthcare providers as changes in the delivery system bring about closer integration to achieve greater efficiencies that improve quality and reduce costs, benefiting patients and their communities. Continuing our roadmap series, four functional streams have been identified for CINs and ACOs to address throughout their efforts to launch and manage their new organizations.

Figure 27. Roadmap 2: Navigating the Antitrust/Regulatory Landscape

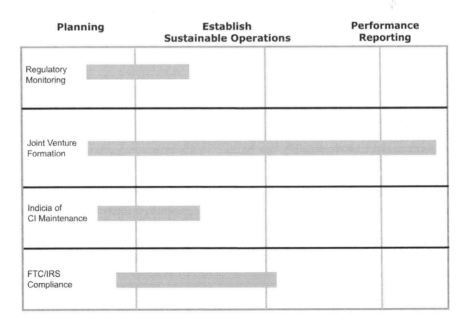

A primary functional stream is formation and ongoing management of the joint venture. Oversight from the CIN or ACO's executive governance board, with physician leadership and involvement of all key participants, is required to ensure compliance and manage change.

Regulatory monitoring is critical, especially in the formative stages of these organizations. A complete understanding of complex regulations is important to be compliant with the most current rules of federal, state and local government agencies. One product of this activity should be a comprehensive antitrust action plan early in the design stage. Third is clinical and financial integration. Elements of clinical integration were identified earlier as 1) staff for care coordination and case management; 2) adoption of practice standards and protocols; 3) use of EHR to ensure patient data exchange; and 4) having staff in place to monitor standards and protocols. In addition, future disruptive innovations may result in new requirements for clinical integration that result in procompetitive effects of higher quality and lower costs.

Last is compliance with FTC, DOJ, DHHS, CMS, IRS, and other government regulatory bodies. This functional stream is an ongoing initiative that ensures continued compliance over time.

Planning for these areas should involve the CEO, senior executives, legal counsel, government affairs experts, and other staff from across the CIN/ACO. Typically this planning requires board involvement and establishment of a regulatory compliance committee coordinated by a government affairs expert and a compliance officer.

INFOCUS: **Challenges Ahead**

Changes to federal and state laws and regulations will continue to have a significant impact on the evolution of CINs and ACOs. To be successful, organizations must build and maintain clinical integration programs that have both positive economic impacts and improve the quality of healthcare. As joint ventures are proposed among competitors (horizontal) and partners throughout the healthcare supply chain (vertical) in the development of CINs and ACOs, federal and state agencies will monitor markets for anticompetitive behavior[197] to ensure that procompetitive effects of improved quality and lower costs mitigate any potential economic harm to consumers.

As these market changes tale place, federal and state regulators should evaluate the implications of allowing the "effects of monopoly extraction"[198] (reducing competition in some regions to stimulate innovation for the benefit of all) over against ensuring the "effects of monopoly extension."

The proposed waiver of federal tax laws, fraud and abuse laws, and the new antitrust statements should be monitored as final rules emerge and supplement the analyses in this book. Clinical integration programs are essential to the structure of ACOs, and will continue to evolve. Those who are involved in developing new relationships among physician practices, hospital organizations,

---

[197] Besanko D, Dranove D, Shanley M, Schaefer S. Competitors and competition. In: *Economics of Strategy*, 3rd ed. Hoboken, NJ: John Wiley and Sons, Inc., 2004, pp. 218–223.

[198] Raskovich A, Miller NH. Cumulative innovation and competition policy. Department of Justice Economic Analysis Group Discussion paper, September 2010. Accessed online July 27, 2011, at http://www.justice.gov/atr/public/eag/262643.pdf.

and other suppliers of services and products should ensure that key staff members are in place to deal with the challenges and risks that will continue to emerge with future changes in federal and state laws and regulations.

Table 26. Chapter 5 Challenges and Risks

Challenges	Risks
Ensuring that clinical operations across CIN/ACO participants demonstrate the indicia of clinical integration established by the FTC.	If indicia of clinical integration are not met, the FTC or DOJ can rule against the formation of a CIN and or ACO and unwind the makings of the network.
Moving quickly enough to remain competitive in a market amidst the changing landscape of federal safe harbors and state antitrust laws.	Loss of opportunities to form the best non-exclusive joint ventures for the benefit of the local patient and beneficiary population.
Maintaining tax-exempt status of a Medicare ACO and keeping service lines that generate unrelated business income at arms length from the ACO.	Loss of tax-exempt status would result in significant federal and state tax burdens on shared savings distributions.
Maintaining government affairs resources to ensure regulatory compliance and monitor the changing landscape of regulations for the Shared Savings Program, HITECH Act, HIPAA, and other laws.	Lack of insights for CIN and ACO leaders on regulatory matters and risk of loss of competitive balance in geographic markets with the potential of creating anticompetitive practices.
Potential Mitigation Strategies	
√ Conduct an antitrust and regulatory readiness assessment that includes the areas of clinical, legal, financial, and administrative operations.	
√ Engage legal counsel with expertise in antitrust matters, IRS Code implications, and state regulatory issues pertinent to CIN/ACO legal and contractual arrangements.	
√ Monitor changes in federal and state laws and regulations as they are released.	
√ Develop a strategy for clinically integrated networks that are needed to meet the formative requirements for the Medicare ACO.	
√ Develop an antitrust and regulatory action plan to ensure compliance across the framework of federal and state antitrust laws and regulations.	

Chapter 6. Technology Advancement

...IT must play a central role in the redesign of the health care system if a substantial improvement in health care quality is to be achieved during the coming decade. [199]

Institute of Medicine

2001 Report. Crossing the Quality Chasm

The IOM envisioned over a decade ago that health information technology would be essential to eliminate medical errors and improve the quality of care delivered in the United States. Health information technology infrastructure for CINs and ACOs will help meet the continuously evolving requirements for higher quality and affordability by getting the right information to the right place at the right time. Section 3022 of the Affordable Care Act specifies that the Medicare ACO must have "clinical and administrative systems," and use "telehealth, remote patient monitoring, and other such enabling technologies" to report cost and quality measures as well as coordinate patient care activities.[200] These same requirements will likely apply to Medicaid pediatric ACOs and private payer ACO models as well.

The availability and adoption of health information technology has grown rapidly over the past three decades. The need for these systems as prerequisites for healthcare and reimbursement reforms has increased interest in their adoption. Such other initiatives as EMR implementation incentives, the conversion to International Classification of Diseases tenth edition (ICD)-10 coding, and efforts to establish nationwide health information exchanges (HIEs) have reinforced the importance of technology in healthcare. For CINs and ACOs,

---

[199] Institute of Medicine, Committee on Quality of Health Care in America. Using Health Information Technology. In: *Crossing the Quality Chasm: A New Health System for the 21st Century*. Washington, DC: National Academies Press; 2001. p. 164.
[200] H.R. 3590, Patient Protection and Affordable Care Act, §3022(b)(2)(F) and (G). Requirements for ACOs (2010).

health information technologies serve important functions of giving teams real-time access to patient records; stratification and identification of patients requiring treatment or intervention; collaboration and coordination across the continuum of care, monitoring and measuring quality and outcomes; and improving quality and affordability of both ambulatory and inpatient care.

The importance of EMRs has been demonstrated in many ways throughout the last decade. These systems bring tremendous potential for increased patient safety and improved care, but also carry new risks that must be mitigated. In 2004 the federal government led the cause when then-President George Bush issued a mandate for EMRs to be implemented across the nation within 10 years to support the establishment of a national health information network.[201] Since 2004, the Obama Administration guided ARRA and the HITECH Act through Congress, launching CMS's meaningful use of electronic health records program and setting in motion the largest reform of the health care system since 1965. A wide range of laws and programs requiring the adoption of health information technology accompanied the acts.

Many potential benefits come with the implementation of EMRs, including improved safety through elimination of medical errors, reduction of unnecessary procedures and tests, improved care coordination, and the potential to achieve better health outcomes as well as nationwide savings in healthcare costs. Healthcare industry observers, however, have noted that adoption of EMRs was slow through 2009 in light of capital requirements for initial system purchases; difficulty validating projected returns on investments; anticipated maintenance requirements; and resistance on the part of healthcare provider organizations and physicians to make the transition from paper medical records to the EMR environment.[202] As financial incentives increase along with access to funding for procurements and implementations, some of these monetary barriers will be lowered for many health service providers and practices. In response to the need to understand the status of EMR implementations across the country, the

---

[201] Ford EW, Menachemi N, Peterson LT, Huerta TR. Resistance is futile: but it is slowing the pace of EHR adoption nonetheless. *J Am Med Inform Assoc.* 2009;16(3):274–281.
[202] Jha AK, DesRoches CM, Campbell EG, et al. Use of electronic health records in U.S. hospitals. *N Engl J Med.* 2009;360(16):1628–1638.

Healthcare Information and Management Systems Society's (HIMSS) Analytics subsidiary created the EMR Adoption Model[SM] which has been recognized as a significant barometer of the national status of EMR implementations.[203]

A snapshot of the model with results from 2009 through 2010 illustrates the progress of adoption across the country.

Figure 28. HIMSS Analytics EMR Adoption Model

		2009 Final	2010 Final
Stage 7	Complete EMR; CCD transactions to share data; Data warehousing; Data continuity with ED, ambulatory, OP	0.7%	1.0%
Stage 6	Physician documentation (structured templates), full CDSS (variance & compliance), full R-PACS	1.6%	3.2%
Stage 5	Closed loop medication administration	3.8%	4.5%
Stage 4	CPOE, Clinical Decision Support (clinical protocols)	7.4%	10.5%
Stage 3	Nursing/clinical documentation (flow sheets), CDSS (error checking), PACS available outside Radiology	50.9%	49.0%
Stage 2	CDR, Controlled Medical Vocabulary, CDS, may have Document Imaging; HIE capable	16.9%	14.6%
Stage 1	Ancillaries – Lab, Rad, Pharmacy – All Installed	7.2%	7.1%
Stage 0	All Three Ancillaries Not Installed	11.5%	10.1%

©2011 HIMSS Analytics   Data from HIMSS Analytics™ Database   N =   5,235 / 5,281

The data used by the model to evaluate hospitals are self-reported by several thousand hospitals across the country. The model tracks the rate of adoption based on a number of different statistics and variables.[204]

A number of health systems and hospitals have achieved Stage 7 of the model, showing progress across the country with EMR adoption.[205]

[203] HIMSS Analytics. EMR Adoption Model. Accessed online June 17, 2011, at http://www.himssanalytics.org/hc_providers/emr_adoption.asp.
[204] Hersh W, Wright A. What Workforce is Needed to Implement the Health Information Technology Agenda? Analysis from the HIMSS Analytics™ Database. *AMIA Annu Symp Proc*. 2008:303–307. Published online 2008.
[205] HIMSS Analytics. Stage 7 Hospitals. Accessed online June 17, 2011 at http://www.himssanalytics.org/hc_providers/stage7Hospitals.asp.

Table 28. Stage 7 Hospitals and Health Systems

Health System	Locations	No. of Sites	No. of Beds
Children's Hospital Boston	Boston, MA	1	397
Children's Medical Center	Dallas, TX	1	487
Children's Medical Center	Plano, TX	1	72
Citizen's Memorial Healthcare	Bolivar, MO	1	74
Kaiser Permanente	California	34	7,654
Mayo Clinic	Minnesota	2	1,951
NorthShore University HealthSystem	Evanston, IL	4	858
Sentara Healthcare	Norfolk, VA	6	1,587
Seoul National University Bundang Hospital	Bundang, South Korea	1	910
Stanford Hospital and Clinics	Palo Alto, CA	1	613
Tucson Medical Center	Tucson, AZ	1	612
University of Pittsburgh Medical Center	Pittsburgh, PA	1	296
University of Wisconsin Hospital and Clinics	Madison, WI	2	570

These organizations comprise a select group that has achieved a standard of excellence with health information technology integration in their care delivery settings. They have established a new standard in their cultures for utilization of EMRs to improve patient care, by moving their care provider teams from paper-based medical records to the paperless EMR-driven care setting.

Recognizing challenges faced by the industry, the Joint Commission issued a report at the end of 2008 regarding safety concerns related to health information technology implementation, and suggested 13 suggested actions to help improve patient safety and mitigate risks.[206] A number of issues were cited in the commission's report; however, the one to emphasize here is unintended adverse consequences. In a study of five hospitals and their computerized provider order

---

[206] Joint Commission. Sentinel Event Alert, December 11, 2008. Safely implementing health information and converging technologies. Accessed online July 20, 2011 at http://www.jointcommission.org/assets/1/18/SEA_42.PDF.

entry system, Ash, Sittig and their colleagues defined and provided a detailed analysis of a set of nine unintended adverse consequences.[207] The unintended adverse consequences noted by the team include:

- More work or new types of work for physicians and other clinicians
- Workflow complications
- System demands
- Communication breakdowns
- Persistence of paper medical records
- Emotional repercussions
- New types of errors
- Shifts in power in the care environment
- Overdependence on technology

The issue of workflow redesign is crucial to both computerized physician order entry and implementation of every EMR. EMR implementation requires the engagement of clinicians, physicians, and IT staff along with vendors to ensure successful transition to the new EMR-driven environment is successful. The involvement of staff members in EMR implementation and workflow redesign minimizes the occurrence of unintended adverse consequences, e-iatrogenesis (defined as "patient harm caused at least in part by the application of health information technology"),[208] and other events that may negatively affect the quality of patient care.

With legislative and regulatory reforms accelerating ACO and clinical integration program development among hospitals and physician practices, ensuring interoperability among EMRs will support accurate and timely bilateral

---

[207] Ash JS, Sittig DF, Poon EG, Guappone K, Campbell E, Dykstra RH. The extent and importance of unintended consequences related to computerized provider order entry. *J Am Med Inform Assoc.* 2007;14(4): 415-423; Campbell EM, Sittig DF, Ash JS, Guappone K, Dykstra RH. Types of unintended consequences related to computerized provider order entry. *J Am Med Inform Assoc* 2006;13(5):547-556.
[208] Weiner JP, Kfuri T, Chan K, Fowles JB. e-Iatrogenesis: the most critical unintended consequence of CPOE and other HIT. *J Am Med Inform Assoc.* 2007;14(3):387-388.

health information exchange between hospitals and office-based EMRs. Interoperability in turn will ensure the efficient coordination and continuity of care offered by any CIN or ACO. In light of these issues, CMS announced its final criteria for its meaningful use of electronic health records incentive program on July 13, 2010. The criteria provide the set of technical requirements that eligible hospitals and healthcare professionals must meet in order to receive incentive payments and avoid penalties.[209] Establishing health information exchange, clinical decision support and computerized physician order entry capabilities are all requirements that will become increasingly important for ACOs. Organizations have already begun attestation for Stage 1 incentives in 2011. Penalties for entities that do not implement certified EMR technology will not be imposed until 2016. CMS defined Stage 1 requirements as follows:[210]

Stage 1 of the meaningful use program includes both a core set and a menu set of objectives that are specific to eligible professionals or eligible hospitals and critical access hospitals.

Eligible professionals have 25 meaningful use objectives (15 are required). To qualify for an incentive payment, they must meet 20 of the 25 objectives.

♦ 5 additional objectives may be chosen from the list of 10 menu set objectives.

Eligible hospitals and critical access hospitals have 24 meaningful use objectives (14 are required). To qualify for an incentive payment, they must meet 19 of the 24 objectives.

♦ 5 additional objectives may be chosen from the list of 10 menu set objectives.

Stage 2 requirements are in the planning stages. While they were originally scheduled for release in 2011, the Office of the National Coordinator for Health Information Technology (ONC-HIT) Policy Committee has delayed the projected release to mid-year 2014.[211] Stage 2 will reinforce many of the Stage 1 objectives and measures, and will place a stronger emphasis on care coordination.

---

[209] Blumenthal D, Tavenner M.. The "meaningful use" regulation for electronic health records. *N Engl J Med.* 2010;363(6):501–504.
[210] Center for Medicare and Medicaid Services. CMS EHR Meaningful Use Overview. Accessed online June 16, 2011, at http://www.cms.gov/EHRIncentivePrograms/30_Meaningful_Use.asp#TopOfPage.
[211] Mosquera M. Panel endorses delay of stage 2 meaningful use to 2014. Government Health IT. June 8, 2011. Accessed online August 27, 2011, at http://govhealthit.com/news/panel-endorses-delay-stage-2-meaningful-use-2014.

Industry-wide conversion from ICD-9 to ICD-10-CM and PCS is an issue that every healthcare organization in the United States has been preparing for over the last few years. A precursor to this conversion is a required transition for all certified EMR providers to ensure that administrative systems can adhere to the changes in reporting structure from Accredited Standards Committee X12 4010a to 5010.[212] Testing and compliance for healthcare providers on this new capability began in 2009; and will continue across the industry through 2012 in preparation for the ICD-10-CM and PCS conversion. This conversion will affect every healthcare organization in the United States that deals with recording, aggregation, or exchanging of patient health information; it will require significant resources and planning. Resources and planning will also be required to meet the health information management needs of organizations working to implement ACOs and CINs.[213] An important element to ensure successful conversions will be connecting health information management leaders with physician/clinical leaders to address a number of issues:[214]

♦ Adequate training must be provided across the CIN or ACO for staff members responsible for interpreting and using the vastly expanded coding structures (growing from approximately 17,000 codes under ICD-9 to over 155,000 for ICD-10-CM and PCS[215]);

♦ Testing of information technology interfaces must be conducted to ensure accuracy of health data to support efficient health information exchange across all CIN and ACO participants;

♦ Bidirectional mapping involving medical coding experts must be conducted for the transition from ICD-9 to the expanded ICD-10-CM and PCS codes.

These conversions cannot be entirely automated. The magnitude of change that will take place across organizations for physicians, nurses, health

---

[212] CFR Part 162 Health insurance reform; modifications to the Health Insurance Portability and Accountability Act (HIPAA); final rules. *Federal Register* 45; 2009;74:3296–3328.

[213] AHIMA. e-HIM Workgroup on the Transition to ICD-10-CM/PCS. Planning organizational transition to ICD-10-CM/PCS. *Journal of AHIMA*. 2009;80(10):72–77.

[214] Steindel SJ. International classification of diseases, 10th edition, clinical modification and procedure coding system: descriptive overview of the next generation HIPAA code sets. *J Am Med Inform Assoc*. 2010;17(3):274-282.

[215] Raths D. Is ICD-10 a Quality Initiative? Innovators will use ICD-10 to further their business models and clinical capabilities. *Healthc Inform*. 2010;27(9):24-28.

information management professionals and others involved in the medical coding and recording of patient case data along with documenting plans of care and other information will require manual interventions critical for healthcare delivery and system transformation. A recent article in the Journal of the American Health Information Management Association identified key points to understand in preparing for future conversions to ICD-10, which are outlined below in Table 29. It is important to recognize that these transitions will not happen in a vacuum and will have to be phased in over multiple years––much as the industry experienced with other major transformations, including what will be experienced with the move to the ACO model of care and meeting the three stages of Meaningful Use criteria.

Table 29. Other Key Points for ICD-10 Conversions[216]

Conversion Issue	Point to Consider
Conversions cannot be totally automated.	They will require active engagement of collaborative subject matter experts on the new code sets.
Conversions are not individual isolated events.	They are multi-phase processes that will take a number of years to complete.
Translating from ICD-9 to ICD-10.	All purposes valid translations cannot be created for use in impact analyses.

As the healthcare industry implements EMRs and embark upon the ICD-10 conversion, achieving interoperability between disparate systems will further aid in achieving the long-term goals of having more complete and accurate records of patient histories.

Why Should I Share?

It was reported in the *Archives of Internal Medicine*[217] in January 2011 that "poor communication between primary care physicians and specialists on referrals and consultations is an all-too-common problem that has real repercussions on patient care...It can lead to duplicate lab tests, repeat procedures, wasted time

---

[216] Butler R, Mills R, Averill R. Reading the Fine Print on ICD-10 Conversions. *Journal of AHIMA*.2011:82(6);28–31.
[217] O'Malley AS, Reschovsky JD. Referral and Consultation Communication Between Primary Care and Specialist Physicians: Finding Common Ground. *Arch Intern Med*. 2011 Jan 10;171(1):56–65.

and resources, conflicting prescriptions, and potential harm to patients." That study proceeded to report that "even though **69.3%** of primary care physicians said they send specialists notification of a patient's history and the reason for the consultation all or most of the time, just **34.8%** of specialists said they routinely receive such information. Meanwhile, **80.6%** of specialists say they send consultation results to the referring physician all or most of the time, but only **62.2%** of primary care physicians say they ever get that information.

The concept of sharing patient data and health information outside the four walls of a healthcare enterprise is anathema to many hospitals and health systems. It is driven by a multitude of factors, ranging from fiercely competitive markets to paranoia regarding data privacy and security. It is essential, however, to the management and operation of a successful CIN/ACO initiative that data be easily shared amongst all caregivers in a patient-centered, clinically integrated coordinated care model in order to deliver care more efficiently and effectively and to ensure that all caregivers have the most up-to-date information about their patients at all times.

It is this level of patient-centered care coordination and collaboration among providers that is the key to truly managing the health of individual patients, patient populations, and achieving improvements in quality and affordability at the heart of the ACO and CIN model. Establishing an electronic exchange infrastructure is complex, however, not only because of the heterogeneous information systems spread across the care continuum – hospital information systems, ambulatory EHR's and practice management systems, and the like––but also because many ACOs and CINs will span organizational boundaries beyond the walls of a single enterprise or entity. Because the CIN/ACO may be comprised of multiple organizations, establishing the electronic connections when the CIN/ACO doesn't "own" all the pieces and parts (e.g. hospitals, physician practices, imaging centers, reference labs, etc.), requires a flexible architecture for data exchange that can create a virtual integrated delivery network.

Virtualizing the Clinically Integrated Delivery Network

When asked by David Burda, the editor of *Modern Healthcare*, whether he would want to join an ACO if he were a new physician just starting out, Jay Crosson, the Permanente Medical Group senior adviser for health policy and former chair of the Medicare Payment Advisory Commission, answered, "I absolutely would."[218]

Why such a definitive response? Because Dr. Crosson experienced firsthand the value to for both patient and provider when the hospital, physician, and payer are closely aligned during his work as a physician within the Kaiser Permanente system for more than 30 years. Wherever a patient goes within the Kaiser system, be it a hospital or physician's office, each authorized provider—from nurses to primary care physicians to one or more specialists—has an overall understanding of the patient's history and health status based on their ability to review every interaction the patient has had with every member of the care team. This holistic and coherent approach—a 360-degree view—ensures that care is coordinated and congruent with the protocols and guidelines for that particular patient. In other words, the highest-quality care is delivered at the lowest cost.

Kaiser Permanente has spent billions of dollars over many years on "bricks and mortar" infrastructure to achieve this level of coordination, including buildings, people, and health information technology. From an information technology perspective alone, Kaiser has spent billions on a hospital and ambulatory information system to ensure every physician across acute and ambulatory settings is using the same system; and as a result, he or she has the most recently updated information about every patient.

There is no doubt that the integrated delivery network model as exemplified by Kaiser and such others as Intermountain Healthcare, Geisinger Health System

---

[218] Video interview: former MedPAC chairman Jay Crosson on ACOs. *Modern Healthcare*, August 9, 2010. Accessed online July 20, 2011 at http://www.modernhealthcare.com/article/20100809/VIDEO/308099999.

and Mayo Clinic, has achieved the greatest degree of success in improving care collaboration and reducing the cost of care. On the other hand, a model that requires a single or common ownership and substantial capital resources to build or purchase the infrastructure necessary to replicate an experience like Kaiser's is not realistic for nationwide or even regional CIN/ACO implementation, because a central goal of a CIN/ACO is to lower the cost of care, not increase it. Moreover, as CIN/ACOs take shape, many will be joint ventures that include participants and stakeholders who are not part of the same physical or legal organization—requiring a virtual network to accomplish their work. The expectation that every provider use the same information system is simply unrealistic, given human behavior, organizational dynamics, cost, and the nature of cross-organizational workflow. Hence the value of new interoperability standards that will increasingly allow for information exchange at a lower cost of implementation.

Meanwhile integration vendors are working to assist providers in virtualizing health care records. This work is intended to help create the integrated delivery network experience and achieve the level of coherence experienced by Kaiser's providers without having to own all the pieces and parts and requiring everyone to be part of the same organization using the same information system. While data standards and interface development are complex, and while the currently available information is often limited compared to single source systems, it is the reality of healthcare today. Because of the current, episodic nature of an ACO's bundled payment and shared savings model, it presents complex issues of care coordination.

To successfully coordinate care on more than an episodic basis, distribute funds accurately, and improve quality as measured against benchmarks; community-wide coordination of patient information in a clinically integrated model is essential. HIE technology is the underlying connection of all stakeholders and participants in a CIN/ACO across organizational boundaries and disparate information systems, so that information can be shared community-wide and care coordination enabled. Participants require a range of connectivity in an ACO: HIE technology can help meet and support those needs.

Figure 29: Spectrum of Connectivity for ACO Participants

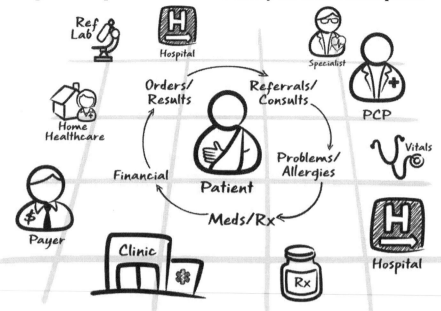

While we are specifically addressing the integrated delivery network type ACO, this spectrum of participants applies to each of the other four ACO models and the CIN defined in Chapter 3.

Defining HIE: Noun or Verb?

Before entering too deeply into the technology required to manage a successful CIN/ACO, it is important to define "health information exchange" because users of HIE often use the term in different contexts. HIE as a noun commonly refers to a third-party nonprofit organization formed to enable information sharing among multiple healthcare entities. Examples of this type of HIE are the regional health information organization and the health information organization. These entities and HIE are used interchangeably to refer to *publicly* funded initiatives serving either a local geographic region or a state. Some statewide initiatives, such as the Delaware Health Information Network and the Colorado Regional Health Information Organization are ARRA-qualified state-designated entities eligible to receive federal funds to support their operations. In the case of such regional initiatives as the Mississippi Coastal Health Information Exchange, there are a variety of funding mechanisms, both public and private, in place to support business operations. In addition to these HIE initiatives many others are at various stages of formation and operation across the country.

Whether an HIE initiative is statewide or regional, its value in supporting a CIN or ACO and powering comprehensive clinical integration hinges to a great extent on the quality and completeness of the data contributed by participating stakeholders. The resources of the federal State Health Information Exchange Cooperative Agreement Program are provided to designated state agencies and organizations that focus on engaging the right participants and allocate funds to create and strengthen infrastructure and capacity for health information exchange across and among healthcare providers in each state.

For a third-party HIE to fully support ACO operations, all providers—not only physicians and hospitals—participating in an ACO must also be participants in that HIE. This participation, however, is usually not the case. In a public regional or state HIE, the primary focus in the first few years is connecting hospitals and physician practices. In the future mature ACO model, *all* stakeholders involved in delivering care to a patient will be connected: hospitals and physician practices as well as long-term care facilities, community health teams, nurse care managers, home health agencies, physical therapists, reference labs, imaging centers, and the like. It is therefore less likely that an HIE (in its noun form) will be able to fully support the information exchange needs of an ACO in the near term.

HIE as a *verb* commonly refers to the *activity* of exchanging health information across disparate information systems and multiple locations of care, both acute and ambulatory. The third-party HIE introduced above employs the verb usage of the term when it deploys HIE technology to enable the active sharing of information among its participants. Similarly, there are hundreds of local private information exchanges already in operation nationwide, sponsored by such community hospitals as Hoag Hospital and El Camino Hospital in California, and such health systems or integrated delivery networks as Intermountain Healthcare in Utah, and CHRISTUS Health, with care locations across seven states and Mexico. Each of these self-funded private HIE organizations has deployed

HIE technology to actively exchange health information to all members of the care team across acute and ambulatory care settings. In the private HIE setting, hospitals and health systems have a much stronger influence over stakeholder participation. As a result, the private HIE has a much higher likelihood of being able to support a CIN/ACO comprehensively by engaging all stakeholders beyond its hospitals and physician practices. This point can be illustrated to show some of the various channels through which information must flow.

Figure 30: HIE as a Verb -- Active HIE Among ACO Participants

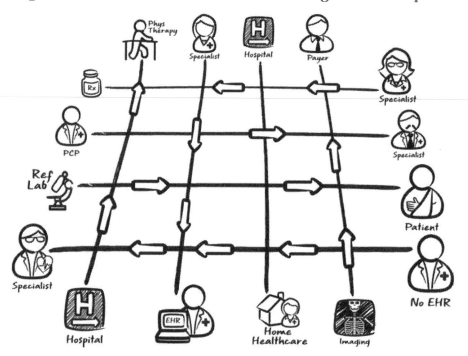

In the end, both the noun and verb forms of HIE are describing the same thing: the exchange of health information. The differences lie in the organizational structures, funding and sustainability mechanisms, goals of the entity, and stakeholder participation. The technology required for exchanging health information is essentially the same and in either case is necessary in managing a CIN/ACO.

HIE Deployment Framework for Clinical Integration and ACO Management

Successful CIN and ACO initiatives must possess an HIE infrastructure with specific competencies to support governance, operations, and clinical quality measurement, and financial goals and objectives. The Vermont Blueprint for Health project discussed in Chapter 2 serves as an example of HIE as a critical component of both medical home and ACO implementation in that state. HIE technology is critical to coordinate care, bridge the gap across acute and ambulatory settings, collect data, identify gaps in care and sentinel events, facilitate analysis for timely feedback and measuring progress toward quality or outcome goals, and track payment distribution. In addition to the multiple underlying technologies required to manage an CIN/ACO, particularly those at the source that gather, store, assimilate, codify, or process data, there are several HIE-related technologies that are also needed.

When it comes to deploying HIE capabilities however, there is no "one-size-fits-all" model because as discussed in Chapter 3, there are multiple types of ACOs. Therefore, the HIE framework must be flexible, adaptable, scalable and deployable in a model that adds capabilities incrementally to achieve the clinical integration objectives and goals of an ACO initiative. A flexible and incremental HIE deployment framework for ACO and CIN initiatives can be depicted as flowing through a number of levels.

Figure 31: Flexible and Incremental HIE Deployment Framework

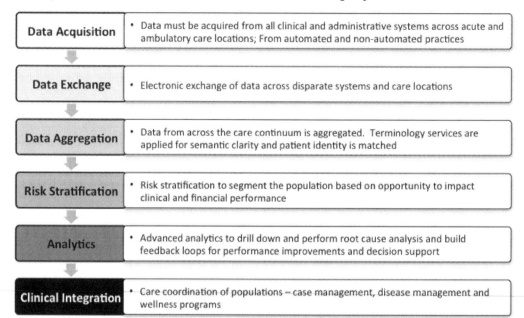

Data Acquisition	• Data must be acquired from all clinical and administrative systems across acute and ambulatory care locations; From automated and non-automated practices
Data Exchange	• Electronic exchange of data across disparate systems and care locations
Data Aggregation	• Data from across the care continuum is aggregated. Terminology services are applied for semantic clarity and patient identity is matched
Risk Stratification	• Risk stratification to segment the population based on opportunity to impact clinical and financial performance
Analytics	• Advanced analytics to drill down and perform root cause analysis and build feedback loops for performance improvements and decision support
Clinical Integration	• Care coordination of populations – case management, disease management and wellness programs

Nontraditional IT Competencies

As noted in the deployment framework above, a CIN/ACO requires a sophisticated technology infrastructure at its foundation to facilitate its objectives of sharing health information among all stakeholders in order to improve quality and reduce costs. The most essential feature of this infrastructure is the ability to share information and coordinate care across organizations in a virtual integrated delivery network-like infrastructure, also described earlier in this chapter. In fact, as Glaser and Salzberg noted in *Hospitals and Health Networks*, "While applications such as the EHR and the patient health record are important, data may be the most important ACO information technology asset."[219] We would suggest that what you do with the data, such as applying clinical intelligence and delivering at the point of care, is even more important.

---

[219] Glaser J, Salzberg C. Information technology for accountable care organizations. *Hospitals and Health Networks*, September 2010. Accessed online July 23, 2011, at http://www.hhnmag.com/hhnmag_app/jsp/articledisplay.jsp?dcrpath=HHNMAG/Article/data/09SEP2010/090610HHN_Weekly_Glaser2&domain=HHNMAG.

Such traditional healthcare applications as EMRs, hospital information systems, emergency department information systems, office-based practice management systems, laboratory and radiology information systems, and patient administration applications are designed to record patient care information during an episode of care and are limited in scope to that care setting's organizational boundaries. While each discrete solution is important, many of these non-office-based technologies were not designed to provide output that could support the innovative coordination of care model needed for ACOs and CINs, which extends beyond the four walls of a hospital, an emergency department, an imaging center or a lab for example.

To be successful, we believe a CIN/ACO requires technology that can seamlessly integrate information and data across organizational boundaries spanning many discrete technologies, apply such clinical intelligence as advanced clinical decision support and analytics, and deliver knowledge at the point of care. Because the participants in the CIN/ACO likely will be affiliated with disparate organizations—and unlike Kaiser, not all will be using the same information system—support technology for the CIN/ACO will need to facilitate virtualization of the patient's record and make it available to the care team by connecting to disparate systems across multiple care locations and integrating data with local systems and technologies already in use. An illustration of the electronic virtual care team shows the bilateral flow of patient information that is needed to facilitate effective HIE actions:

Figure 32: Electronic Virtual Care Teams

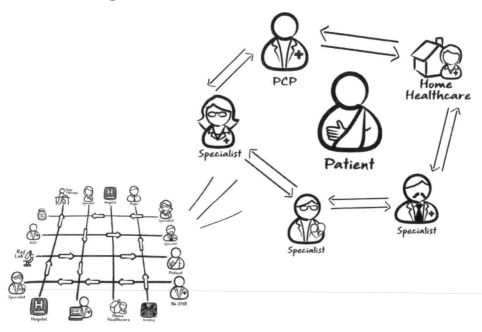

As discussed in Chapter 1, Section 3502 of the Affordable Care Act calls for the development and initiation of new community health teams to support medical homes (recognized as part of the foundation of ACOs). The efforts of these teams will be enabled by HIE capabilities that positively effect coordination of care and support the physicians and care teams delivering patient care in geographically dispersed locations throughout the regions they serve.

Supporting Every Provider of Care

While ARRA and the HITECH Act are focused on enabling physicians to adopt EMRs, the reality is that many physicians still rely on paper records for patient care and use electronic data mainly for billing purposes.[220] According to the CDC's 2009 National Ambulatory Medical Care Survey[221], only about 44 percent of physicians answering a mail survey reported using all or partial EMR systems

[220] President's Council of Advisors on Science and Technology. Report to the President realizing the full potential of health IT to improve healthcare for Americans: the path forward. December 8, 2010, 25. Video of full presentation available at: http://www.wellsphere.com/healthcare-industry-policy-article/realizing-the-full-potential-of-health-it-to-improve-healthcare-for-americans-the-path-forward/1299758.
[221] Hsiao C, Hing E, Socey TC, Cai B. Electronic Medical Record/Electronic Health Record Systems of Office-based Physicians: U.S., 2009 and Preliminary 2010 State Estimates. Center for Disease Control and Prevention. December 2010. Accessed online July 10, 2011 at http://www.cdc.gov/nchs/data/hestat/emr_ehr_09/emr_ehr_09.pdf.

(not including systems solely for billing) in their office-based practices. Of this 44 percent, about 21 percent reported having systems that met the criteria of a basic system, with only 6.3 percent having an extensive and fully functional electronic record system.[222] This assessment means that more than half of all physicians in the United States still maintain paper-based practices. Within those practices, some physicians are comfortable using such electronic technology as e-mail and a Web browser, while others still prefer a paper chart and are reluctant to participate in ARRA incentives. Nevertheless, many of these same physicians will need to participate in a CIN/ACO model as these entities continue to expand in markets across the country. Educating these late-adopter physician(s) on the benefits and needs for health IT adoption will be especially important as CIN/ACO start-ups get underway. This is particularly true because the meaningful use incentives, although going a long way toward encouraging adoption of EMR technology, will take years to reach critical mass.

The adoption of an EMR to record data electronically is only part of the equation. Data must be "harvested" from every care location, clinical intelligence applied, and knowledge exchanged with each member of the patient care team, which will likely be across a virtual integrated delivery network-like environment. This integration means that the HIE platform must support one-to-one, one-to-many, and many-to-many communications in a *multi-directional, inbound and outbound* active exchange framework. These data must be available to the provider in their native workflow––as discrete data in the EMR if it exists or via a browser-based application in their practice. The EMR must be able to "outbound" data as discrete elements or in the form of a continuity-of-care document, so that it is consumable by other information systems in use across the care continuum. Similarly, in a non-automated care location, the browser-based application must not only display data, but enable the gathering and recording of data as an "EMR-lite," so that it can be exchanged with and accessible by other non-automated locations, as well as consumable in the form of a continuity-of-care document or as discrete elements by the heterogeneous information systems across acute and ambulatory care settings.

---

[222] Centers for Disease Control and Prevention. Electronic medical record/electronic health record use by office-based physicians: U.S., 2008 and preliminary 2009. Accessed online July 23, 2011 at http://www.cdc.gov/nchs/data/hestat/emr_ehr/emr_ehr.htm.

Many "traditional" HIEs are data aggregation platforms only, with a Web-portal application attached, so that participants can access information that has been centrally stored in contrast to an active exchange infrastructure. The portal-based health information application is fundamentally different from an active HIE.

Figure 33: HIE and the Portal-based Health Information Application

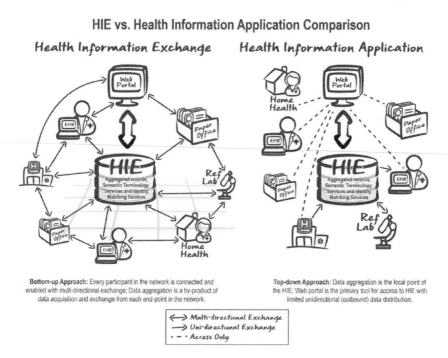

HIE vs. Health Information Application Comparison

Health Information Exchange — Health Information Application

Bottom-up Approach: Every participant in the network is connected and enabled with multi-directional exchange; Data aggregation is a by-product of data acquisition and exchange from each end-point in the network.

Top-down Approach: Data aggregation is the focal point of the HIE; Web portal is the primary tool for access to HIE with limited unidirectional (outbound) data distribution.

⟷ Multi-directional Exchange
⟶ Uni-directional Exchange
- - - Access Only

One of the fundamental differences between the health information application and the active HIE is the effect on a provider's workflow. If a provider has adopted an EMR, the traditional portal-based HIE solution requires the provider to work outside of their new workflow, which was specifically redesigned to support an EMR-based environment and electronic record keeping. Experience shows that if a provider has gotten over the "hurdle" of adopting an EMR, then the most effective HIE solution is the multi-directional active exchange infrastructure model, which enables a provider to stay in their native EMR-based workflow, while still enabling the active exchange of information––orders, results, consultations, and referrals––with other EMR-based providers as well as with non-automated practices. The health information application model requires the provider to exit their native EMR-based workflow and log onto a separate health information application portal-type solution, which is only for accessing the information. Most health information application-type solutions have the ability to export discrete data into EMRs; and if so, it is only in a unidirectional model as displayed above.

So the fundamental difference between the portal-based health information application and the active HIE, is that health information application is an information access model and is not an active exchange. To support clinical integration programs and ACOs, active exchange across organizational boundaries is required, with seamless integration into any EMR, while also enabling Web-based access to data for providers who are still in paper-based practices and furthering the exchange with the ability to harvest data in each endpoint of the network. In this manner, the inbound-outbound, multi-directional active HIE model ensures data are synchronized across all caregivers.

While the number of HIE vendors is expanding, certification and interoperability requirements have conversely forced consolidation in the office-based EMR vendor market. Consequently some physicians are finding themselves with unsupported products or outdated technologies that need replacement. Others work in markets where a handful of vendors predominate or in environments where local health systems are assisting with single or selected vendor implementations. While the idea of a single-vendor world is appealing, as mentioned earlier, it is not contemporary reality. Consequently, any sustainable CIN/ACO initiative likely will need to be interoperable with a number of different EMR/EHR solutions requiring health information exchange.

Of course a CIN/ACO could be developed in the absence of such technologies; online registry reporting, for example, would quickly enable large groups of providers to populate a common Web-based system in which limited analytics could be run and from which improved care management might be delivered. We recognize this type of system as a starting point, however, and not a sustainable state of operation––especially for newer models of care delivery requiring quality monitoring, rapid clinical process improvement, and financial performance measurement. As such, the technology needed to support a

CIN/ACO would need to be vendor-agnostic and simultaneously support the workflow of the provider wherever he or she stands on the technology adoption curve from a paper-based environment to a fully automated practice.

Technology and Continuity of Care

One of the greatest challenges for physicians is being able to see what all the members of the patient's care team are doing, from visits to other practitioners and specialists to trips to emergency rooms and urgent care centers. The following case illustrates the complexities of a typical cross-provider care episode successfully facilitated under the active HIE deployment framework.

Mr. Johnson is a 59-year-old construction worker with a long history of diabetes. He has documented early retinopathy and hypertension but no evidence of other end-organ changes from his chronic diabetes. He presents to his primary care physician, Dr. Clark, with fever, acute shortness of breath, and rales and wheezing in the left lower lobe. Dr. Clark diagnoses Mr. Johnson with acute pneumonia (confirmed on a chest x-ray) and admits him to Metro Community Hospital (MCH).

In the hospital, Mr. Johnson is newly diagnosed with renal disease (elevated serum creatinine, proteinuria, and mild acidosis). At discharge, he is placed in an intensive home care program for strict monitoring of sodium and protein intake along with diabetes monitoring. He is discharged to the MCH home care agency to be seen by a visiting RN. His discharge medications include insulin, an oral antibiotic, and two new medications—a brand-name diuretic and a new ACE inhibitor for renal disease and hypertension.

During the visiting RN's third visit to Mr. Johnson, she becomes concerned by his rising blood pressure, weight gain, and general lethargy. She calls Dr. Clark to order new laboratory tests, which she then draws and delivers to the lab herself. The nurse questions Mr. Johnson, who insists he is compliant with his medication program.

Because MCH, the home care agency, Dr. Clark's practice, the local laboratory, and Bayside Pharmacy, which fills Mr. Johnson's prescriptions, all belong to an ACO, their clinical findings on Mr. Johnson are published in a common electronic community health record powered by HIE technology. This community health record features an innovative patient management "dashboard" displayed electronically to all authenticated members of Mr. Johnson's care team.

The home care nurse consults the dashboard and notices the list of medications from the MCH discharge summary does not reconcile with the list from Bayside Pharmacy. During further discussions with Mr. Johnson, she learns that he filled the two inexpensive generic prescriptions but not the expensive new diuretic and ACE inhibitor. With the recent decline in the construction business, Mr. Johnson's income has been severely reduced and he admits he cannot afford to take the two medications for his renal disease.

The nurse also receives Mr. Johnson's recent laboratory test results via the dashboard. The results show a deterioration of renal function with increased serum creatinine levels and electrolytes, suggesting a recurrence of metabolic acidosis. She contacts Dr. Clark, who switches Mr. Johnson to an alternative generic medication for his renal disease. Dr. Clark then sends an electronic referral to a new nephrologist to see Mr. Johnson emergently so that he can receive more intensive evaluation of his worsening renal disease.

Because the visiting RN and Dr. Clark were part of a CIN/ACO with active HIE technology that supports high-quality care and efficient practice, they were able to intervene quickly with use of real-time and accurate patient health data to prevent another admission to the hospital. Without the collaborative capabilities provided by the technology framework and active exchange infrastructure, such a successful outcome would be in doubt and, at the very least, considerably less efficient and more expensive. Multiple bilateral connections can exist across organizations for the purposes of improving connectivity across the network of CIN/ACO participants.

Figure 34: A Virtual IDN

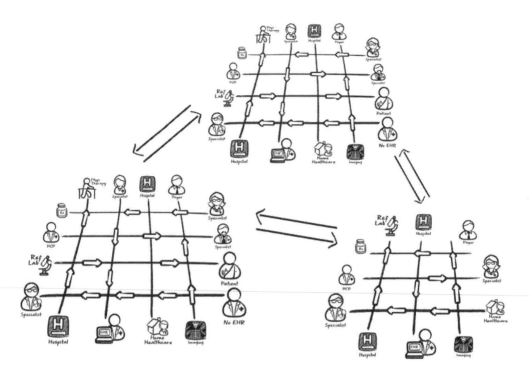

Health data exchange across boundaries leads to improvement in the quality and continuity-of-care information shared in a timely manner among the members of the virtual care team. It enables care collaboration across multiple providers and organizations and is critical for the CIN/ACO to achieve optimal levels of clinical integration and population health management, as well as the required quality and affordability improvements. Technological solutions needed to support such continuity of care and enhanced provider collaboration include:

- Data and workflow integration across disparate information systems and settings;
- A unified view of the patient across organizations and care locations;
- Real-time updates from participating entities and alerts of such updates to ensure timely care synchronization across all accountable parties;
- Clinical decision support, such as risk stratification to identify care opportunities, and clinical alerts to ensure adherence to care guidelines and protocols;

- Aggregation of patient information to enable analysis and formulation of business intelligence on patient populations for the purpose of clinical quality monitoring, outcomes and performance measurement, and financial outcomes management.

Semantics of Future Care

Readers familiar with the telephone game or sharing workplace water-cooler gossip have likely noted the often-amusing outcomes of miscommunication. In healthcare, however, garbled communication can mean the difference between life and death. How is it possible, then, to share patient data across multiple physician practices, health systems, and allied health providers effectively and efficiently when their health information technology systems don't even "speak the same language"? Moreover, how do we make the underlying data actionable for managing the CIN/ACO?

The ability to create coherence between systems that do not "speak the same language" is an HIE function called semantic interoperability; it is vital to realizing the potential of sharing information across the continuum of care. Semantic interoperability establishes a seamless exchange of data between two or more systems or healthcare networks, ensuring that health data are not only understandable within their original context but also capable of supporting clinical decision-making, care collaboration, public health reporting, clinical research, health service management, and more.

From Logical Observation Identifiers, Names, and Codes to Systematized Nomenclature of Medicine (SNOMED), ICD-9, ICD-10, National Drug Codes, and Current Procedural Terminology (to name just a few), there are a multitude of code sets and terminologies requiring semantic interoperability in the contemporary CIN/ACO environment. Add the subtle nuances of clinician-friendly terminology and free text from physician dictation and one begins to comprehend the semantic challenges of health information exchange.

Consider, for example a simple description of an infected tympanic membrane as recorded in the chart of a patient with acute otitis media. Such terms as *erythematous*, *injected*, *inflamed*, or *reddened* all describe essentially the same clinical finding. To enable consistent data sharing across such variations in terminology and disparate code sets, an effective terminology services platform is needed to meet sophisticated mapping process requirements. The result: a unified view of the patient from multiple data contributors, enabling decision support, trending, analytics, and effective care.

In addition to resolving differences in terminology across the disparate data sources in the care continuum, a similar semantic problem exists with patient identity. A provider in the emergency department who is caring for a patient for the first time needs the most up-to-date information about that patient as a member of the CIN/ACO's patient population—particularly in cases in which the patient comes from outside the contracted payer patient population. This type of scenario poses a challenge. In each of the information systems at the endpoints of the network—hospital systems, ambulatory EMRs, practice management systems, and others—the patient has a unique medical record number. In situations in which the physicians or hospitals are using different systems (the far more likely scenario in most locations) data aggregation becomes a complex and limiting problem. Creating interfaces, developing common patient identity management systems, and doing so in a HIPAA-secure environment are only a few of the challenges to aggregating relevant data on behalf of improved patient care.

Further, in the silo-oriented U.S. healthcare system, the multiple encounters are not linked via a unique common patient identifier across organizational boundaries and information systems. This problem does not exist in most developed countries with national health systems because every patient has a single national medical record number, thereby linking together multiple care encounters related to an episode of illness. To effectively manage a CIN/ACO, it is essential for HIE technology to correlate, link, and assimilate multiple encounters, so that when a patient presents in the emergency department, the physician can quickly search for all historical data about that specific patient from any previous visit in any care location or from a provider who is a participating stakeholder in the CIN/ACO. Ensuring that "John Doe is John Doe" is extremely important as we seek to improve the quality of care and enhance patient safety in the United States.

Figure 35: Semantic Interoperability and Identity Management Across Organizations and Systems

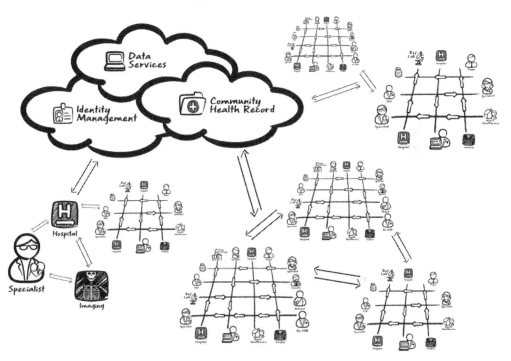

Because semantic interoperability facilitates collaboration, decision support, reporting, and detecting trends—meaningful uses of actionable data can result from effectively implementing an active HIE that accounts for both this language and patient identification issues. In light of this crucial requirement, ensuring that it is achieved for all ACOs will be critical to the success of healthcare delivery system transformation.

Connecting the True "Last Mile"

While much of the attention of HIE is focused on establishing electronic connections between hospitals and physicians, the true "last mile" of connectivity is reaching the patients themselves. For a CIN/ACO to be maximally effective, it is essential for its patients to be active participants in managing their health. While generally classified under the category of "patient engagement" technologies, there are two primary solutions for connecting patients to the HIE:

Personal Health Records. The most basic tool for electronically exchanging information with the patient is a secure messaging system in which the patient and their clinical team can dialog and share information. This provider-controlled system is highly desirable and a solid place in which to develop a patient centric care model and is discussed further below under patient portals. Alternatively, there is the advent of the personal health record or PHR. The PHR takes the relationship to a new place in which the patient controls and maintains an independent database of clinical information that they, the patient, consider appropriate. Think of the PHR as a copy of the medical record that the patient or guardian maintains independently and therefore edits and manages over time. Personal health records usually offer electronic access to their health information exchanged through the HIE, via a Web-based or mobile application.

There are many free and subscription-based personal health records available in the market today offered by vendors, payers and providers. While initially thought to be a panacea, only a small percentage of the American public has visited and created a personal health record, even when it is free; and less than half of those have returned to use it. Consequently it is no surprise that Google recently announced it is leaving this market. That said, for some patients and guardians, the personal health record will offer a convenient and increasingly easy-to-use capability for tracking key information like prescriptions, or managing chronic conditions and also offer tools and content for managing one's health.

Patient Portals. Patient portals, unlike PHRs, are a way in which to enable the patient to converse securely with the health care team. This provider-controlled access tool may be sponsored by hospitals and/or physician practices in a "tethered" (containing information unique to that organization) or "untethered" form––in which case it contains multiple provider and organizational information. A patient portal offers a number of advantages over a personal health record, not the least of which is confidence by the health care team in the accuracy of the information it contains. Other technical advantages can include things such features as Web-based, integrated voice reminders or mobile access to health information exchanged by the HIE, in a bi-directional exchange with their providers. In contrast a personal health record is unidirectional. At the base level, patient portal, patients with a patient portal have electronic access to such critical information such as lab results, medications, allergies, and immunizations exchanged through the HIE. Like a personal health record, patients can present new information to their existing records exchanged via the HIE; however the information would be seen and reviewed by the health care team and added on their behalf.

In addition, the portal has such other more advanced capabilities as secure communication with providers, appointment scheduling, and electronic bill-payment. Some patient portals go further to provide such valuable content as lifestyle, fitness, and nutritional coaching.

The most advanced patient portals have clinical decision support capabilities that monitor data exchanged via the HIE, constantly looking for information like potential drug interactions or notifying the patient about treatment options that might be useful, based on their medical history. With outcomes-based reminders and alerts generated by the patient portal and leveraging data exchanged via the HIE, patients can take a more proactive role in managing their health.

Whether through a personal health record or a patient portal, empowering patients with electronic access to their health information aligns and engages patients with their providers and supports the CIN/ACO goals of improved outcomes at a lower cost.

HIE Strategy for The Future Care Environment

Active HIE technology is central to achieving three factors for CIN/ACO success: stakeholder collaboration; an end-to-end care delivery network; and a strong technology infrastructure that brings together health records, patient populations, and clinical decision support.

Ensuring progress is, however, a challenge. A clear and logical HIE strategy can support effectively building and managing a CIN/ACO, yet many organizations do not know where to begin. One of the limiting factors to having independent physician groups band together as provider service organizations and forming ACOs and or CINs in various markets is funding. Working together with other organizations that can assist in capitalizing the HIE development work is one way to climb across this barrier. In addition to the financial challenges there are also operational and technical limitations. The most proven strategy for deploying HIE technology builds a solid exchange on a basic foundation. Additional functions can be layered according to specific needs and timelines, taking into consideration the workflow and technological maturity of the CIN/ACO's participants.[223]

An incremental bottom-up approach to deploying HIE is an effective way to produce both immediate and lasting value for the CIN/ACO. The bottom-up approach involves first connecting hospitals, physician practices, and such critical ancillary service providers as reference laboratories and imaging centers and "liquefying" transactions at a local level. This approach is in contrast to a traditional top-down regional health information organization approach to HIE that attempts to connect all possible stakeholders at once and aggregate all data simultaneously.

The first step is to engage physicians and other healthcare providers where care is delivered, connecting disparate information systems and automating clinical messaging and workflow to create a solid and well-adopted HIE foundation. The HIE can then build upon that foundation and provide greater value over time by adding other functions and services. An important aspect of this first step is automating core healthcare transactions: ordering tests, referring patients among providers, and coordinating information among care teams. In

[223] Agency for Healthcare Research and Quality, National Resource Center for Health Information Technology. Webinar. May 14, 2010. Building and maintaining a sustainable health information exchange (HIE): experience from diverse are settings.

accomplishing this critical step, the basic HIE connects core hospital systems (that is, the laboratory, radiology, transcription, security, emergency department), EMRs, practice management systems, and other entities in such a way that information flows securely across the HIE infrastructure. Automating core transactions yields the following benefits:

- Creates immediate value for hospitals, physicians and other providers: improved information quality and savings in time and money, leading to user satisfaction and high early-adoption rates.
- Enables a lower-cost and more rapidly deployable approach than common methods of building an HIE, which require extensive and expensive infrastructure to accomplish the same goal.
- Establishes connections to all stakeholders participating in the CIN or ACO and fosters rapid coordination of care and collaboration.
- As the level of connectivity across participants increases and the HIE grows from the bottom up, its additional functions may include:
- Aggregating patient records and health information from all connected stakeholders to create a longitudinal record of care.
- Applying identity management services to ensure identification of a patient's correct longitudinal health record.
- Applying terminology services to ensure data are semantically correct across all data sources connected to the CIN/ACO participants via HIE technology.
- Harvesting data from ambulatory care settings to establish registries and apply advanced clinical decision support, such as risk stratification, disease management and population management tools for information retrieval, proactive and personalized care management, and analytics.
- Engaging patients through electronic connections via the HIE to personal health records or a patient portal, thereby empowering the patient to take a proactive role in managing their own health, and helping clinicians achieve their outcomes performance metrics.
- Deploying gateway services to exchange information with such external networks as the national health information network, other HIEs, and public health agencies.

The bottom-up approach, which focuses first on system integration and exchange at a local level with local systems presently used by providers, has proven successful in a wide range of environments. It delivers significant value in a short time frame and at a lower cost than traditional "build it and they shall come" models of HIE deployment. Certainly efforts to standardize and aggregate normalized data in a centralized manner are the ideal; however, they are also time-consuming and complex endeavors. Rather than compete with such systematic approaches, bottom-up HIE leverages those initiatives and will better position ACO development and management activities.

Thus a good HIE strategy is based upon established standards while simultaneously ensuring flexibility and adaptability over time. The rapidly evolving contemporary environment does not adhere to any one specific standard or approach. Many methods are used, and even such common "standards" as HL7 come in several flavors. The HIE solution must be "future-proof," complying with privacy, security, and communication standards while still being open and adaptable to future standards as they evolve. The definitive component in the strategy is selecting technology that enables providers to always keep the patient in focus and empowers all authorized providers to actively participate, collaborate, and proactively coordinate care.

Beacon Communities and Impact on ACOs

The Beacon Community Cooperative Agreement Program (Beacon Program) is a national program launched and administered by the ONC-HIT in 2010, in which where 17 communities (with involvement from various integrated delivery networks, hospitals, physician practices, government agencies, safety net organizations, patients, etc) were granted $265 million to support the implementation of new advancements in health information technology throughout their communities and regions. Each community's needs were considered different but their program goals were to enable health system improvements.[224] As such, the Beacon Program will provide new health

---

[224] White House Press Release. Vice President Biden, HHS Secretary Sebelius Announce Selection of 15 Health IT Pilot Communities through Recovery Act Beacon Community Program. May 4, 2010. Accessed online July 23, 2011, at

information technology roadmaps, lessons learned, and a multitude of best practices for CINs and ACOs to expand their health information technology infrastructure and capabilities. The Beacon Program supports awardees in helping them build and strengthen their health information technology and exchange capabilities to improve care coordination, increase the quality of care, and slow the growth of healthcare spending.[225] This initiative directly supports CMS's Three Part Aim.

ACOs and CINs will face numerous challenges associated with the development of an effective health information technology. These challenges include: implementation of an EHR across the organization: health information exchange across a diverse group of stakeholders; multidirectional active exchange; clinical decision support; identifying and acting upon care opportunities; monitoring and measuring performance; and the successful achievement of meaningful use by at least 50% of the CIN and or ACO's primary care physicians.

The results and lessons learned from the Beacon communities will help overcome these challenges. Beacon communities must define, track, and report on their progress toward measurable health and efficiency performance goals, similar to requirements for ACOs and CINs. The resulting findings will also support health care organizations' efforts to meet meaningful use requirements.

The goals of select Beacon Program communities illustrate how health care providers may benefit from the experience of the Beacon communities.

http://www.whitehouse.gov/the-press-office/vice-president-biden-hhs-secretary-sebelius-announce-selection-15-health-it-pilot-c; Department of Health and Human Services Press Release. Cincinnati, Detroit selected as final health IT pilot communities under innovative HHS Recovery Act Beacon Program. September 2, 2010. Accessed online July 23, 2011, at http://www.hhs.gov/news/press/2010pres/09/20100902a.html.

[225] Office of the National Coordinator for Health Information Technology. BEACON Community Program Introduction. Accessed online May 29, 2011, at http://healthit.DHHS.gov/portal/server.pt?open=512&objID=1805&parentname=CommunityPage&parentid=2&mode=2&cached=true.

Table 30. High Level Goals of Beacon Community Programs[226]

Community	Goal
Bangor Beacon Community	Improve health of patients with diabetes, lung disease, heart disease, and asthma by strengthening care management; improving access to, and use of, adult immunization data; preventing unnecessary ED visits and hospital readmissions; and using health information technology to expand access to patient records.
Beacon Community of the Inland Northwest	Expand care coordination for patients with diabetes in rural areas and expand the existing HIE to provide greater connectivity throughout the region.
Southern Piedmont Beacon Community	Increase use of health information technology, including HIE among providers and increased patient access to health records to improve care coordination, encourage patients' involvement in their own medical care, and improve health outcomes while controlling cost.
Central Indiana Beacon Community	Expand the country's largest HIE to new community providers in order to improve cholesterol and blood sugar control for diabetic patients and reduce preventable readmissions through telemonitoring of high-risk chronic disease patients after hospital discharge.
Delta BLUES Beacon Community	Improve access to care for diabetic patients through the meaningful use of EHRs and HIE by primary care providers in the Mississippi Delta, and increase the efficiency of healthcare in the region by decreasing healthcare costs for diabetic patients through the use of EHRs.

Each of these Beacon Program communities seeks to introduce or expand health information technology, enabling interventions needed to improve the cost, quality of, and access to health care services. In addition, each Beacon community must have a strong governance structure in place that will involve multiple stakeholders within their community.[227] These similarities further illustrate how Beacon Program sites can provide valuable lessons for ACOs and CINs.

---

[226] Office of the National Coordinator for Health Information Technology. BEACON Community Program Goals. Accessed online May 29, 2011, at http://healthit.DHHS.gov/portal/server.pt?open=512&objID=1805&parentname=CommunityPage&parentid=2&mode=2&cached=true.

[227] Mckethan A, Bramer C, Fatemi P, Kim M, Kirtane J, Kunzman J, Rao S, Jain SH. An Early Status Report On The Expand Beacon Communities' Plans For Transformation Via Health Information Technology. *Health Aff (Milwood).* 2011 Apr;30(4):782–8.

The Road to Interconnectivity and Data Exchange

The road to establish an HIE deployment framework starts with engaging physicians from the CIN/ACO in process design to ensure their buy-in, and help identify information they need to support population health management. As HIE efforts mature, establishment of an oversight committee focused on all elements of HIE will be important to provide leadership and guidance to cross-functional implementation teams and to set strategic objectives for long-term success of the ACO's HIE initiative.

The last element of our roadmap concerns strategic benefits realized for the ACO at the community level. Implementation of effective, active HIE will accelerate the ACO's ability to support requirements for data needed by physicians and other clinicians in population health advanced clinical decision support, population stratification, patient care identification, disease and care management, quality monitoring, and performance measurement. Ultimately, each CIN or ACO's roadmap will vary to some degree depending on the participants involved and the model being implemented.

Clinical Data Reporting Systems

As EMRs and information exchange systems mature and come into being, a critical and parallel discussion needs to center around clinical data reporting systems (CDRS). These systems provide the business intelligence for which the CIN or ACO needs to operate. They are an essential component of what was missing in the 80s to support PHOs that largely failed. Understanding population health management, and truly managing down to the provider level with clinical and financial data will be necessary for successful health systems to manage clinical and financial risk. Modeling software that begins to identify how best to manage populations of patients continues to be developed and is expected to be a major area of focus in the coming years.

With nearly 20 current vendors competing in the CDRS market space, there are a number of factors to consider when picking a system to aid in data reporting down to the physician level.

- Whether or not the system can accept discrete data;
- Whether or not the vendor has experience with the source systems;
- Whether a registry is available;
- Whether or not the reporting components can be modified by the end user organization or whether they require code changes.

All of this and more should be taken into consideration for these important vendor selection and system acquisition decisions. Many large systems are looking at implementing full data warehouses. While the nature of this is beyond the scope of this book, many clinical data reporting systems may be eclipsed by more mature reporting systems over time. If this is the local tactical approach, then the CIN/ACO will have to weigh the value of the short term reporting system in the context of realizing its cost and relative shelf life. In all cases, some type of clinical data reporting system will be necessary and likely need to be implemented well before health information exchange is fully matured. As such the CIN/ACO leadership will need to define a limited number of metrics from which to start as the new organization is built and the competencies and technologies become increasingly available.

INFOCUS: Challenges Ahead

CINs and ACOs depend on the ability to share and act on information about specific patients and population groups through peer-to-peer and peer-to-patient communications in a highly secure network. Physicians, clinical care teams, hospitals and health systems involved in delivering care to a patient need a complete picture of a patient's past care and current needs in order to more effectively reduce the potential for medical errors, eliminate redundant tests and procedures, improve provider-to-provider coordination, streamline workflow, improve patient and provider satisfaction, reduce administrative inefficiencies, improve quality, and lower the cost of care. Collaboration and coordination among physicians and other healthcare providers delivering patient-centered care is one of the critical elements needed to truly achieve meaningful health information exchange and effectively managing a CIN/ACO.

Provider care coordination is made possible in the real world of healthcare through collaboration and coherence: connecting information, systems, services, and people in a significant way that enhances their ability to work together and provide a complete view of patient health—effectively virtualizing the integrated delivery network.

An additional challenge is clinical decision support and analytical tools for both hospital and physician practice settings. Having robust but non-taxing advanced clinical decision support is known to be a critical problem across the industry. As vendors continue to improve the clinical intelligence of these tools, the capabilities to support the information requirements of the healthcare delivery workforce will be strengthened. As the field of analytics continues to build momentum, along with advances in modeling and simulation capabilities, new tools will enhance monitoring measurement and alerting capabilities for total population- and patient-level health management. One study noted the importance of such tools in the field of pharmacotherapy to reinforce a hospital pharmacy staff's ability to predict potential drug interactions and reduce the risk of adverse events.[228] The healthcare industry is rapidly catching up with other industries in the field of data analytics as a result of dedicated research and development initiatives. Research is yielding benefits for the transformation of care delivery. Challenges remain, however, in the fields of analytics and clinical decision support that will continue to fuel research and development efforts.

Advances made in technology are making the virtual integrated delivery network model possible by bridging information, systems, services, and people to create a coherent collaborative care model. Collaborative care keeps the patient in focus at all times, connecting cloud services; brick-and-mortar clinical, administrative, and financial services; and such local applications as clinical

---

[228] Barrett JS, Mondick JT, Narayan M, Vijayakumar K, Vijayakumar S. Integration of modeling and simulation into hospital-based decision support systems guiding pediatric pharmacotherapy. *BMC Med Inform Decis Mak.* 2008;8(6). Accessed online August 27, 2011, at: http://www.ncbi.nlm.nih.gov/pmc/articles/PMC2254609/pdf/1472-6947-8-6.pdf.

decision support systems and EMRs with the community of people who care for the patient. These advances enable organizations, affiliated providers, and other allied caregivers who work together but are not part of the same entity, to collaborate on a platform and create a high level of coordinated care, much as in the top integrated delivery networks across the United States. ACO and CIN success will hinge on continued industry progress with adoption of EMR systems, proactive efforts to ensure seamless transitions to ICD-10 coding, and selecting HIE technology that extends beyond regulatory and physician organizational boundaries to create that end-to-end virtual integrated delivery network. Challenges and risks should be identified, evaluated, and mitigated for ACO or CIN implementation.

Table 31. Chapter 6 Challenges and Risks

Challenges	Risks
Aggregation of patient health information from disparate systems at different levels of maturity.	Inefficient interfaces between EMRs and other health information technology across CIN/ACO participants. Creates potential for patient data corruption and breakdown in data transfer with patient transitions.
Selecting and implementing a CDRS to meet the business intelligence needs of CINs and ACOs.	Implementing CDRS in an environment in which true integration and HIE does not truly exist is a large challenge for the industry.
Enabling the HIE deployment framework to benefit all CIN/ACO participants.	Occurrence of technology incompatibilities; inability to stratify risk across participants; and insufficient clinical decision support that negatively impacts quality of patient care.
Meeting Stage 2 and 3 criteria (yet to be defined) for CMS Meaningful Use of EHRs program.	May put future incentive payments to eligible providers and hospitals at risk.
Instituting coordinated network-wide ICD-10 conversion plans.	Not planning sufficiently for ICD-10 conversion could result in negative impact to CIN/ACO revenue cycle and disrupt continuity of care.

Table 31. Chapter 6 Challenges and Risks, cont.

Potential Mitigation Strategies
√ Knowing the customer and focusing on physician workflow and clinical decision support needs.
√ Ensuring effective project implementation of semantic terminology and conversions.
√ For CDRS carefully define the near term reporting needs and limit the scope of work to definable elements that will reap the greatest value to the CIN/ACO.
√ Establishing cross-functional committees to manage HIE implementations.
√ Ensuring that all health data elements and disparate systems are accounted for in HIE required interfaces.
√ Engaging an HIE oversight council with C-level executives who make key decisions to mitigate strategic risks and set priorities to establish the HIE deployment framework.

Chapter 7. The Quality Continuum- Continuous Improvement

Systems awareness and systems design are important for health professionals, but they are not enough. They are enabling mechanisms only. It is the ethical dimensions of individuals that are essential to a system's success.

Avedis Donabedian, MD, MPH
(1919–2000)
Professor of Public Health, University of Michigan

Landscape of Issues

Establishing the framework of performance monitoring and measurement for evaluating the effectiveness of program and population health management is a critical issue for the success of ACOs. This is true for all CIN/ACO initiatives, including the Medicare ACO program, private payer ACOs, Medicaid pediatric ACOs, and clinically integrated networks––not only for outcomes and performance reporting but also to understand their performance record as they evolve. In 2001 the IOM acknowledged a need to strengthen capabilities in performance measurement in both operational performance and health outcomes. Redesign challenge #6, "Performance and Outcome Measurement for Quality Improvement and Accountability" (Figure 7) targeted this need, and the industry has responded with numerous healthcare quality management tools and initiatives focused on improving both process and system capabilities. However, as Dr. Donabedian indicated, putting the systems in place is not enough. In order to reach the goals that underlie this challenge, the nation needs people, both physician leaders and other clinicians motivated by an ethical imperative to improve our nation's health system. Leaders who develop and utilize the skills and traits defined in Chapter 3 will be best equipped to help their organizations adhere to these design principles and meet the Three Part Aim as set forth by CMS.

A number of measurement areas are important to evaluate on a regular basis for both public and private payer ACOs. These measurement areas are identified below, and are consistent with the original topics in Section 1899(b)(3)(A) of the Social Security Act in the description of the Medicare Shared Savings Program.[229]

Figure 36. Measurement Areas for ACOs

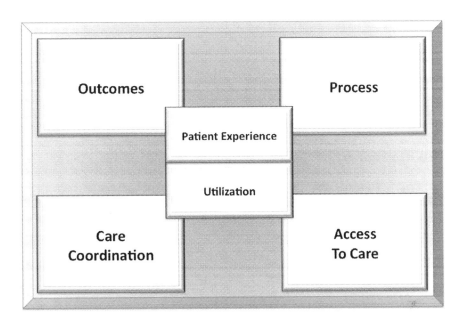

There are challenges to establishing and maintaining performance measures across these different areas. Some of these challenges include:

♦ Regional variation in conditions and procedures to treat designated populations;

♦ Investment of time and financial resources to develop and test new measures;

♦ Applicability of measures based on patient demographics (such as geriatric vs. pediatric populations);

♦ Accounting for risk adjustment factors that include demographics, severity or co morbidity of conditions, geographic variation, and provider factors;

♦ Setting appropriate spending targets;[230]

---

[229] Social Security Act. Shared savings program. Section 1899(b)(3)(a). Accessed online June 21, 2011, at ttp://www.ssa.gov/OP_Home/ssact/title18/1899.htm.
[230] Berenson R. Shared savings program for accountable care organizations: a bridge to nowhere? *Am J Manag Care.* 2010;16(10): 721-726. Accessed online July 20, 2011, at http://www.ajmc.com/issue/managed-care/2010/2010-10-vol16-n10/AJMC_10oct_Berenson_721to726.

◆ Linking structure and process measures to health outcomes.[231]

As measures are defined and implemented, and challenges addressed, an important next step will be an accurate understanding of the correlations across measures. This step includes understanding both positive and negative effects of changes in operations and patient care. The recognition that there may be setbacks as well as improvements will enhance the value of insights that CIN/ACO leaders obtain on the effectiveness of organizational transformation initiatives and the ways in which continuous quality improvement requires flexibility to adapt during the transition.

In addition, we must consider the issue of how information is codified and reported. Two seemingly competing, but actually compatible, fields are involved: administrative claims and clinical data. The preponderance of quality reporting for the past twenty years has been performed with claims-based billing system information. This source is often considered inaccurate and is contested by some physicians and providers. Billing data is often not specific enough and inherently leave out certain conditions and relevant information from the analysis. For example, claims or billing data can tell you whether a blood test was billed, but may not provide the results of the test or its relevance to patient care. Clinical reporting systems can obtain test results, the clinical interventions that were made, and sometimes relevant outcomes. Clinical reporting systems are, however, far less mature than their billing counterparts; do not contain all information from disparate systems; are usually data repositories missing key data, and have basic rules for clinical decisions--if they have rules at all. Moreover, claims data have been worked for decades, allowing clinicians to make adjustments for their shortcomings and create a rich longitudinal data source. In fact, CMS uses claims data for most analysis, including performance of Medicare ACOs. Thus the industry remains dependent on claims data, while simultaneously developing new clinical systems.

---

[231] Kerr EA, Krein SL, Vijan S, Hofer TP, Hayward RA. Avoiding pitfalls in chronic disease quality measurement: a case for the next generation of technical quality measures. *Am J Manag Care*. 2001;7(11): 1033-1043. Accessed online July 20, 2011 at http://www.ajmc.com/media/pdf/AJMC2001novKERR1033-1043.pdf.

Equally or perhaps more important is codification of the clinical record itself. The Inefficiencies are inherent in clinician-produced point-and-click, structured documentation. Such systems as SNOMED use exhaustive libraries to codify what they can recognize from within the record and are far more specific to clinical conditions than the more rudimentary billing system codes. ICD-10 coding is a movement to close that gap, with greater amounts of more detailed data. Meanwhile, such increasingly smart technologies as Natural Language Processing software are beginning to automate the recognition of free text entries and voice-to-text conversions allowing codification of the medical record without the workflow intrusion of point-and-click documentation. Until these systems mature, however, and are more fully deployed, we remain dependent on claims data and a number of manual and direct data entry systems for quality reporting requirements. Moreover, the entire U.S. healthcare system will be challenged with the transition in 2013 to ICD-10 coded data. The new ICD-10 diagnostic codes will increase specificity in many ways as seen in the next two tables.[232]

Table 32. Differences between ICD-9 and ICD-10 Diagnostic Codes

ICD-9	ICD-10
3-5 characters	3-7 characters
Approximately 13,000 codes	Approximately 68,000 codes
Space limitation to increase codes	Flexible system with increased # of codes
Lacks specificity	Increased level of specificity
Lacks laterality	Codes include laterality (right vs. left)

In addition to new diagnostic codes, the ICD-10 transition introduces new procedure code sets. These code sets are used to report services and procedures in ambulatory care and physician office settings.

---

[232] American Medical Association. Fact Sheet 2: The Differences Between ICD-9 and ICD-10. 2010. Accessed online June 24, 2011, at http://www.ama-assn.org/ama1/pub/upload/mm/399/icd10-icd9-differences-fact-sheet.pdf.

Table 33. Differences between ICD-9 and ICD-10 Procedure Code Sets

ICD-9	ICD-10
3–5 characters	7 characters
Approximately 3,000 codes	87,000 codes with availability to expand
Lacks specificity	Increased level of specificity
Lacks laterality	Codes include laterality (right vs. left)
Based on outdated technology	Reflects current medical and device-related terminology
Uses generic terminology for body part references	Has more specific terminology for body part references
Lacks descriptions of methodology and approaches for procedures	Will have expanded descriptions of methodologies and approaches to procedures
Inadequate definition of procedures	Precisely defines procedures with detail regarding body part, approach, any device used, and other qualifying information

It will be crucial for a number of reasons for CIN/ACOs to ensure that a seamless transition takes place with these conversion projects. First, the level of detail and specificity in patient health data will increase exponentially as a result of this transition. As CIN/ACOs accept greater degrees of accountability and risk for the quality of care delivered, ICD-10-coded health records will provide new levels of information to help identify gaps in care, track effectiveness of treatment plans and measure health outcomes. Second, as CIN/ACO operations focus on improving performance measurement and reporting, these new code sets will increase the industry's quality of health data and awareness of clinical root causes, diagnoses, and plans of care, yielding greater detail in reports from departments of clinical quality and health information management. The basic ICD-10 codes were originally endorsed through the World Health Organization's World Health Assembly and have been in use in 25 other countries since 1994. This shift clearly places an administrative burden on the industry, but it is necessary in order to clarify our understanding of health data originating from both inpatient and ambulatory care settings and thereby improve quality of care across the country.

Legislative Guidance: The Affordable Care Act and the Proposed Rule

Affordable Care Act Section 3022[233] contains initial guidance for the industry regarding the quality measures, collection and reporting processes to be reported for the Medicare Shared Savings Program (Medicare ACO). It is important to note that the Medicare Shared Savings Program is a single-payer ACO, with standard requirements and quality measures. There are many differences between a Medicare ACO and a multi-payer or private (commercial) ACO. The latter two types of ACOs have more latitude to design their quality measures based on their actual quality and population underwriting experience. In addition, the CMS Innovation Center demonstrations do not have to follow the same requirements as the Medicare ACO. It remains to be seen whether the regulatory constraints placed on Medicare ACOs will help to protect the Medicare program more than they foster innovations in health finance and delivery.

With release of the Proposed Rule substantial guidance was provided for quality measures, the intended use of such measures, and their scoring methodology.[234] Sixty-five measures were proposed, and it is important to note that they are proposed only for initial reporting and the Year One performance period. These measures are presented in Appendix G including each measure's applicable domain, title and description, and type of measure (e.g. outcome, process, or patient care experience). Measures for the second and third years of the three-year program will be determined in future federal rule making.

The use of nationally recognized quality measures is important, and there are several organizations that develop quality measures, including the National Quality Forum, National Committee on Quality Assurance, Joint Commission, American Medical Association, and medical specialty societies. Although physicians and hospitals have reported "static" quality measures to CMS and the Joint Commission, most are not experienced with reporting a large number of care management and outcome measures especially since provider technology

---

[233] H.R. 3590, Patient Protection and Affordable Care Act, §3022(b)(3)(A)(i-iii). Shared savings program quality measures criteria (2010).
[234] Fed. Reg. Vol. 76, No. 67. April 7, 2011. II(E)(2). Proposed Measures To Assess the Quality of Care Furnished by an ACO. pp. 19569-19570.

has not fully matured in data capture and reporting. As a result, organizations are looking at more fully developed claims data to monitor and report managed care and outcomes measures. In any case, maintaining the integrity and accuracy of the data and quality measures will be important in order to accurately monitor, evaluate, and report ACO performance.

The proposed measures span five domains, and may be conveniently categorized under two components of the Three-Part Aim.
- **Aim 1: Better Care for Individuals**
    - Patient/Caregiver Experience
    - Care Coordination
    - Patient Safety
- **Aim 2: Better Health for Populations**
    - Preventive Health
    - At-Risk Population/Frail Elderly

Aim 3, lower growth in expenditures, is an ultimate goal of all the measures proposed, and will be realized in financial performance and shared savings. Within these five proposed quality domains, the final set of measures are also aligned with the IOM's six aims of quality improvement identified in Chapter 1 and the priorities of the new National Quality Strategy.

As previously mentioned, a number of other quality and performance metrics assess health outcomes, healthcare processes, gaps in care, patient experiences, the operational performance of healthcare facilities, and office-based physician office care. Consideration was given in the selection of measures for the Proposed Rule to ensure alignment with other government incentive programs that include the Physician Quality Reporting System (PQRS), Electronic Prescribing Incentive, Meaningful Use of EHRs, and the Hospital Inpatient Quality Reporting Program, along with requirements of Medicaid and private- sector quality initiatives.[235] The final performance measures for the first performance

---

[235] Fed. Reg. Vol. 76, No. 67. April 7, 2011. II(E)(2)(b)(2). Scoring Methodology. pp. 19569-19570.

period will have some degree of correlation between the Shared Savings Program measures and these other programs.

Part of the reason for alignment or harmonization among the performance measures is to reduce the burden of reporting and collection requirements; however, in some cases it may not be advantageous to Medicare ACO participant organizations to have strong alignment with other requirements--especially where static, mandatory regulatory reporting metrics focus on areas of little importance to an organization's patient population or areas identified as needing quality improvement. This issue of alignment will be determined through the final rule making process.

Stakeholders were engaged in the definition and selection of measures for the Proposed Rule. As Medicare ACO initiatives move toward a multi-payer structure, lessons learned and best practices will emerge from other ACO programs in the private sector and such government programs as the Pioneer ACO Model. Participants in advanced government pilot programs and private sector ACOs will bring new insights to the industry on the structure, process, outcome and patient experience measures that will be important to improve quality and affordability.

There are three other sections of the Affordable Care Act to note: Section 3013 on quality measure development; Section 3014 on quality measurement; and Section 3015 on data collection and public reporting.

Section 3013

The Affordable Care Act authorized $75,000,000 for fiscal years 2010–2014 to identify gaps in quality measures and the need for new development of measures used in Federal health programs. This process is to be carried out at least every three years. Factors in the identification and design of potential new measures include: 1) gaps where no quality measures exist; 2) improvement of existing measures; 3) pediatric quality measures identified in Section 1139A of the Social Security Act; and 4) measures identified in Section 1139B of the Social Security

Act in the Medicaid Quality Measurement Program.[236] Section 3013 also identifies several priorities summarized below.

Table 34. Priorities for Quality Measure Development[237]

No.	Description
1	Health outcomes and functional status of patients.
2	Management and coordination of healthcare across episodes of care and care transitions for patients across the continuum of providers, care settings and plans.
3	Experience, quality, and use of information provided to and used by patients, caregivers, and authorized representatives in shared decision making about treatment options.
4	Meaningful use of health information technology.
5	Safety, effectiveness, patient-centeredness, appropriateness, and timeliness of care.
6	Efficiency of care.
7	Equity of health services and disparities across populations and geographic areas.
8	Patient experience and satisfaction.
9	Use of innovative strategies and methodologies.
10	Other areas identified by DHHS.

The priorities set forth in the table above serve as guidelines to address the four factors that are critical in future quality measure design and endorsement. Such organizations as the National Quality Forum and the National Committee for Quality Assurance are two recognized industry-leading organizations that focus on the design, validation and endorsement of quality measures. In 2010 DHHS contracted with the National Quality Forum's National Priorities Partnership that has 48 member organizations, listed in Appendix H. The efforts of the National Priorities Partnership have supported DHHS in facilitating the development of and consensus on national priorities for the new National Quality Strategy. In March 2011 DHHS released its report to Congress titled, *National Strategy for*

---

[236] H.R. 3590, Patient Protection and Affordable Care Act, §3013(b). Identification of quality measures (2010).
[237] H.R. 3590, Patient Protection and Affordable Care Act, §3013(c)(2). Prioritization in the development of quality measures (2010).

Quality Improvement in Health Care. A number of national aims and priorities were identified in this report.

Table 35. National Aims and Priorities for National Quality Strategy[238]

National Aims
Better Care: Improve overall quality by making health care more patient-centered, reliable, accessible, and safe. **Healthy People/Healthy Communities:** Improve the health of the U.S. population by supporting proven interventions to address behavioral, social and environmental determinants of health in addition to delivering higher-quality care. **Affordable Care:** Reduce the cost of quality health care for individuals, families, employers, and government.

National Priorities
1. Making healthcare safer by reducing harm caused in the delivery of care. 2. Ensuring that each person and family is engaged as partners in their care. 3. Promoting effective communication and coordination of care. 4. Promoting the most effective prevention and treatment practices for the leading causes of mortality, starting with cardiovascular disease. 5. Working with communities to promote the wide use of best practices to enable healthy living. 6. Making quality care more affordable for individuals, families, employers, and governments by developing and spreading new healthcare delivery models.

For CIN/ACO participant organizations, understanding the Three Part Aim established for CMS by Administrator Berwick provides insight into subsequent efforts linking it to the Medicare Shared Savings Program in the Proposed Rule; and the policy framework of quality aims and priorities provides the context for DHHS and CMS's perspective on the quality landscape. The policy pronouncements of these aims, goals, and priorities provide a more strategic view than is used by ACOs, CINs, and other healthcare service provider organizations in tactical quality measurement and performance improvement activities.

---

[238] Department of Health and Human Services. *National Strategy for Quality Improvement in Health Care.* March 2011. Accessed online June 21, 2011, at http://www.healthcare.gov/center/reports/nationalqualitystrategy032011.pdf.

If an organization decides to become a Medicare ACO, its physician leaders must understand and attempt to reconcile, the two different approaches. Static mandated quality reporting for regulatory compliance, developed for strategic policy reasons outside the context of a specific hospital or physician office experience, may require different metrics than advanced clinical decision support used for tactical disease management that has been shown to produce real cost savings and quality improvements and depend on the hospital-specific quality improvement context. In many cases, hospitals and physician offices may have to deal with both sets of metrics. This task should not be too difficult, as it is a conundrum health care organizations deal with daily; but it does create additional work and demonstrates how difficult public payer programs can be with their additional requirements and regulatory burdens and barriers.

The design and validation of quality and performance measures is a complex, costly and resource-consuming process; however, their development will allow the industry to gain keener insights into the quality and effectiveness of care, and assist with continuous improvement for these new ACO and CIN organizations and their programs.

Healthcare is moving away from paying for individual episodes of care toward reimbursing for care across the continuum of services for a patient—and even paying for physicians and hospitals to take care of entire populations. As this paradigm shift takes place and care is coordinated by multidisciplinary teams, the industry will be better able to track, measure, evaluate and pay for total population health and patient-centered care across multiple settings.[239] This holistic approach to the patient and entire populations is similar to the shift sparked by the work of Avedis Donabedian in the 1960s, away from minimum quality standards and toward optimal quality care. The Joint Commission in their refocus on entire organizations and their clinical processes, rather than

[239] American Medical Association. Response to the Centers for Medicare and Medicaid Services regarding request for information on accountable care organizations and the Medicare shared savings program. December 2, 2010. p. 8. Accessed online July 20, 2011 at http://www.ama-assn.org/ama1/pub/upload/mm/399/cms-aco-comment-letter-2dec2010.pdf,

individual service lines and static measures took up that change, considered revolutionary at the time.[240]

Optimal care is also reflected in coordinated care that is patient centered, follows the patient across the continuum, and is designed to be more efficient and effective. Efficiency is important not only to improve the quality of care for the patient but also the quality of life for the physician and other clinicians. The ongoing industry transition to higher volumes in ambulatory care will cascade as the Affordable Care Act floods waiting rooms with newly insured persons. Efficiency and efficacy may then become not only a requirement of payers, but also a demand placed on physicians. These concerns will no doubt affect the way we set up and evaluate CINs and ACOs as clinicians begin to see the value of greater coordination. As innovations are developed and tested through the CMS Innovation Center, new forms of care delivery and quality measurement will be developed. For now, however, addressing each of the government's quality priorities presents unique challenges due to the complexities of regulatory requirements and the interconnectivity of structure, process, and outcome performance measures. But overcoming these challenges will improve delivery of healthcare as well as our ability to establish CINs, ACOs and other new initiatives arising from health reform in the United States.

Sections 3014 and 3015

Section 3014 of the Affordable Care Act calls for convening multi-stakeholder groups (usually healthcare trade associations), through voluntary participation and public nominations.[241] The purpose of convening these groups is to obtain input into the selection of consensus-developed quality measures. The DHHS is required to compile this public input and publish an annual report each year, starting in 2012. This annual report is supposed to identify gaps in quality measures for government-funded programs based on priority areas and the new National Strategy for quality measures.

---

[240] Daniels R. Nursing Fundamentals: Caring & Clinical Decision Making, Clifton Park, NY: Thomson Learning; 2004, pp. 492-494.
[241] H.R. 3590, Patient Protection and Affordable Care Act, §3014(a). New duties for consensus-based entity (2010).

This compilation and reporting is intended to formalize the current process of maintenance and phasing-out of government mandated measures required to be reported under government regulations.[242] The sum of $20,000,000 was appropriated from Medicare trust funds for these activities.[243]

Section 3015 identifies sources of grant funding for the collection and aggregation of measures for quality and resource use. This section also requires funding and development of websites to publicly report provider-specific information on quality and performance measures.

Organizations Engaged in Measure Development

A number of nonprofit industry organizations are involved in the identification, design, and validation of quality measures for the healthcare industry. Each organization has a primary focus, however, as healthcare has evolved over the past decade, their need to collaborate has increased. Individual, private sector companies also identify, design, and validate quality measures for a variety of reasons. Health insurance plans are the most actively involved in this effort, as they store and analyze huge quantities of data on care delivery, and are legally accountable and financially at risk for the quality of care delivered. Data mining techniques, quality improvement programs, and actuarial services have been pioneered by these organizations as they work to improve the quality and affordability of care.

An important issue that has emerged in recent years is the need to harmonize the many different measures. This need has become more pressing as government regulations increasingly require reporting of static measures, which may collide with internal efforts for continuous quality improvement that are usually focused on different metrics. These different measures may have overlapping population segments; track performance for complementary or competing quality measurement organizations; or require seemingly identical measures of conditions or diseases but use different data, exclusions,

---

[242] H.R. 3590, Patient Protection and Affordable Care Act, §3014(b). Multi-stakeholder group input into selection of quality measures (2010).
[243] H.R. 3590, Patient Protection and Affordable Care Act, §3014(c). Funding (2010).

numerators, or denominators. In 2010 the National Quality Forum issued a report that identified several issues justifying the need for improved harmonization. Problems noted with the current lack of coordination include "inconsistent focus, inconsistent target population and/or exclusions, and inconsistent scoring/computation."[244] As CINs and ACOs begin operations and develop measures by which they will be evaluated and paid, we can see the importance in harmonizing measures to reduce the cacophony of often-conflicting quality metric requirements, and streamlining the evaluation and payment of physicians and hospitals for their services.

Some of the government and private nonprofit organizations involved in quality measures include:

♦ **Centers for Medicare and Medicaid Services (CMS)**: CMS requires mandatory reporting of quality measures by hospitals, physicians, and other providers of products and services. CMS's Measures Management System[245] provides a standardized process for ensuring "that CMS will have a coherent, transparent system for measuring quality of care delivered to its beneficiaries." This system has been developed in coordination with the other organizations mentioned in this section. CMS collaborates with such private nonprofit organizations as The Joint Commission and the American Medical Association to develop quality measures required for regulatory compliance, including the Hospital Outpatient Quality Data Reporting Program, the Physician Quality Reporting System, and Hospital Compare.

♦ **Agency for Healthcare Research and Quality (AHRQ):** AHRQ is an agency within DHHS providing a clearinghouse for quality measures, coordination of evidence-based guidelines, and annual reporting of clinical quality measures at the national level. It also manages the Consumer Assessment of Healthcare Providers and Systems (CAHPS) patient satisfaction surveys.

♦ **National Committee for Quality Assurance (NCQA):** The NCQA is one of the primary certification and accreditation organizations for patient-centered

---

[244] National Quality Forum (NQF), *Guidance for Measure Harmonization: A Consensus Report,* Washington, DC: NQF; 2010. p. 15.
[245] Centers for Medicare and Medicaid Services. Measures management system. Accessed online July 16, 2011, at http://www.cms.gov/MMS/Downloads/QualityMeasuresDevelopmentOverview103009.pdf.

medical home initiatives, health plan accreditations, disease and case management, and other healthcare provider certification and recognition programs. The NCQA provides and governs the development of the Healthcare Effectiveness Data and Information Set (HEDIS) ambulatory care measures. In the fall of 2010 the NCQA issued an extensive document for public comment outlining potential measures for ACOs.[246] While the Proposed Rule does not call for credentialing of ACOs, the NCQA is pursuing development of an ACO accreditation program.[247]

- **National Quality Forum (NQF):** The NQF focuses on building consensus on national healthcare priorities and goals for quality measurement and performance improvement. It is the leading endorsement organization in the industry for development and approval of quality measures. As new quality measures are developed and tested for ACOs the NQF will play a vital role in validating these measures prior to their official use and application.

- **American Medical Association (AMA):** A national association for physicians, the AMA convened the Physician Consortium for Performance Improvement® (PCPI) in 2000. Since that time, the PCPI has grown to include participants from over 130 organizations and has identified 270 measures across 43 measure sets. The PCPI is working to develop measures on patient-centeredness, covering a range of disciplines and multiple chronic conditions and potentially useful to ACOs.[248]

- **The Joint Commission (TJC):** Hospitals and health systems all maintain TJC accreditation regarding their clinical care processes, ability and performance on specific quality measures and standards of care. TJC has been involved in performance measurement since the mid-1980s and launched its ORYX initiative in the late 1990s as the first national program for "measurement of hospital quality, which initially required the reporting only of non-

---

[246] National Committee for Quality Assurance. Appendix A: ACO measure grid. Accessed online July 16, 2011, at http://www.ncqa.org/portals/0/publiccomment/ACO/Appendix%20A_ACO_Measure_Table.pdf.
[247] National Committee for Quality Assurance. Successful Pilot Tests Clear the Way For July Debut of ACO Standards. Press Release. April 18, 2011. Accessed online June 27, 2011, at http://www.ncqa.org/tabid/1330/Default.aspx.
[248] American Medical Association. Response to the Centers for Medicare and Medicaid Services regarding request for information on accountable care organizations and the Medicare shared savings program. p. 8. December 2, 2010. Accessed online July 16, 2011, at http://www.ama-assn.org/ama1/pub/upload/mm/399/cms-aco-comment-letter-2dec2010.pdf,

standardized data on performance measures."[249] TJC has established sets of standardized core performance measures for hospital operations and contributes to the national strategy for improving transparency of healthcare quality through its quality check website and its annual report on the status of healthcare quality in America's hospitals. The Joint Commission announced in its 2010 report a new focus on "accountability measures-- measures of evidence-based care closely linked to positive patient outcomes."[250]

◆ **Utilization Review Accreditation Commission (URAC)**: The URAC is a healthcare quality accreditation organization for health plans, provider organizations, and physician practices with 28 accreditation and certification programs. The programs include healthcare utilization reviews, patient-centered health care homes (PCHCH), pharmacy benefits management, healthcare website maintenance, claims management, and disease management among others. In additional, the PCHCH program consists of 28 essential standards that are aligned with the Joint Principles of the patient centered medical home program discussed earlier in Chapter 2. These accreditations serve an important purpose for insurance commissioners, state and federal legislators, employers, and consumers because they are a sign of high quality and represent the accredited healthcare organization's ability to meet acceptable levels of performance metrics.

Industry Quality Measure Reporting Initiatives

A number of quality measure initiatives drive performance evaluation of the operations of physician offices and healthcare organizations. Figure 37 is an example of five important industry quality measurement programs.

---

[249] Chassin MR, Loeb JM, Schmaltz SP, Wachter RM. Accountability measures--using measurement to promote quality improvement. *N Engl J Med*. 2010 Aug 12;363(7):683–8.
[250] The Joint Commission. Improving America's Hospitals. The Joint Commission's Annual Report on Quality and Safety. 2010 Annual Report. p. 4. Accessed online August 22, 2011, at http://www.jointcommission.org/assets/1/18/2010_Annual_Report.pdf.

Figure 37. Select Industry Quality Measure Initiatives Related to Future ACOs

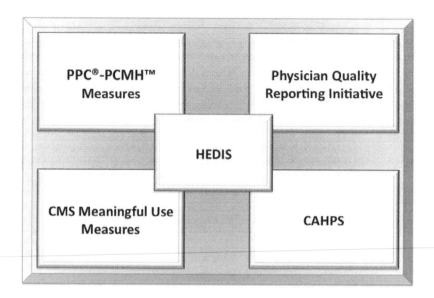

One of the key challenges for physician practices, hospitals and integrated delivery systems is the need to meet multiple reporting requirements, some of which are mandatory reporting required by government regulation and based on static metrics of health services and patient populations. Harmonization of the measures as well as automation of data collection and reporting requirements will be essential to support the industry's continued need for reducing administrative workload and costs.

HEDIS

The Healthcare Effectiveness Data and Information Set (HEDIS), "is a tool used by more than 90 percent of America's health plans to measure performance on important dimensions of care and service."[251] The NCQA governs the development of HEDIS quality measures, which undergo a process that may take as long as 28 months.[252] NCQA also oversees the measurement and reporting of HEDIS measures. These metrics are used by private employers and CMS to

---

[251] National Committee for Quality Assurance. HEDIS and quality measurement. Accessed online July 16, 2011, at http://www.ncqa.org/tabid/59/Default.aspx.
[252] National Committee for Quality Assurance. HEDIS measures development process. Accessed online July 16, 2011, at http://www.ncqa.org/Portals/0/HEDISQM/Measure_Development.pdf.

provide quality rankings for health plans based on their performance achieved in partnership with provider organizations and physicians. There are 71[253] HEDIS performance measures identified across eight domains.

Table 36. HEDIS Domains of Care

Number	Title
1	Effectiveness of care
2	Access to / availability of care
3	Satisfaction with the experience of care
4	Use of services
5	Cost of care
6	Health plan descriptive information
7	Health plan stability
8	Informed health care choices

As HEDIS measures are updated and have new measures issued annually, harmonization with the CMS measures is an industry priority. With industry movement toward multi-payer ACO models, both HEDIS measures and others developed for government programs will be needed to meet the evaluation requirements of public and private ACOs.

PPC®-PCMH™ Measures

The NCQA has created industry standards for the establishment and operation of medical homes. While there are several reporting indices, standard number six calls for reporting of standardized measures. These measures may be derived from any number of NQF-endorsed quality measures (either outcome- or process-related), or HEDIS measures from the NCQA.

---

[253] National Committee for Quality Assurance. What is HEDIS? Accessed online July 16, 2011, at http://www.ncqa.org/tabid/187/default.aspx.

CMS's Meaningful Use of EHRs program is a three-stage initiative focused on the structure aspect of the Donabedian triad (structure, process, outcome). The meaningful use program looks at the level of usage, standardization, and interoperability of EHRs. Started in 2010, the program is scheduled to be fully phased in by 2015. Eligible hospitals and providers can capture incentive payments for meeting objectives and criteria specified by CMS in each of the three phases. Starting in 2016, eligible providers and hospitals[254] that do not meet the requirements will be assessed a penalty against their Medicare or Medicaid payments. Measures for Stage 1 were made final and announced in July 2010. For eligible professionals 20 of 25 **Objectives** AND six clinical quality **Measures** must be met in Stage 1. Eligible hospitals and critical access hospitals are required to meet 19 of 24 objectives. Figure 38 provides an example of the reporting path for eligible professionals.

Figure 38. Stage 1 Meaningful Use Reporting for Eligible Professionals

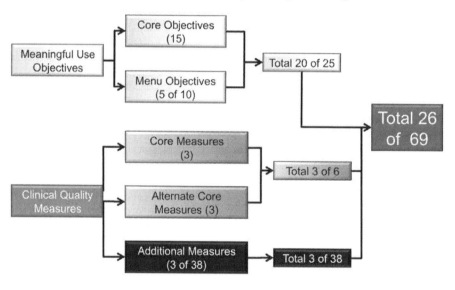

The 25 objectives for professionals consist of a number of outcome and process topics, such as patient demographics, vital signs, problem lists, clinical decision support, and health information exchanges. Although labeled "process"

---

[254] Centers for Medicare and Medicaid Services. Overview of eligibility criteria for providers and hospitals. Accessed online July 16, 2011, at http://www.cms.gov/EHRIncentivePrograms/15_Eligibility.asp#TopOfPage.

and "outcome" the topics are really surrogates because they measure whether the structure is in place to provide data that could improve outcomes; however, but they do not actually measure outcomes. Details of the 44 clinical quality **measures** can be found on the CMS website[255] and relate more directly to patient care outcomes and the individual- and population-based levels. Eligible professionals are only required to meet only six of the 44 measures; however, this requirement is certain to increase in Stages 2 and 3.

Providers must choose to participate in either the Medicare or the Medicaid track. Two important distinctions are the annual incentive payments available (Medicare = $44,000 and Medicaid = $63,750); and for the Medicare program, the groups of eligible professionals are restricted to doctors of medicine, osteopathy, dental surgery/medicine, podiatry, optometry, or chiropractics. Under the Medicaid program eligible professionals also include nurse practitioners, certified nurse-midwives, and physician assistants. Having effective and meaningful adoption of EHRs is important for both ACOs and CINs to track, measure, and report on health care and quality, so this program is significant to support ongoing operations as well as evaluation leading to proper reimbursement.

Consumer Assessment of Healthcare Providers and Systems (CAHPS)

CAHPS is a set of surveys CMS uses to obtain consumer and patient feedback on services provided by hospitals, in-center hemodialysis units, Medicare Advantage insurance, and plans, and nursing homes. These surveys could provide feedback for CINs and ACOs on the patient experience aspects of quality. As with many areas of quality measurement, these surveys are not designed to utilize any electronic record systems data. This is a critical area in which the government and private sector are working to help obtain the data needed by physicians, hospitals, and other service providers to support the timely collection and analysis of patient experiences. Such information will also be important for future CINs and ACOs to measure, and the electronic capture of these data will

---

[255] Centers for Medicare and Medicaid Services. Meaningful use clinical quality measures. Accessed online August 21, 2011 at http://www.cms.gov/QualityMeasures/03_ElectronicSpecifications.asp.

improve efficiency of data collection, reducing operational and regulatory burdens.[256]

Physician Quality Reporting System[257]

The Physician Quality Reporting System (PQRS) was initially launched as a pilot initiative in 2007 as the Physician Quality Reporting Initiative or PQRI. When the Affordable Care Act made the initiative permanent, it was renamed by CMS as PQRS. Originally enacted through the 2006 Tax Relief and Health Care Act, PQRS was a voluntary reporting program. This program presently allows eligible providers to report individual quality measures or measure groups to CMS. Practices that meet the reporting requirements have the opportunity to capture an incentive payment of up to "2% of their estimated Medicare Part B PFS allowed charges." The PQRS measures are also endorsed by the NQF, with some having been developed by the AMA and NCQA.

Active Quality Measurement and Advanced Clinical Decision Support

These various quality measurement programs appear interrelated. CMS, The Joint Commission, AMA, NQF and other standards bodies make great efforts to collaborate. Most of the measures, however, are static because they report a specific measure at a point in time but do not give its context or sufficient meaning to allow for care or disease management. Improving outcomes and performance is very difficult using static quality metrics.

For example, a high hemoblobin A1c (HbA1c) measure indicates that a specific person has diabetes at a given point in time. This metric is commonly required by government regulations to be reported by hospitals and physicians (PQRS Metric #1, NQF Metric #575, AMA HOQR DM-4). But the measure by itself does not tell why the person has diabetes (the person may have high blood sugar due to

---

[256] American Medical Association. Response to the Centers for Medicare and Medicaid Services regarding request for information on accountable care organizations and the Medicare shared savings program. December 2, 2010. p. 7. Available at: http://www.ama-assn.org/ama1/pub/upload/mm/399/cms-aco-comment-letter-2dec2010.pdf,
[257] Centers for Medicare and Medicaid Services. Physician Quality Reporting Initiative (PQRI). Accessed online July 16, 2011, at http://www.cms.gov/PQRI/01_Overview.asp#TopOfPage.

pregnancy, or taking certain medications such as corticosteroids), or the risk of the condition's worsening. Such additional information, such as tobacco use and obesity can help identify the risk and how bad it is. That is how basic clinical decision support works. Active quality metrics, and the associated advanced clinical decision support, go much further by linking all available data (clinical and claims) together in a longitudinal patient record, thereby indicating what can be done about the condition and when (opportunities for intervention and impact).

In the case of the person with a high HbA1C, if he or she has such other co-morbidities, such as hypertension or borderline hyperlipidemia, and pre-diabetes indicators that include metabolic syndrome, obesity and tobacco use, the patient is the classic "ticking time bomb" with low current risk of poor outcomes but high future risk and high impact on health. Immediate outreach and intervention can immediately improve both the static metric and the long-term clinical and financial outcomes. A similar case of high HbA1C, in an older person with such different co-morbidities as retinopathy, ESRD, and no lifestyle issues with controlled HbA1c would look the same in terms of the HbA1c metric, and basic clinical decision support might identify the person as high-risk. But combining all data and applying advanced clinical decision support would recognize that all future outreach and interventions would have no impact because the diabetes has already taken its toll, the patient has learned the lessons of self-care and is now in maintenance.

Due to the lack of automated systems across the industry and the incomplete adoption of quality measures, regulatory reporting and basic decision support programs have been burdensome and ineffective over the past decade. With the implementation and increased pace of adoption of EHRs, convergence of claims and clinical data, and the use of related active quality measurement and advanced clinical decision support technology, however, the gap is closing, new measures are being defined, and new capabilities are being launched across the industry to support ACOs and CINs.[258]

---

[258] Jenrette, J. and Yale, K. "ACO Technologies: Performance and Reporting Tools," ACO West Conference, San Diego, CA, November 19, 2010.

Quality Measurement from Demonstrations and Pilots

CMS's Physician Group Practice Demonstration Project had a well-defined set of measures used to monitor and evaluate the impact of changes made in the participating physician group practices' operations and the way they delivered care. Since that program began in 2000, other healthcare organizations have started forming private payer-based ACOs to verify their impact on quality improvement and their economic impact. The results of CMS's Physician Group Practice Demonstration project are summarized below.

Table 37. Results of Physician Group Practice Demonstration (through 12/2010)[259]

Performance Year	Type of Results	Description
1	Clinical quality	All 10 physician groups improved clinical management of diabetes patients achieving benchmarks for at least 7 of 10 diabetes clinical quality measures.
1	Shared savings	Two physician groups shared $7.3M in savings (out of $9.5M total for Medicare).
2	Clinical quality	All 10 physician groups achieved benchmarks at least 25 of 27 quality measures for patients with diabetes, coronary artery disease and congestive heart failure. Five groups achieved benchmark on all 27-quality measures.
2	Shared savings	Four physician groups shared $13.8M in savings (out of $17.4M total for Medicare).
3	Clinical quality	All 10 physician groups continued to improve quality of care and achieved benchmarks on at least 28 of 32 quality measures for patients with diabetes, coronary artery disease, congestive heart failure, hypertension, and cancer screening. Two groups achieved benchmark performance on all 32 measures.
3	Shared savings	Five physician groups shared $25.3M in savings (out of $32.3M total for Medicare).

---

[259] Centers for Medicare and Medicaid Services. Physician group practice demonstration project fact sheet, updated December 2010. Accessed online July 16, 2011, at https://www.cms.gov/DemoProjectsEvalRpts/downloads/PGP_Fact_Sheet.pdf.

Performance Year	Type of Results	Description
4	Clinical quality	All 10 physician groups continued to improve quality of care and achieved benchmarks on at least 29 of 32 quality measures for patients with diabetes, coronary artery disease, congestive heart failure, hypertension, and cancer screening. Three groups achieved benchmark performance on all 32 measures.
4	Shared savings	Five physician groups shared $31.7M in savings (out of $38.7M total for Medicare Trust Fund).

Methods to Effect Performance Improvement

ACO performance improvement teams will need to employ new tools and methods to identify opportunities for intervention that will help achieve measurable improvements in quality along with lower costs. Healthcare organizations ranging from hospitals, integrated delivery networks, physician groups, and private and public payer organizations have employed quality improvement tools and techniques for several decades.[260] One of the industry's pioneers in healthcare quality improvement, Avedis Donabedian, MD, MPH, gave us his quality framework, which analyzes quality improvement in the three areas depicted below.

---

[260] McIntyre D, Rogers L, Heier E. Overview, history, and objectives of performance measurement. *Healthcare Finance Review*. 2001;22(3):7-21. Accessed online July 16, 2011, at http://www.cms.gov/HealthCareFinancingReview/Downloads/01springpg7.pdf.

Figure 39. Donabedian's Quality Framework[261]

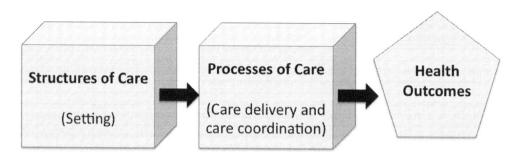

A number of quality improvement tools and methods have emerged since Donabedian's work was published and adopted across the industry decades ago. In today's environment of quality management and performance measurement, Six Sigma methodology and techniques have served as one of the tools used to assess performance, redefine clinical and administrative processes, eliminate waste, and allow continuous improvement. This methodology has demonstrated its value in facilitating necessary innovations and continuous improvement efforts in support of the implementation and ongoing management of ACOs and CINs.

Healthcare facility performance improvement teams have traditionally focused on rigorous analysis of clinical and administrative processes to identify waste and areas for improvement along with opportunities to improve health outcomes. At its core Six Sigma provides healthcare organizations with a systematic set of techniques for identifying strategic process improvements and new product and service lines for development. Six Sigma techniques utilize statistical methods to effect change and make reductions in "customer defined defect rates."[262] Six Sigma uses various methodologies including "work outs," "Define, Measure, Analyze, Design, Verify," and "Define, Measure, Analyze,

[261] McDonald KM, Sundaram V, Bravat DM, et al. *Closing the Quality Gap: A Critical Analysis of Quality Improvement Strategies.* Rockville, MD: Agency for Healthcare Research and Quality; 2007. AHRQ Technical Review 9, §5b. Methodological approach, model 2: Donabedian's quality framework. Accessed online July 16, 2011, at http://www.ncbi.nlm.nih.gov/bookshelf/br.fcgi?book=hstechrev&part=A25445; Donabedian A. Evaluating the quality of medical care. *Milbank Quarterly* 2005;83(4):691-729. Reprinted from *Milbank Memorial Fund Quarterly* 1966;44(3):166–203. Accessed online July 16, 2011, at http://www.milbank.org/quarterly/830416donabedian.pdf.
[262] Vest J, Gamm L. A critical review of the research literature on Six Sigma, Lean and Studer Group's Hardwiring Excellence in the U.S.: the need to demonstrate and communicate the effectiveness of transformation strategies in healthcare. *Implementation Science.* 2009;4(35):1-9. Accessed online July 16, 2011, at http://www.implementationscience.com/content/pdf/1748-5908-4-35.pdf.

Improve, Control." An entire community of Six Sigma experts has emerged to assist the healthcare industry with use of these tools. Such formalized process improvement methodologies such as these will continue to be heavily relied upon to advance the quality agenda.

One tool that many projects rely on is the core Six Sigma DMAIC roadmap.[263] The five DMAIC roadmap steps are as follows:

1. **Define**: Establish the performance improvement project's goals and the customer's requirements.

2. **Measure**: Evaluate the current level of performance.

3. **Analyze**: Determine the root cause of poor performance.

4. **Improve**: Eliminate defects to improve efficiency, reduce waste, and achieve cost savings or increase revenue.

5. **Control**: Establish new procedures, policies, and use of new tools to monitor and maintain performance.

Performance improvement projects are conducted in all areas of healthcare operations (e.g. finance, risk management, surgery, pharmacy, radiology, rehabilitation) and have been shown to improve patient safety, increase revenue cycle performance, redesign clinical and administrative workflow, and achieve cost savings. In some cases, projects have been combined with Lean Thinking methodology, which focuses on waste elimination and the application of value stream mapping[264] to illustrate the current state of processes, establish the resources required for various steps; and provide quality improvement teams with a roadmap to create a more efficient healthcare service organization. Applying these methods to the formative design stage of ACOs and CINs will be important to their success.

---

[263] iSix Sigma. DMAIC roadmap. Accessed online July 16, 2011, at http://healthcare.isixsigma.com/index.php?option=com_k2&view=item&layout=item&id=1477&Itemid=372
[264] Schroeder R. Just-in-time systems and lean thinking. In: *Operations Management: Contemporary Concepts and Cases.* 3rd ed. New York, NY: McGraw-Hill Irwin; 2007;408–411.

While many healthcare organizations today have assembled and deployed Six Sigma resources to improve the quality and lower the cost of care, there is evidence that challenges the effectiveness of the methodologies, and more research is needed to fully understand how Six Sigma works best in a healthcare organization. Dellifraine and colleagues conducted a literature review of studies published on Six Sigma and Lean in the Thinking in the healthcare industry between 1999 and June 2009, which concluded there has is "very weak evidence" that the use and application of Six Sigma and Lean Thinking methodologies have led to overall improvement in healthcare quality.[265] Out of 177 total studies, the researchers identified only 34 empirical studies that had performance data; only 11 of these studies conducted statistical analyses to determine whether there was statistically significant improvement after the intervention was implemented. Last, only one of the 34 studies "adequately reported outcome results." There researchers also noted that none of the studies discussed the costs associated with implementation of these methodologies, which include hiring and training staff, the use of consultants, and cultural transition––all of which should factor into the overall value to healthcare organization embarking upon use of these tools.

Future Paths

A number of organizations are actively involved in improving quality measures and programs needed to support the changing landscape of healthcare delivery in the United States. ACOs and CINs, which focus on innovation, performance improvement, clinical quality, health outcomes, and financial performance, will help to redefine and further the advancement and measurement of quality. The roadmap for quality measurement emphasizes five functional streams, all of which involve various stakeholders in the process of evaluating performance at the micro and macro levels. Underlying these five functional streams is the issue of new and emerging quality measures. As new models of care take shape, the need for new measures will continue, to provide insights necessary to better understand the quality of care delivered and improvements in health outcomes.

---

[265] DelliFraine JL, Langabeer JR 2nd, Nembhard IM. Assessing the evidence of Six Sigma and Lean in the health care industry. *Qual Manag Health Care*. 2010 Jul-Sep;19(3):211–25.

Figure 40. Roadmap 5: Quality Continuum- Momentum for Improvement

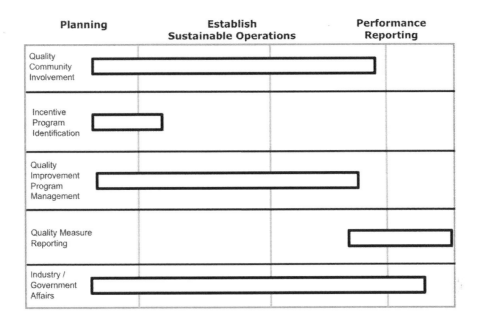

The first stream illustrated is quality community involvement. To set up a CIN or ACO, quality metrics must be identified, both for regulatory reporting and individual facility improvement. Moreover, involvement of physicians is important to obtain buy-in and identify areas in need of improvement. As measures evolve it is crucial to continue to engage executives and staff to understand the new requirements and to participate actively engaged in defining and developing new measures. Each healthcare organization, while having many elements in common and sharing a common purpose, has evolved over time and has any number of different systems in place.

Next is incentive program identification. Organizations will have to make choices about the metrics they emphasize to maximize quality and performance improvement and obtain incentives for their stakeholders. Programs like the CMS PQRS and Meaningful Use of EHRs programs will all have varying requirements: and participation in these programs may need to be balanced with participation in public and private sector ACOs. Each will involve additional reporting requirements, which create administrative burdens. Management of quality improvement program is an essential function, regardless of the size of the organization or the number of its stakeholders. Once measures have been identified and associated financial performance incentives established, ongoing work will be required monitor and track performance against metrics, correct course as needed, and create new policies and procedures that encourage new behaviors to meet the quality metrics. Quality improvement is a continuous activity that becomes more important when financial incentives are at stake. As new performance evaluation models and methods are tested, there will also be a need for rollout of these new programs.

Quality measure reporting involves clinical outcomes and economic impact through the efforts of the ACOs and CINs. Giving stakeholders a clear perspective on the potential economic benefits is essential in helping governance teams assess progress and institute further changes to workflow design, clinical care, and administrative processes and systems to improve quality for the population and community served and improve revenue for the ACO or CIN.

The last functional stream identified is industry/government affairs. These new programs will require additional regulatory compliance and result in additional government scrutiny. Maintaining good relations, at both federal and state levels, will be critical. Mistakes can be costly, especially when government agencies are not clear about implementation of new programs and can change their minds after the fact. Good record keeping, along with verification of new instructions, will help keep the public payer ACO out of trouble. CMS also continues to seek out innovations that improve the quality of care delivered. Good relations with CMS can also allow the organization to better understand how CMS is changing their programs and identify new opportunities for funding. It is also important to monitor changes in CMS quality metrics. Many CMS quality measures will continue to be refined through future federal rule making.

INFOCUS: Challenges Ahead

Many challenges lie ahead in the field of quality measurement and performance evaluation for ACOs and CINs. Pilot programs and demonstrations have produced documented results on which to build; however, the new Medicare ACO goes much further in terms of number of quality measures and other requirements. As CMS makes final the Proposed Rule, organizations considering becoming a Medicare ACO must figure out how the rule aligns with other industry quality programs and performance assessment tools. A critical challenge across the industry will be meeting the data collection requirements and reporting on static quality measures that may not produce quality or performance improvements. As the NQF, NCQA, AMA, TJC, and CMS collectively work to standardize and harmonize measures used for evaluating healthcare operations, more work is needed across the industry to continue automation of the data collection and identify measures of structure, process, and outcome that truly improve quality and affordability of care.

Table 38. Chapter 7 Challenges and Risks

Challenges	Risks
Factoring in local variations in populations, patient conditions and service utilization for comparative performance measurement and reporting.	Having incomplete and potentially inaccurate comparisons of ACOs and CINs clinical outcomes performance.
Meeting reporting requirements for multiple programs whose measures are not yet harmonized.	Conflicting Meaningful Use, HEDIS, PQRS, and other measures may create burdensome workloads and unnecessary stress on physician practices thus increasing the potential for variations inaccuracies in reported clinical and financial results.
Fully evaluating patient and caregiver experience and linking responses to specific episodes of care.	Not capturing sufficient data to evaluate the qualitative perception of patients on the care received and of physicians or nurses on the care delivered.
Ensuring sufficient training is put in place and attended by physicians and clinicians on the transition from ICD-9 to ICD-10.	Not factoring in ICD-10 transition to quality measure trends post 2013 may result in inaccuracies in evaluating CIN/ACO performance on health outcomes.
Focusing on reporting of static, regulatory required metrics, rather than identifying the underlying root cause and forgetting to make continuous quality improvements.	Meeting all quality metrics, but having no improvement in quality or reductions on cost, thereby missing out on shared savings or other incentives.

Table 38. Chapter 7 Challenges and Risks, cont.

Potential Mitigation Strategies
√ Support requests for input to federal rule making processes with meaningful and well-constructed ideas to assist legislators in crafting new or refined laws.
√ Implement advanced clinical decision support tools that are integrated with harmonized performance reporting. Engage physicians in quality metric development and performance improvement teams to identify opportunities to improve processes, reduce waste, and achieve cost savings that effect transformation around the structure of care, process of care, and health outcomes at the population level.
√ Upgrade the quality management team with sufficient resources so that team members can not only monitor and report but can also measure and improve structure, process, and outcomes.

Chapter 8. Comparative Effectiveness – Advancing the Model

Comparative effectiveness research provides important guidance for health care innovations and patient treatment decisions based on quality outcomes and value.

Ronald A. Williams, MD, Chairman and CEO, Aetna, Inc.
"Addressing Insurance Reform,"
Testimony before the United States Senate, March 24, 2009

Comparative effectiveness research (CER) evaluates different medical therapies to determine what works best in healthcare.[266] Health information technology could play a significant role in CER activities. In fact, government policy makers and legislators recognize the link between greater availability of data through health information technology and potential improvements in CER.[267] Various technology tools are needed to conduct CER, including technology for sharing data sets that will be transformed into value-adding knowledge in the research infrastructure.[268] To meet the needs of CER proposed by the federal government, significant resources will be needed, and they may include the use of EHRs and other clinical databases to compile source data and information for CER studies and evidence compilation.[269]

So what does CER mean for clinically integrated networks and accountable care organizations? That is an issue that we will explore in this chapter. If a provider-based organization is accountable or at-risk for a population of patients, there may be greater interest on the part of hospitals and physicians to identify which treatments are more effective and efficient. Comparative effectiveness

---

[266] Concato J, Lawler EV, Lew RA, Gaziano JM, Aslan M, Huang GD. Observational Methods in Comparative Effectiveness Research, *Am J Med*. 2010 Dec;123(12 Suppl 1):e16-23. CER may also compare different delivery models, such as primary care physician compared to hospitalist care, or clinically integrated networks versus patient centered medical homes, but the main focus of this chapter is on comparison of therapies.

[267] Department of Health and Human Services Recovery Funding Page. Comparative Effectiveness Research. Accessed online July 15, 2011, at http://www.hhs.gov/recovery/programs/cer/index.html.

[268] Navathe A. and Conway P. Optimizing Health Information Technology's Role in Enabling Comparative Effectiveness Research. *Am J Manag Care*. 2010;16(12):SP44-SP47. Accessed online August 12, 2011, at http://www.ajmc.com/supplement/managed-care/2010/AJMC_10dec_HIT/AJMC_10decHIT_Navathe_SP44-47.

[269] Etheredge L. Creating A High-Performance System For Comparative Effectiveness Research *Health Aff (Millwood)*. 2010. 29(10):1761–1767.

research may provide some clues, but there are other methods more widely used in practice to identify effective treatments such as comparisons with evidence-based medicine that takes evidence-based consensus guidelines, which may be enhanced with comparative effectiveness and other medical research to develop best practice protocols. Gaps in care may be identified and corrected when clinical practice is compared to these best practice protocols. This application of evidence-base medicine is one of the practical results of medical research, and is widely used to improve the quality and affordability of care.

Who performs comparative effectiveness research, how the research is conducted, and the use of the results are questions being asked as the field of comparative effectiveness research grows in visibility and importance. In addition, established methodologies comparing present physician practices to evidence-based medicine and identifying gaps in care will expand as providers become more accountable for care and seek out best practices.

Introduction

CER is generally used to refer to any work that compares different medical devices, drugs, and treatment methods to determine which are more effective in treating a disease or condition. Essentially, CER attempts to determine "what works best" in healthcare by comparing different therapies meant to treat the same disease or condition.[270] There is an established medical research infrastructure and a growing part of that infrastructure looks at the relative effectiveness of different treatments. The field of comparative effectiveness research has received increasing attention with the burgeoning availability of new medical technologies and the increasing cost of healthcare. Practical application of comparative effectiveness research includes use of evidence-based medicine and best-practice protocols. Patient preferences and preferred outcomes are also becoming increasingly important considerations.

---

[270] Concato J, Lawler EV, Lew RA, Gaziano JM, Aslan M, Huang GD. Observational Methods in Comparative Effectiveness Research, *Am J Med*. 2010 Dec;123(12 Suppl 1):e16–23.

The term comparative effectiveness research currently encompasses a wide range of activities and is almost as diverse as the universe of medical therapies being studied.[271] Payers, consumers, patients, providers, and other caregivers are increasingly interested in the technologies that provide the greatest value. Value may be defined as the technologies, medicines, or treatment techniques that are most effective at treating diseases and disorders that provide the greatest benefits while causing the least clinical harm, and provide them at the lowest economic cost. With reforms in the finance and delivery of healthcare, and perspectives brought by such new players as the Patient-Centered Outcomes Research Institute, the field of comparative effectiveness is growing and becoming increasingly important.

Comparative effectiveness may examine relative clinical benefits or harms (therapeutic effectiveness), and may include discovery of relative cost-effectiveness. There is ongoing debate among industry observers and policy makers as to whether cost-effectiveness should be included when comparing different treatments, especially for government-funded research––in part because of concerns about restricting the availability of costly treatments that benefit only a subpopulation or have marginal benefits over existing treatments. Restrictions on services with marginal clinical benefits and higher costs may satisfy government budget examiners, but clinicians and patients who see some benefit might object. There seems to be a general consensus among health services researchers about the importance of pursuing clinical comparative effectiveness while and leaving cost considerations to those in government and the private sector responsible for making decisions on how best to finance care.[272] As CINs and ACOs continue to advance as new models of care delivery, their interest in CER will increase as the benefits and drawbacks of specific treatment options are identified. CER may become even more important as models of performance evaluation continue to shift toward quality of care and value thus affecting reimbursement and compensation.

---

[271] Private discussion with Sean Tunis, Director, Center for Medical Technology Policy, May 2011.
[272] Wilensky GR. The Policies And Politics of Creating A Comparative Clinical Effectiveness Research Center. *Health Aff (Millwood)*, 2009 Jul-Aug;28(4):w719–29.

Clinical efficacy is sometimes confused with comparative effectiveness, but they are different activities with different purposes. Efficacy, according to the Food and Drug Administration (FDA), is a measure of whether a device or drug works better than doing nothing. Efficacy is usually determined through tightly structured and controlled clinical trials that compare a new drug or device to a placebo, although in some situations comparison may be made to existing treatments (such as pre-market notification for certain medical devices). Comparison to a placebo is a low threshold to meet and is not intended to compare different medical therapies that treat the same disease or condition. The FDA also weighs clinical benefits and risks of a new drug or device to determine its safety. Safety and efficacy must be proven before a drug or device is allowed by the FDA to be marketed and made available to the public.[273] Once safety and efficacy are established to the satisfaction of the FDA, the drug or device may be marketed to the public, even if the long-term effects of the treatment are unknown. This is a potentially fertile area for CER studies that can follow treatments after they are marketed, especially by using such health information technologies as EHR, and identify side effects not evident in the narrowly focused clinical trials used for FDA approval.

ARRA and the Affordable Care Act created new CER programs with substantial increases in funding. Different approaches to CER, the wide range of activities related to comparative effectiveness, and confusion between efficacy and cost-effectiveness led to a need to define CER. The Institute of Medicine (IOM) Committee on Comparative Effectiveness Research Prioritization defined comparative effectiveness research as:

...the generation and synthesis of evidence that compares the benefits and harms of alternative methods to prevent, diagnose, treat, and monitor a clinical condition or to improve the delivery of care. The purpose of CER is to assist consumers, clinicians, purchasers, and policy makers to make informed decisions that will improve health care at both the individual and population levels.[274]

---

[273] Tunis SR, Stryer DB, Clancy CM. Practical Clinical Trials: Increasing the Value of Clinical Research for Decision Making in Clinical and Health Policy, *JAMA*. 2003 Sep 24;290(12):1624–32.

[274] Institute of Medicine. Committee on Comparative Effectiveness Research Prioritization. *Initial National Priorities for Comparative Effectiveness Research*. Washington, DC: The National Academies Press. 2009. pp. 2–10.

It is not insignificant that the definition of CER adopted by the IOM does not specifically mention cost-effectiveness, because of the sensitivities of focusing on cost at the expense of quality.[275] Moreover, legislation increasing federal government funding has specifically mandated that findings of federally funded research cannot be used for coverage decisions.[276] It remains to be seen how long federally funded CER can be kept separate from economic effectiveness considerations in federal government health care programs (e.g. Medicare and Medicaid, etc). In addition, the IOM definition favors applied research, rather than basic research. This emphasis reflects Congressional interest in care delivery and wide dissemination of research findings that could directly inform consumer and provider clinical decision-making.[277]

Because of the lack of emphasis on cost-effectiveness, government-funded CER initiatives may not be immediately useful to new provider care models that focus on the financial impact of clinical actions, such as CINs and ACOs. All CER research findings, however, can help increase the body of knowledge of evidence-based medicine, improve best practice protocols and quality, and be used to strengthen clinical decision support for physician and patient benefit. It is unlikely that an individual hospital or physician will have the resources necessary to conduct research that compares different medical therapies. Nevertheless, new and more accountable provider organizations will make decisions on appropriate care, and look to reduce inappropriate care. As the ACOs and CINs models evolve and these organizations gradually assume greater degrees of risk essentially operating more like health insurance payers, they may become more involved in medical coverage decisions, benefit design, and appeals of decisions about care provided. These decisions require an understanding of both therapeutic effectiveness and cost-effectiveness. Fortunately, there is a large body of work in this field and other organizations have developed evidence-

---

[275] Wilensky GR. The Policies And Politics of Creating A Comparative Clinical Effectiveness Research Center. *Health Aff (Millwood)*, 2009;28(4):w719-w29.

[276] H.R. 3590, Patient Protection and Affordable Care Act, §6301(i) and (j), Patient-centered Outcomes Research . Rules and Rules of Construction. p. 620. (2010).

[277] H.R. 3590, Patient Protection and Affordable Care Act, §937(a)(1), Dissemination and Building Capacity for Research. p. 621. (2010).

based medical protocols and clinical decision support tools useful to ACOs and CINs as they face these decisions.[278]

History of Comparative Effectiveness Research

Research into the comparative effectiveness of medical drugs, devices, and treatment methodologies has been performed by a wide range of organizations and individuals for many different reasons.[279] Life science companies (manufacturers of drugs and medical devices), health plans, healthcare providers, and other private sector organizations perform a variety of CER-related programs. Independent, private organizations have also been established to organize, support, or conduct such research.[280] Governments may compare different treatments for a variety of purposes, including basic scientific research to increase knowledge; identify the highest-value product or service (best outcome and quality for the cost) for government reimbursement; or fulfill legislative fiat. Increasingly, federal government policy makers are looking to patients as the ultimate judges of value, and to patients' preferences as an important consideration in comparative effectiveness research.

Research into comparative effectiveness in the United States has been limited for a number of reasons. First, research is expensive to conduct, especially randomized, controlled trials that are believed to be more accurate and valid but are also very expensive to organize. An organization would have to see a return or benefit for the investment made, such as a manufacturer of a drug or device who may benefit directly from a study's positive findings. If an organization does benefit--or worse, if the results show harm--the results may be proprietary and kept confidential, limiting the value to society of such research. Second, once results of CER are in the public domain, they may benefit other organizations that

---

[278] A description of one such service, and the results obtained can be found in Javitt JC, et al. Using a Claims Data-based, Sentinel System to Improve Compliance with Clinical Guidelines: Results of a Randomized Prospective Study. *Am J Manag Care* 2005;11:93-102; see also Javitt JC, Rebitzer JB, Reisman L. Information technology and medical missteps: Evidence from a randomized trial. *J Health Econ* 2008;27(3):585–602.

[279] See Congressional Budget Office, Research on the Comparative Effectiveness of Medical Treatments, Publication 2975, December 2007, pp. 7–9.

[280] For example, the Center for Medical Technology Policy, Cochrane Collaboration, Drug Effectiveness Review Project, ECRI Institute, Hayes, Inc., Institute for Clinical and Economic Review, Technology Evaluation Center at BCBS Association, ActiveHealth Management, and Tufts Medical Center Cost-Effectiveness Analysis Registry.

did not pay for the research and eliminate any return on the investment anticipated by the organization originally funding the research. Furthermore, advances in healthcare may cause the technology or medicine being researched to become obsolete before effectiveness can be compared or established, especially for more costly but potentially more valid research methodologies that take years to complete. For these and other reasons, CER is thought to be a public good, requiring government funding.[281]

The federal government has conducted CER but only sporadically. The National Center for Health Care Technology was created in 1978 to research and compare health care technologies. It evaluated a number of technologies and made coverage recommendations to the Medicare program, but was controversial and no longer received funding after 1981. At the same time the Congressional Office of Technology Assessment evaluated the costs and benefits of a variety of technologies but lost funding in 1995.[282]

As of 2011 a number of federal government agencies support or perform some form of CER, including the AHRQ), National Institutes of Health (NIH), CMS, FDA, Centers for Disease Control and Prevention (CDC), Department of Defense (DOD), and Department of Veterans Affairs (VA). Each agency has its own legislative requirements for conducting research, which is usually tied to its core mission.[283] For example, the VA compares various treatment options for recipients of Veterans Health Affairs services. This specification helps ensure that veterans receive proper treatments that are cost-effective and within budget limits. The NIH has a broad mandate to fund basic research and has occasionally sponsored research to compare treatments. CMS has funded research comparing different treatments but usually to determine clinical effectiveness or whether to pay the same amount for two different treatments. It is outside the legislative authority

---

[281] Congressional Budget Office, Research on the Comparative Effectiveness of Medical Treatments, Publication 2975, December 2007, p. 8.
[282] Congressional Budget Office, Research on the Comparative Effectiveness of Medical Treatments, Publication 2975, December 2007, p. 9.
[283] Institute of Medicine. Committee on Comparative Effectiveness Research Prioritization. *Initial National Priorities for Comparative Effectiveness Research.* Washington, DC: The National Academies Press. 2009. pp. 2-13 to 2-17.

of CMS to look at cost-effectiveness. A vast number of activities and resources are available from the federal government related to comparative effectiveness.[284]

ARRA increased total federal government funding for CER by an additional $1.1 billion. The funding was divided among AHRQ ($300 million), NIH ($400 million), and the Office of the Secretary of DHHS ($500 million). The amount given to the Office of the Secretary of DHHS is discretionary funding that can be used for a variety of comparative effectiveness programs. The ARRA funds were targeted to CER within the government (intramural) or outside government (extramural). In addition, $268 million of the funds were required to be used to encourage development and use of "clinical registries, clinical data networks, and other forms of electronic health data that can be used to generate or obtain outcomes data." This financial support to develop and use health information technology to generate and capture data in CER programs demonstrates the importance of new technologies to the future of CER and the importance of coordinating with other government health information technology programs.[285] ARRA also funded the IOM to consult with stakeholders and report on priorities for comparative effectiveness research.[286]

AHRQ has the broadest mandate for comparative effectiveness studies; however, until 2009 only $15 million of the entire $300 million AHRQ budget was targeted to programs related to comparative effectiveness. Before 2009 AHRQ had run a national clearinghouse for medical guidelines, helped fund a number of "evidence-based practice centers," sponsored an "Effective Health Care" program, and funded private sector research. ARRA's funding increase to AHRQ doubled the entire AHRQ annual budget thereby strengthening substantially its emphasis on CER. Programs created or expanded by the new funding include "horizon scanning" for new and emerging issues: synthesis of evidence to compare effectiveness of medical treatments; identification of gaps in research; translation and dissemination of CER findings; coordination and prioritization of

---

[284] Health Services/Technology Assessment Texts, National Library of Medicine, 1994. Accessed online August 11, 2011 at http://www.ncbi.nlm.nih.gov/books/NBK16710/.
[285] Department of Health and Human Services. Comparative Effectiveness Research Funding. Accessed online July 5, 2011 at http://www.hhs.gov/recovery/programs/cer/index.html.
[286] Institute of Medicine. Committee on Comparative Effectiveness Research Prioritization. *Initial National Priorities for Comparative Effectiveness Research.* Washington, DC: The National Academies Press. 2009.

comparative effectiveness projects; training and career development; and a program to formally engage stakeholders.[287] As these new initiatives gain momentum at the same time ACO and CIN programs are maturing in the coming years, opportunities to leverage insights will materialize to help provider improve patient care.

Government agencies are subject to Congressional and public scrutiny, so great caution is exercised by these organizations to mitigate controversial actions or initiatives. In fact, AHRQ lost funding in the mid-1990s when research into back surgery resulted in controversial guidelines that were opposed by orthopedic surgeons.[288] Concern about the effect of CER, and the potential to use such information to make reimbursement decisions, has led to restrictions on the use of CER results. For example, the Affordable Care Act established a tax-exempt, private nonprofit organization called the Patient Centered Outcomes Research Institute (PCORI). PCORI is separate from the government to reduce the potential for political intervention and manipulation. In addition, PCORI research findings may "not be construed as mandates for practice guidelines, coverage recommendations, payment, or policy recommendations," nor may they be used for coverage or reimbursement decisions by "any public or private payer."[289]

The Patient Protection and Affordable Care Act of 2010

PCORI was created by the Affordable Care Act to identify priorities for comparative effectiveness research and fund research comparing "health outcomes and clinical effectiveness, risks, and benefits of two or more medical treatments, services, or items."[290] PCORI takes a patient-centered approach, and is designed to improve the interaction between patient and provider by increasing the availability of valid evidence-based medical information to enable meaningful discussion between patient and the clinician. The "patient

---

[287] Department of Health and Human Services. American Recovery and Reinvestment Act.
Agency for Healthcare Research and Quality: Comparative Effectiveness Research Program Summary. Accessed online July 5, 2011 at http://www.hhs.gov/recovery/reports/plans/pdf20100610/AHRQ%20CER%20June%202010.pdf, See also http://www.ahrq.gov/fund/cerfactsheets/
[288] Gray BH, Gusmano MK, Collins SR. AHCPR and the Changing Politics of Health Services Research. *Health Aff (Millwood)*, 2003 Jan-Jun;Suppl Web Exclusives:W3–283–307.
[289] H.R. 3590, Patient Protection and Affordable Care Act, §6301(d)(8), Release of Research Findings. §6301(i). Rules. (2010).
[290] H.R. 3590, Patient Protection and Affordable Care Act, §6301(a)(2)(A), Comparative Clinical Effectiveness Research; Research. (2010).

preference" approach is central as some policy makers believe most of medical decisions fall somewhere between 25 percent of care that is based on evidence and 10 percent of procedures that should never be done. It is this middle 65 percent, according to industry observers, where information can be applied to better inform patient preference. According to a governing board member, PCORI expects to bring about a new era in which both patients and their caregivers have access to the best information, and the tools to turn that information into knowledge allowing both patient and clinician to make the best decisions.

The PCORI website describes the organization as:

> ...an independent organization created to help patients, clinicians, purchasers and policy makers make better informed health decisions. PCORI will commission research that is responsive to the values and interests of patients and will provide patients and their caregivers with reliable, evidence-based information for the health care choices they face.[291]

The description is decidedly focused on patients and decision making, which may limit the ability of the organization to fund or participate in basic research that increases scientific knowledge unless there is a connection with consumer health decisions. Of course, the argument can be made that all basic research increasing scientific knowledge should be related to consumer health decisions. In addition, PCORI may not "mandate coverage, reimbursement, or other policies for any public or private payer,"[292] limiting the organization's ability to keep from being involved in considerations of cost-effectiveness––a concern for organizations paying the costs of care, such as government health programs, employers, health insurance companies, and partially capitated CINs, or ACOs. Nevertheless, the output of PCORI will add to medical knowledge, and if valid the results will be used by healthcare stakeholders.

PCORI is required to establish and carry out a research agenda that focuses on "priority areas" of research. It is governed by a board of governors appointed by the U.S. Government Accountability Office from public nominations, and must

---

[291] Patient Centered Outcomes Research Institute home page. organizational description. Accessed online July 15, 2011, at http://www.pcori.org/home.html.
[292] H.R. 3590, Patient Protection and Affordable Care Act, §937(a)(1), Dissemination and Building Capacity for Research (2010).

appoint advisory panels and a methodology committee. PCORI does not itself perform research; rather it supports research through a variety of activities, including funding, collaborating with other government agencies, establishing a peer-review process for primary research, adopting research priorities, standards, processes and protocols, and disseminating and publishing research findings. PCORI is required to submit annual reports to Congress, the Administration, and the public; and there are a number of requirements that increase the transparency of the work performed by PCORI—which helps to increase the validity of the process and projects funded).[293]

Funding for PCORI comes from a new Patient-Centered Outcomes Research Trust Fund that receives monies from several sources, including Medicare trust funds, private sector health plans, self-insured plans, pharmaceutical companies, and general funds of the federal government. While funding will slowly increase from 2010 to 2019, it is expected to rise to $500 million by 2014. The amount of funding available to PCORI depends on a complex set of formulas tied to the number of persons covered by public and private health care.[294] Some believe PCORI annual funding could be as much as $650 million, depending on the amount brought in by the health coverage surtax, and total $3 billion over 10 years.[295]

National Institute for Health and Clinical Excellence

A number of organizations in other countries sponsor or perform comparative effectiveness research. This factor is important as it not only shows that comparative effectiveness is a global issue but also because it provides lessons learned from comparative effectiveness activities in other countries. In the United Kingdom (UK) the National Institute for Health and Clinical Excellence (NICE) is widely recognized as a pioneer in comparative effectiveness research. NICE was created in 1999 by the government of the United Kingdom to evaluate

---

[293] H.R. 3590, Patient Protection and Affordable Care Act, §6301(i) and (j), Patient-centered Outcomes Research. Rules and Rules of Construction. (2010).

[294] Clancy C, Collins FS. Patient-Centered Outcomes Research Institute: The Intersection of Science and Health Care. *Sci Transl Med.* 2010 Jun 23;2(37):37cm18.

[295] Leonard, D. Time for PCORI's Implementation, at http://www.npcnow.org/Public/Newsroom/E-newsletter/2010_e-newsletters/April_2010_EVI/Time_for_PCORI's_Implementation.aspx.

the clinical and cost effectiveness of various drugs, devices, and procedures. Part of the UK National Health Service (NHS), NICE organizes systematic reviews of existing comparative effectiveness research (meta-analyses), and develops cost effectiveness models to arrive at cost-benefit conclusions. It does not fund primary research, nor does it directly decide which treatments to cover or how much to pay. If a drug, device, or methodology is approved by NICE as effective, it must be covered for reimbursement by the NHS health program. But the NHS decides how much to pay, and if a medical therapy is not approved by NICE it is not automatically rejected by the NHS. With a staff of 200 and a budget of approximately $60 million, NICE does not have extensive resources and it takes awhile to develop studies and produce results. NICE has published about 250 recommendations on procedures, over 100 studies on specific technologies, and 60 treatment guidelines. It is up to local government authorities to make coverage decisions on treatment technologies and methodologies that are not studied by NICE. Australia, Canada, France, and Germany have government agencies similar to NICE. All of these countries have some form of centralized government-funded and controlled health care finance and delivery system, perhaps making NICE and similar organizations not directly applicable to the U.S. healthcare system.[296]

Commercial Comparative Effectiveness Research

A number of private sector comparative effectiveness programs currently operate in the United States. Life science companies, such as drug and device manufacturers, commission CER to determine the effectiveness of their products to gain a competitive advantage, identify improved uses for their products, and potential new uses. As reimbursement becomes more restrictive and the market becomes more competitive, life science companies may find it increasingly important to engage in comparative effectiveness studies to understand cost and benefits of their products. Health plans, self-insured employers, and government payers are interested in CER to determine the quality of drugs, devices, and procedures, and to better understand their overall value to patients. Hospitals and health systems review treatment methodologies in their pharmacy and therapeutic committees and quality committees to assist with quality and risk management, determine pharmacy formularies, and make capital allocation for new devices. As integrated delivery networks, physician-hospital organizations, and physician groups assume increased risk and greater responsibility for quality and cost in such new provider organizations such as CINs and accountable care arrangements, CER and evidence-based medicine will increase in importance.[297] In addition as this shift occurs the federal government may re-examine regulations governing the use of comparative effectiveness studies to better align with such reformed delivery entities as ACOs, CINs, and other new models of care delivery.

Medical drug and device manufacturers are required by the FDA to conduct clinical trials in developing their products to demonstrate safety and efficacy, and in some cases to show how one device compares to another. These studies focus on safety and efficacy, but not relative clinical or cost effectiveness. Manufacturers are beginning to study clinical and cost effectiveness through CER and application of pharmacoeconomics mainly to inform the design and content of package inserts but also to determine how their products compare with competitors as they prepare to go to market and help identify differentiators in the marketplace. This activity will become more critical as drugs and devices lose their patent protections and the protected drug and device portfolios of large companies shrink. In addition, the FDA is beginning to use the results of CER in the regulation of products. Comparative effectiveness is also becoming more critical for manufacturers, as payers increasingly perform comparative studies to find drugs and devices that provide greater value. Providers, consumers, health plans, self-funded employers, governments, CINs and ACOs are interested in proof that a more costly drug or device results in a commensurate increase in clinical benefit for patients.[298]

---

[297] Miller J. Aetna Manages Cancer Care. *Managed Healthcare Executive*. July 2011;21(7):18-21. Accessed online August 17, 2011, at http://managedhealthcareexecutive.modernmedicine.com/mhe/Thought+Leadership/Aetna-manages-cancer-care/ArticleStandard/Article/detail/728450.

[298] Institute of Medicine. Committee on Comparative Effectiveness Research Prioritization. *Initial National Priorities for Comparative Effectiveness Research*. Washington, DC: The National Academies Press. 2009. pp. 2–17.

Health insurance plans have an interest in CER as they strive to improve quality and affordability. Not only are health insurance plans at risk for the cost of care, they are also legally accountable for the quality of care, required to justify coverage decisions, and must work with patients or physicians who challenge these decisions and adjudicate their appeals. Health plans also use the results of CER to increase their knowledge of evidence-based medicine, develop best practice clinical protocols, and provide clinical decision support tools and technologies to physicians, nursing care managers, and patients. These technologies are used for predictive modeling and risk stratification, care management, disease management, total population registries, quality measurement, specific care recommendations, and personal health records.[299] Many of these technologies and tools may be leveraged by CINs and ACOs as the industry evolves and these organizations are increasingly interested in evidence-based medicine.

While CINs and ACOs will assume more accountability and risk for the outcomes of care, and pay-for-performance programs are taking greater responsibility for care the reality is that in most areas of the country today, health plans are the predominant bearers of risk and have the greatest experience and largest array of tools for risk mitigation and care management. As a result, health insurance plans are at the forefront of researching the quality and effectiveness of various medical drugs, devices, and procedures, and they have sophisticated infrastructure for reviewing the findings of medical research and making decisions.[300] The result has been identification of optimal treatment methodologies[301] and processes that assist patients and physicians in understanding appropriateness of different treatment options. Many health plans publish the results of their research as medical coverage policies.[302] As the market expands around risk-sharing between providers and health insurance plans, observers anticipated that many of these risk mitigation and care management strategies and tools may be shared with providers.[303] As CINs and ACOs become more experienced in managing and improving care outcomes, they

---

[299] Juster IA. Technology-Driven Interactive Care Management Identifies and Resolves More Clinical Issues than a Claims-Based Alerting System. *Dis Manag* 2005;8(3):188–97,

[300] Kongstvedt, PR, ed. Essentials of Managed Health Care, 5th ed. Sudbury, MA: Jones and Bartlett Publishers. 2007. pp. 47–50.

[301] Javitt JC, et al. Using a Claims Data-based, Sentinel System to Improve Compliance with Clinical Guidelines: Results of a Randomized Prospective Study. *Am J Manag Care* 2005;11:93–102

[302] For example, see Aetna Clinical Policy Bulletins, which are detailed, technical documents explaining how decisions are made: http://www.aetna.com/healthcare-professionals/policies-guidelines/clinical_policy_bulletins.html

[303] See "Aetna and Carilion Clinic Announce Plans to Collaborate on Accountable Care Organization," Accessed online August 17, 2011, at http://www.aetna.com/news/newsReleases/2011/0310_Aetna_and_Carilion.html.

may become key players in the U.S. healthcare system's larger framework of comparative effectiveness capabilities.

Many of the provider organizations outlined in Table 11 in Chapter 3 use comparative effectiveness techniques to assist with quality and risk management, determine pharmacy formularies, and make capital allocations. Such new business models for healthcare delivery and finance as medical homes, CINs, and ACOs require providers to take greater clinical and financial responsibility and risk in the process of ensuring that optimal care is delivered for their patients. As these organizations refine their business practices, their perspective on clinical effectiveness may become broader, looking not only at the quality of care but affordability as well. Managing these new models of care delivery will require providers to have greater awareness of the relative benefit and harm of different treatment methodologies. This information will increase the importance of and demand for CER and related evidence-based medicine and clinical decision support services.[304]

Life science companies, provider organizations, health plans, and other commercial entities also support such broader efforts in CER, as the government-funded PCORI, which focuses on increasing the ability of patients and physicians to make better informed treatment decisions and improve overall quality and affordability. Government policy makers maintain that the current health finance and delivery system allows treatments with marginal clinical benefit relative to their cost. They see the current situation as contributing to unsustainable cost growth requiring greater information and transparency on clinical effectiveness and cost of care to address this national problem. It is therefore natural that a wide range of stakeholders support such organizations as PCORI and other private sector efforts to obtain up-to-date, objective, and credible information on the effectiveness and value of health care services.

---

[304] Miller J. Aetna Manages Cancer Care. *Managed Healthcare Executive*. July 2011;21(7):18-21. Accessed online August 17, 2011, at http://managedhealthcareexecutive.modernmedicine.com/mhe/Thought+Leadership/Aetna-manages-cancer-care/ArticleStandard/Article/detail/728450.

Comparative Effectiveness and Coverage Decisions

Organizations with the responsibility and burden of risk for clinical and financial outcomes of care have an interest in comparing both clinical and cost effectiveness. These comparisons are used to determine benefit design and decide which therapies are covered in the benefit package. Coverage decisions are made by all organizations accountable for care of a defined population, including government agencies that fund health programs (e.g. Medicare, Medicaid, state indigent care and children's health programs, Veterans Health Administration, and the like.), unions, self-insured employers, health insurance plans, and ACOs. All these organizations have developed a wide range of activities to determine which treatments provide the best clinical outcomes for the resources expended.

A variety of comparative effectiveness services have been created to assist with decisions on clinical and cost effectiveness. The Blue Cross and Blue Shield Association has operated the Technology Evaluation Center whose clients include many of the Blue Plans and the CMS.[305] Other organizations that support or perform clinical effectiveness research include the Center for Medical Technology Policy, Cochrane Collaboration, Drug Effectiveness Review Project, ECRI Institute, Hayes, Inc., Institute for Clinical and Economic Review, and Tufts Medical Center Cost-Effectiveness Analysis Registry.[306]

CMS is the largest payer of health care services and products in the United States, with a total budget for fiscal year 2011 of $782 billion. Given the size of its budget, and continued growth of its programs administered, funded, and regulated by CMS (e.g. Medicare, Medicaid, State Children's Health plans, and the new health insurance exchanges), CMS has a substantial interest in CER.[307] An example of a coverage decision-making process, which includes comparative

---

[305] Wilensky GR. The Policies and Politics of Creating A Comparative Clinical Effectiveness Research Center. *Health Aff (Millwood)*, 2009 Jul-Aug;28(4):w719-w29.
[306] Institute of Medicine. Committee on Comparative Effectiveness Research Prioritization. *Initial National Priorities for Comparative Effectiveness Research*. Washington, DC: The National Academies Press. 2009. pp. 2-17 to 2-18; and Congressional Budget Office, Research on the Comparative Effectiveness of Medical Treatments, Publication 2975, December 2007, p. 8.
[307] Wilensky GR. The Policies and Politics of Creating A Comparative Clinical Effectiveness Research Center. *Health Aff (Millwood)*, 2009 Jul-Aug;28(4):w719-w29.

effectiveness input from external technology assessment resources is shown in Figure 34.[308] The Medicare National Coverage decision-making process illustrates the level of complexity in evaluating medical therapies for coverage decisions.

Figure 34. Medicare National Coverage Process[309]

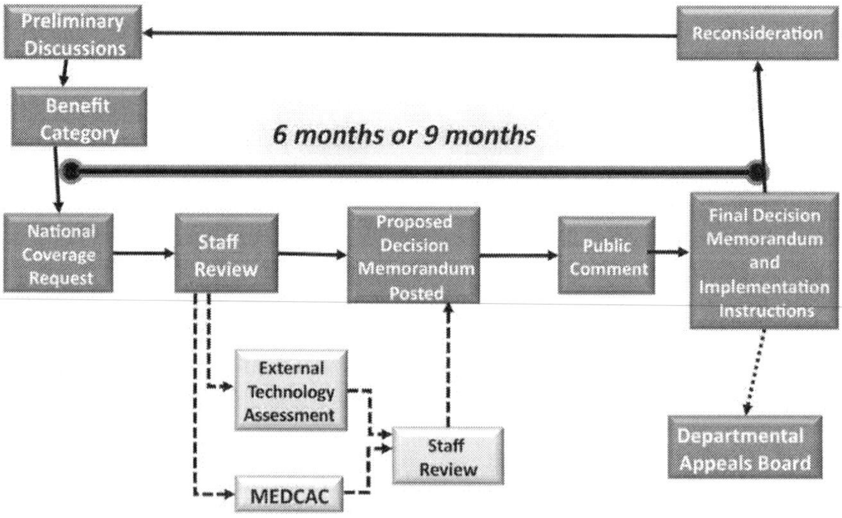

Source: Center for Medicare and Medicaid Services

Decisions rendered through this process are for items and services required for the diagnosis and treatment of an illness or injury covered by Medicare. The underlying methodology and program is run as an evidence-based process that allows opportunities for public participation.[310] As CINs and ACOs continue to grow in their tolerance of clinical and financial risk and acceptance of responsibility, they will be more attuned to the decisions made by such payer organizations such as CMS in their national and local coverage processes, and may even begin to adopt these coverage determinations.

[308] Jacques, LB, The Stakeholder Perspective, presentation at the third DEcIDE Symposium on Comparative Effectiveness Research Methods, June 6, 2011.

[309] From "Evidence for Decisionmaking, A Medicare Perspective" presentation by Louis B Jacques, MD, Director, Coverage & Analysis Group, Centers for Medicare and Medicaid Services, third DEcIDE Methods Symposium: Methods for Developing and Analyzing Clinically Rich Data for Patient-Centered Outcomes Research, Monday June 6, 2011, Rockville, MD.

[310] Center for Medicare and Medicaid Services. Overview of Medicare Coverage Determination Process. Accessed online July 6, 2011, at https://www.cms.gov/DeterminationProcess/.

Comparative Effectiveness Research Methods

A variety of methods are used to research the effectiveness of medical therapies, and arrive at conclusions about the best treatment for a condition. Each method has strengths and weaknesses and requires different levels of rigor and validity. Here we look at two different categories of research methods--randomized controlled trials and observational studies-- and their usefulness in comparative effectiveness research.

The randomized controlled trial (RCT) is considered the gold standard of research methods. In an RCT, an experiment is designed in which research subjects are chosen and randomly assigned to a treatment group or a control group, and the effects of treatment are then isolated and observed. The research subjects are chosen to minimize differences in their health status, and all other aspects of the study are controlled or accounted for as well as possible so that the only difference between the two groups is the treatment provided. By controlling as many variables as possible in the study, researchers attempt to isolate the cause-effect relationship between the treatment given and outcome recorded.[311]

Observational studies include a variety of research designs in which no experiment is set up in advance with random assignment or controls. Observational studies may be used in situations in which a controlled experiment may not be possible. Controlled trials are not possible, for example, where ethical standards prohibit the use of human subjects (e.g., effects of radon gas or cigarette smoking), or when setting up an RCT is difficult (e.g., rare occurrence of side effects, or lack of resources to get a large enough experimental population). Observational studies make conclusions about the effects of the treatment in question based on educated guesses (inferences) from the data.[312] Observational studies include cohort studies, case-controlled studies, case series, and case reports.[313] Figure 35 illustrates progression through a hierarchy of evidence.

---

[311] Agency for Healthcare Research and Quality. Glossary of Terms, definition of randomized controlled trials. Accessed online September 13, 2011, at http://www.effectivehealthcare.ahrq.gov/index.cfm/glossary-of-terms/?pageaction=showterm&termid=101.
[312] ClinicalTrials.gov Protocol Registration System. Protocol Data Element Definitions (DRAFT), definition of observational studies. Accessed online September 13, 2011, at http://prsinfo.clinicaltrials.gov/definitions.html.
[313] Akobeng, AK, Understanding Randomised Controlled Trials, Arch Dis Child 2005;90:840–844.

Figure 35. Hierarchy of Evidence for Intervention or Treatment Effectiveness [314]

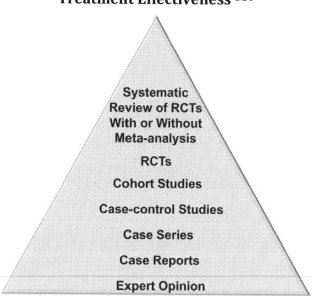

The RCT is considered the most rigorous and valid research design as it attempts to reduce errors, eliminate bias and extraneous effects (also known as confounding variables) by controlling the study as much as possible. A systematic review of a set of randomized controlled trials using meta-analysis may provide additional validity as it assembles results of many RCT and can cover larger populations and filter out weaknesses of individual trials.

There are weaknesses to RCT, however, especially in situations in which decisions that impact a large group of persons must be made quickly, such as coverage decisions that must be implemented in the short-term for a large population in a health plan, CIN/ACO, or clinical formulary decisions by one of these organizations. To begin, RCTs are more expensive to conduct and take much longer to set up, implement, and provide results--in many cases it takes years and millions of dollars. Second, because the population is controlled, the results apply to a defined population and may not be generally applicable. Finally, because the procedures used in a RCT are controlled and the experiment

---
[314] Akobeng, AK. Understanding Randomised Controlled Trials. *Arch Dis Child.* 2005;90(8):840–4.

is carried out under optimal conditions, it may be difficult to replicate or implement in a regular clinical setting.[315]

Observational studies have been criticized as more prone to error as they are perceived to be less rigorous or valid than a RCT. Perhaps not as rigorous as RCTs, observational studies can be designed to reduce errors and improve their validity. The lack of ability to rigorously control the situation and the potential for extraneous variables to affect the results leads to a need for adjustments to observational studies. Once these adjustments are made, the effects of treatment can more reliably be determined.[316] Such techniques as propensity scoring and instrumental variables are used to correct for errors by adjusting observational studies to more closely replicate RCT experiments. Recent studies have shown that properly adjusted observational studies are almost as good as RCTs.[317]

Observational studies have important advantages for application of CER. Because they are less expensive and may use data already collected, they can be completed more rapidly. In addition, observational studies are usually done in real-world clinical settings on actual patients using real interventions rather than strict experimental controls.[318] Thus, the results can be obtained and applied more easily, which is important in situations in which decisions must be made quickly. Future improvements in observational study design will increase the availability of information on better medical therapies, help organizations with decision making on what works best, including which treatments should be used in clinical settings. The selection of one research methodology over another involves a number of issues. Table 40 below provides a summary of some myths regarding each of these methodologies.

---

[315] Concato J, Lawler EV, Lew RA, Gaziano JM, Aslan M, Huang GD.. Observational Methods in Comparative Effectiveness Research, *Am J Med*. 2010 Dec;123(12 Suppl 1):e16-23. Review.

[316] ClinicalTrials.gov Protocol Registration System. Protocol Data Element Definitions (DRAFT), definition of observational studies. Accessed online September 13, 2011, at http://prsinfo.clinicaltrials.gov/definitions.html.

[317] Horwitz RI, Viscoli CM, Clemens JD, Sadock RT. Developing improved observational methods for evaluating therapeutic effectiveness. *Am J Med*. 1990;89:630–638.

[318] Concato J, Lawler EV, Lew RA, Gaziano JM, Aslan M, Huang GD.. Observational Methods in Comparative Effectiveness Research, *Am J Med*. 2010 Dec;123(12 Suppl 1):e16–23. Review.

Table 39. Myths and Evidence on RCTs and Observational Studies[319]

Issue	Myth	Evidence
Gold standard	Randomized, controlled trials are always the gold standard in research design	Randomized trials on the same topic often contradict each other
Unknown confounders	Unknown confounders undermine all observational studies	If a factor is unknown, treatment will not be influenced and confounding is unlikely
Designed to Replicate RCT	Novel strategies in designing and analyzing observational studies can replicate randomization	Purported benefits of new strategies to design and analyze are often conceptual rather than actual
Design vs. Details	Study design matters more than specific details and attributes	Details of patients, interventions, and outcomes are highly relevant

Pragmatic randomized clinical trials (PCTs) have been proposed to combine the validity of RCT with the practical applicability of observational studies. In a PCT the study design is set up specifically to address clinical quality and cost issues of interest to decision makers.[320] The Center for Medical Technology Policy has pioneered PCTs as a way to get provide valid information to all decision makers, including patients, physicians, providers, policy-makers, payers and health care administrators.[321] PCTs are designed to be more applicable and useful in real world situations because they recruit a diverse set of participants from a wide variety of real-world clinical practices and focus on comparing specific medical therapies while collecting a wide range of outcomes.[322]

It is important for CINs and ACOs to understand the implications of these different research methodologies. As the use of CER expands, study results can benefit the patients and providers by bringing new intelligence into the shared

---

[319] Concato J, Lawler EV, Lew RA, Gaziano JM, Aslan M, Huang GD. Observational Methods in Comparative Effectiveness Research, *Am J Med*. 2010;123(12 Suppl 1):e16-23.

[320] Tunis SR, Stryer DB, Clancy CM. Practical clinical trials: increasing the value of clinical research for decision making in clinical and health policy. *JAMA*. 2003 Sep 24;290(12):1624-32.

[321] Center for Medicare Technology Policy. Issue Brief: Pragmatic/Practical Randomized Controlled Trials. Accessed online August 10, 2011, at http://www.cmtpnet.org/comparative-effectiveness/PCT_issue_brief_11-26-08.pdf.

[322] Center for Medicare Technology Policy. Pragmatic Clinical Trials, Center for Medical Technology Policy, accessed online August 10, 2011, at http://www.cmtpnet.org/comparative-effectiveness/pragmatic-trials.

decision-making process. This new information will improve patients' quality of care and ultimately their quality of life.

Health Information Technology and CER

The increasing availability of health information technology is creating tremendous new opportunities to advance knowledge and evidence while strengthening the healthcare industry's ability to study and compare the effectiveness of medical interventions. ARRA recognized the importance of the health information technology data infrastructure in advancing the national CER agenda and allocated $268 million to data infrastructure development.[323] In addition to such existing clinical study methods as RCT and observational studies, health information technology has created opportunities for new analyses by combining such traditional data sources as administrative claims, with clinical information from electronic medical records, registries, and other clinical databases. These new combinations of data and information will enhance CER studies and medical evidence compilation.[324]

Claims data brings a number of advantages to comparative effectiveness studies. There is a large body of literature describing ways to analyze the data, and established methods (such as propensity scoring) to adjust for potential errors. All health plans and self-insured employers have used claims data for years to analyze and improve the quality and affordability of healthcare. As discussed previously, health plans include claims data in their analyses of different treatment options when they develop medical coverage policies. Claims data is also used for a variety of quality, performance improvement, clinical decision support, and care management purposes. Some organizations have taken additional steps to develop sophisticated predictive models and advanced clinical decision support algorithms that yield accurate models of patients and their needed care. These systems are used to improve quality by scanning both claims and clinical data to detect and correct errors in the care delivery process

---

[323] Department of Health and Human Services Recovery Funding Page. Comparative Effectiveness Research. Accessed online July 15, 2011 at http://www.hhs.gov/recovery/programs/cer/index.html.
[324] Etheredge L. Creating a High-Performance System for Comparative Effectiveness Research *Health Aff (Millwood)*. 2010. 29(10):1761–1767.

and deviations from best medical practices.[325] If you combine a clinical trial with subsequent claims data, you can also create a longitudinal record for a patient and continue to follow his or her progress even after the trial is completed. Use of such a longitudinal record could take trials out of the clinic and into daily life, identifying both beneficial and harmful effects in real-life situations.

There are disadvantages to only using claims data as the data may be specific to an episode of care, and lack information necessary to understand the patient's full health status. Without additional information about the patient, it is difficult to identify similar patients or populations and compare the effectiveness of different medical therapies.[326]

Clinical information from such health information technology as electronic health records, personal health records and medical registries, can fill in the elements missing in administrative claims data, providing a more complete picture of a patient or population, and result in a more robust data set for CER. These technologies can provide such important data as medical histories, measures of health status, laboratory test results, and treatment outcomes.[327] The additional data can give sufficient detail to allow proper research methodologies to compare medical therapies, to be compared. Incorporating clinical data with claims data has been described as the "holy grail" of CER, but issues of federal government research priorities, privacy concerns, lack of information technology standardization, and difficulty in aggregating data are roadblocks to such integration.[328,329]

The private sector has advanced its comparative effectiveness research agenda and methodologies at a faster pace than the federal government. It is

---

[325] Javitt JC, Steinberg G, Locke T, Couch JB, Jacques J, Juster I, Reisman L. Using a Claims Data-based, Sentinel System to Improve Compliance with Clinical Guidelines: Results of a Randomized Prospective Study. *Am J Manag Care*. 2005 Feb;11(2):93–02.

[326] Congressional Budget Office, Research on the Comparative Effectiveness of Medical Treatments, Publication 2975, December 2007, pp. 21–22.

[327] Congressional Budget Office, Research on the Comparative Effectiveness of Medical Treatments, Publication 2975, December 2007, pp. 22–23.

[328] Navathe AS, Conway PH. Optimizing Health Information Technology's Role in Enabling Comparative Effectiveness Research. *Am J Manag Care*. 2010 Dec;16(12 Suppl HIT):SP44–7.

[329] Congressional Budget Office, Research on the Comparative Effectiveness of Medical Treatments, Publication 2975, December 2007, p. 22.

already aggregating and integrating administrative claims data with clinical-level data from health information technology. These efforts in time will allow ACOs and CINs to combine quality measures from clinical data with financial performance goals in their claims systems so they can monitor their performance against targets and annual goals in real time.[330]

Comparative Effectiveness and Clinical Decision Support

Clinical decision support (CDS) refers to any methodical process used to assist clinicians or patients with medical decisions. Computer-based CDS is further defined as the use of computers to bring relevant knowledge to bear on decisions about patients' healthcare and well-being.[331] Knowledge relevant to clinical care includes patient data, medical and pharmaceutical claims, clinical data, evidence-based guidelines, the most recent medical literature, personal values, and any other information that could help clinicians and patients make decisions and improve the quality of care. CER is part of the medical literature that goes into CDS.

Basic computer-based CDS technology combines data from a variety of sources, such as medical claims, pharmacy claims, and clinical data from EMRs and translates those data into information and knowledge applied by physicians, other clinicians, and multi-disciplinary caregiver teams to improve the quality of care. The translation of data and resulting conclusions is often accomplished by comparing patient treatments to evidence-based guidelines and identifying gaps in care and sometimes given recommendations on appropriate care according to the evidence-based guidelines used. Comparing treatment recommendations to guidelines is a form of practical comparative effectiveness but has shortcomings.

Many EHRs have basic CDS, which is a requirement for meaningful use under the CMS Meaningful Use of EHRs incentive program.[332] The CMS meaningful use

---

[330] Technology Fundamentals for Realizing ACO Success, Medicity, September 2010, Accessed online July 15, 2011, at http://www.himss.org/content/files/Medicity_ACO_Whitepaper.pdf.
[331] Greenes, R.A. ed. *Clinical Decision Support, the Road Ahead.* Academic Press. Maryland Heights, MO: Academic Press. 2007, p. 6.
[332] Fed. Reg. Vol. 75, No. 144, II(A)(2)(c). Stage 1 Criteria for Meaningful Use. p. 44350. CMS defines CDS in the context of meaningful use, as "HIT functionality that builds upon the foundation of an EHR to provide persons involved in care processes

regulation, however, requires only the implementation of "one clinical decision support rule ...along with the ability to track compliance to that rule" for Stage 1.[333] One rule may be appropriate to prove the concept of delivering CDS, but is inadequate for ongoing decision support across a broad spectrum of diseases and conditions if you are looking for improved outcomes. In addition, studies have shown that current EHRs do not deliver the features needed to improve patient care. Additional technologies are needed for EHRs to be effective, including registries, personal health records, and clinical decision support.[334] A recent study the use of clinical decision support in EHRs from 2005 to 2007 showed "no consistent association between EHRs and CDS and better quality."

Clearly, something is missing; additional clinical information from medical literature and CER is needed to improve and strengthen CDS. Advanced CDS technology is starting to become available, and it addresses the shortcomings of current EHR-based basic CDS by including a variety of additional data, tools, and techniques to improve decision support and care results. Advanced CDS is of great interest to ACOs and CINs as it is more accurate in identifying appropriate care, and allowing providers to mitigate and manage their risk and responsibility for clinical and economic outcomes.

Additional data not currently available to clinically focused EHRs but used in advanced CDS include pharmacy data, claims data, health risk assessments, patient-reported data, disability data, and other medical and demographic information. These additional elements help to provide a more complete picture of the patient, including medical history and future health risk.

Another feature of advanced CDS is the use of more recent medical findings, such as the results of CER. Basic CDS takes clinical information and compares it to evidence-based guidelines. By definition, evidence-based guidelines are consensus standards developed at a given point in time, using the medical

---

with general and person-specific information, intelligently filtered and organized, at appropriate times, to enhance health and health care."

[333] Fed. Reg. Vol. 75, No. 144, II(A)(2)(c). Stage 1 Criteria for Meaningful Use. p. 44328. Requirement for one clinical decision support rule as part of the core set of meaningful use objectives.

[334] Bates DW, Bitton A. The Future Of Health Information Technology In The Patient-Centered Medical Home. *Health Aff (Millwood).* 2010 Apr;29(4):614–21.

literature then available. Industry experts recognize that medical research is constantly advancing, and that "no physician can keep up with the literature and changing medical advances simply with intuition and top-of-mind memory."[335] Advanced CDS technologies, on the other hand, bring the capability to search the latest medical literature; present the latest medical findings identified by a team of experts; and update the evidence in real time—presenting evidence-based medicine practices at the point of care.[336] One drawback of some CDS is the level of effort and cost of human-intensive expert system techniques.[337]

A systematic review of studies of clinical decision support technologies identified specific features of CDS correlated with significant improvements in patient care. These features include: information that fits into clinician workflow; specific care recommendations; information at the point of care; periodic performance feedback; sharing recommendations with patients; and requesting documentation of reasons for not following recommendations.[338] Advanced CDS tools and techniques build in all these features by using real-time care recommendations at the point of care, allowing bidirectional information sharing with the treating clinician and utilizing such patient-facing tools, as personal health records to allow patient self-management.[339]

Comparative Effectiveness and New Provider Organizations

Given current restrictions on government-funded CER, its research results may not be directly useful to such new care models as CINs and ACOs. All CER findings, however, increase general medical knowledge and evidence-based medicine used by these organizations for decision support. Whether directly or indirectly improvements in medical knowledge improve best practice protocols. Thus even government-funded CER with its restrictions increases the body of medical knowledge, indirectly helping physicians and patients make more

---

[335] Miller J. Aetna Manages Cancer Care. *Managed Healthcare Executive*. July 2011;21(7):18–21.
[336] Jenrette, J. and Yale, K. "ACO Technologies: Performance and Reporting Tools," ACO West Conference, San Diego, CA, November 19, 2010.
[337] Greenes, R.A. rd. *Clinical Decision Support, the Road Ahead*. Maryland Heights, MO: Academic Press. 2007 pp. 207-223.
[338] Kawamoto K, Houlihan CA, Balas EA, Lobach DF. "Improving clinical practice using clinical decision support systems: a systematic review of trials to identify features critical to success," *BMJ*. 2005 Apr 2;330(7494):765.
[339] Jenrette, J. and Yale, K. ACO Technologies: Performance and Reporting Tools. ACO West Conference, San Diego, CA, November 19, 2010.

informed decisions about treatment options that improve patient care and quality of life.

CINs and ACOs do have commercially available advanced CDS tools to assist decision-making on appropriate care. As these new provider organizations accept greater responsibility for clinical and financial outcomes, they will find themselves making medical coverage decisions including benefit design, and responding to appeals of care decisions. Fortunately, there is a large body of work in this field and many tools on the market that allow providers to access this information.[340]

The success of such new provider organizations as ACOs and CINs will depend heavily on continued advancements in health information technology. Many organizations are establishing health information exchanges as discussed in Chapter 6 and are deepening their clinical integration in order to have the infrastructure necessary to operate in the new environment. Consider this possibility: properly established CINs and ACOs operating with appropriate health information technology and advanced CDS, and actively exchanging and aggregating data, may contribute to a "rapid-learning health system." Such a system would combine evidence from clinical and comparative effectiveness research with individual patients' information from electronic medical records to determine what works best for a patient.[341]

Another form of CER is comparing different healthcare finance and delivery models. For example, different ACO models (both public and private) could be evaluated and compared as they emerge, their operations become established, and their results and outcomes tested. In fact, the Proposed Rule notes that one of the ways competition could foster improvement would include:

---

[340] A description of one such service and results obtained, can be found at Javitt JC, et al. Using a Claims Data-based, Sentinel System to Improve Compliance with Clinical Guidelines: Results of a Randomized Prospective Study. *Am J Manag Care* 2005;11:93-102.; Javitt JC, Rebitzer JB, Reisman L. Information technology and medical missteps: Evidence from a randomized trial. *J Health Econ* 2008;27(3):585-602.
[341] Etheredge L. Creating a High-Performance System for Comparative Effectiveness Research *Health Aff (Millwood)*. 2010. 29(10):1761-1767.

Provide better benchmarks for quality improvements. For example, although a single ACO might claim that environmental or demographic factors limit what it can achieve in the treatment of certain illnesses, a comparison among multiple ACOs in the same service area could better ensure that the best standards possible under prevailing conditions are being met.[342]

This kind of initiative would focus on the effectiveness of variations in administrative systems, payment reforms, and related compensation models that would tie into opportunities for improving benchmarks to ensure comparability of results and savings achieved against targets. Ideally different health finance and delivery models could be compared, and help advance the study of health care quality, accessiblity and affordability.

INFOCUS: Challenges Ahead

The field of CER covers a broader spectrum that includes federally funded programs and private sector initiatives. While federally funded CER holds promise, it brings challenges to the industry in terms of limits on the use of federal funds and maximizing the utilization of results and findings. Private sector CER studies and programs, such as those funded through the pharmaceutical and biotechnology industry, provide results more quickly, but are usually proprietary and may not be widely publicized. In addition, there may be an element of bias in pharmaceutical and biotechnology CER, especially when the studies are performed for marketing purposes. CER associated with health insurance plans can be more specifically targeted to both clinical and economic outcomes, but may not be readily available to providers unless there is a preexisting relationship.

Finally, health information technology brings additional challenges. New technologies are arriving at a rapid pace, and often faster than industry can keep up with them. There are inherent risks in the development and implementation

---

[342] Fed. Reg. Vol. 76, No. 67. April 7, 2011. I(4)(b). Competition and Quality of Care. p. 19630.

of new technologies, called "technology-related adverse events" by the Joint Commission's 2008 Sentinel Event Report Number 42.[343] EMRs, EHRs, and registries used in CER can pose such risks, as the ability of society to develop new technologies may exceed the capacity of clinicians to use them safely and effectively.

Some of the most important challenges for CINs and ACOs involve effective and permissible use of CER study results to support improvements in the quality of patient care. It remains to be seen whether restrictions on the use of government-funded CER will persist. In addition, providers must consider whether it is worthwhile and economically viable to support CER. As both CER and new provider models continue to shape the future of healthcare services, new challenges will emerge and stakeholders will find ways to meet them for the benefit of providers, patients, and the organizations that fund healthcare.

We need to take medicine from empirical to evidence-based, and not just broad guidelines, but patient-specific medicine.

Janet Woodcock, MD,
Director, Food and Drug Administration,
Center for Drug Evaluation and Research

---

[343] The Joint Commission, "Safely Implementing Health information and Converging Technologies, Issue 42, December 11, 2008. Accessed online July 15, 2011, at
http://www.jointcommission.org/sentinel_event_alert_issue_42_safely_implementing_health_information_and_converging_techn ologies/.http://www.jointcommission.org/SentinelEvents/SentinelEventAlert/sea_42.htm?print=yes[9/20/2010 11:56:01 AM].

Table 40. Chapter 8 Challenges and Risks

Challenges	Risks
Understanding the need for clinical decision support in a CIN/ACO, and how best to use CER results.	Making coverage and clinical decisions without adequate, supporting research findings. Continue "business as usual" without investing in effective decision support.
Ensuring that clinical decision support uses CER to improve evidence-based care.	Decision making without adequate or advanced clinical decision support (i.e., using evidence-based medicine, at the point of care, based on patient-specific requirements).
Understanding capital and actuarial requirements of the ACO, and making decisions based on the best medicine and quality care, rather than educated guesses.	Not doing the right thing for the CIN/ACO and patient due to peer or salesman pressure.
Giving sufficient time and effort to pharmacy and therapeutics (P&T) and Quality Committee work to determine the best clinical pathways to fulfill financial (ACO health plan), clinical (physician), and patient obligations.	Use of incomplete information on various treatment modalities leading to incorrect decisions that violate Hippocratic or fiduciary duties.
Finding appropriate advanced clinical decision support service, whether internally generated or outsourced.	Using existing CER models but learning too late that they do not apply to your patient population.

Table 40. Chapter 8 Challenges and Risks, cont.

Potential Mitigation Strategies
√ Identify appropriate sources of information to make informed coverage and clinical decisions.
√ Build off lessons learned and best practice from various sources, including AHRQ, CMS, and experienced private sector organizations, including non-profit groups and health insurance payers.
√ Maintain vibrant and effective P&T and quality committee processes.
√ Keep track of new developments in government, and private sector comparative effectiveness research. Look for ways to leverage all resources, to reduce the cost of clinical decision support and coverage determinations.

Chapter 9. Financial Perspectives

The test of our progress is not whether we add more to the abundance of those who have much; it is whether we provide enough for those who have too little.

Franklin D. Roosevelt

32nd President of the United States of America

(1882-1945)

Many issues regarding CINs and ACOs have been discussed, including the basic elements of organizational transformation; legislative reforms; the importance of primary care, and clinical integration; clinical decision support; quality measurement; performance improvement; antitrust law and joint ventures; healthcare information technology and health information exchange; and the historical background of the U.S. healthcare system. In this chapter we take a look at health care financing.

The financing of health services is complex. For CINs and ACOs, managing traditional reimbursements and new incentives tied to quality measures and impacted by utilization and costs for specific populations are priorities and challenges for the industry in transforming to clinically integrated networks accountable for quality and cost of care. In light of this situation, a number of issues should be examined from the Affordable Care Act, Proposed Rule and other reform initiatives. These issues involve the Medicare Shared Savings Program; pay-for-performance strategies implemented in pilot programs; and demonstrations; public and private payer financial reform demonstrations; and other financial management issues related to start-up, redesign, or maintenance of healthcare organizations undergoing transformation in the twenty-first century healthcare system in the United States.

Landscape of Financial Challenges

A number of challenges face our nation's primary care physicians and other healthcare providers. Several of these challenges are related to the need for healthcare reform and have resulted in new finance and delivery modes, such as pay-for-performance, CINs, and ACOs. Some of the most pressing challenges include:

- Payment pressures from government-funded programs and unresolved sustainable growth rate adjustments in Medicare payments to physicians and their practices;[344]
- CMS Meaningful Use penalties starting in 2016 for providers who have not achieved compliance with Phases 1 through 3 of the final rules;[345]
- New reporting requirements from CMS in the Physician Quality Reporting System, and payment tied to quality;
- Expansion of the CMS recovery audit contractor (RAC) program to all institutional providers and adoption of the RAC program concept by private payers;[346]
- Rising costs of malpractice insurance;
- Costs of healthcare for the uninsured and underinsured patient population, and the growing costs of uncompensated care;
- Capital outlay requirements for new facilities and enterprise-level health information technology implementation;
- Increasing costs of doing business, including medical technology, commodities, and other regular expenses;
- Rapidly changing reimbursement methodologies, including new value-based purchasing, risk-adjusted DRGs, medical homes, and other initiatives.

The U.S. healthcare system is faced with an unsustainable growth rate that promises to get worse as the baby boomer generation reaches retirement age

---

[344] Simmons J. Medicare payments face another 6.1% cut under SGR. *HealthLeaders Media*, June 28, 2010. Available at: http://www.healthleadersmedia.com/print/FIN-253111/Medicare-Payments-Face-Another-61-Cut-Under-SGR.

[345] Centers for Medicare and Medicaid Services. Meaningful use program overview. Accessed online August 27, 2011, at http://www.cms.gov/EHRIncentivePrograms/.

[346] Centers for Medicare and Medicaid Services. Recovery audit contractor, recent updates. CMS expands FY 2010 RAC ADR limits to all institutional providers, January 29, 2010. Accessed online August 27, 2011 at, http://www.cms.gov/RAC/03_RecentUpdates.asp#TopOfPage.

over the next ten years. Several programs and initiatives in the Affordable Care Act are geared to help mitigate negative effects that hospitals and physician practices face from rampant increases in healthcare costs, continued declines in reimbursement rates by CMS and private payers, and formulary changes affecting prescription drug coverage--especially for chronic conditions.[347] These challenges and others have driven many independent physician practices to either close their small practices or merge with larger medical groups. In addition economic pressures have prompted some medical groups to consider joining or affiliating with large integrated delivery networks to share administrative services (e.g. finance, marketing, risk management, legal counsel, and quality management) and capitalize on interoperable and bidirectional clinical and administrative technologies. Chief financial officers across the country have confronted these challenges, which are further complicated by federal and state regulations, tax requirements, investment management, uncompensated care, nonprofit exemptions, and revenue cycle management issues. All these factors compounded by the current economic turmoil.

Financial reform in healthcare is not new. Several industry-level payment reform initiatives have been started over the last 30 years. The timeline below depicts a number of these key reforms, some of which made significant changes in the financial operations of the U.S. healthcare system. This evolution has led to the emergence of CINs, ACOs, and other innovative models.

---

[347] Center for Healthcare Research and Transformation. Issue brief, July 2010, Health care cost drivers: chronic disease, comorbidity, and health risk factors in the U.S. and Michigan. Accessed online August 30, 2011, at: http://www.chrt.org/assets/price-of-care/CHRT-Issue-Brief-August-2010.pdf.

Figure 41. 30 Years of Health Services Payment Reform Models & Programs

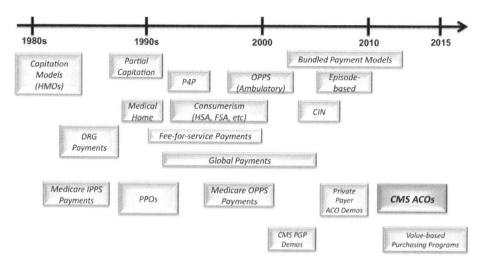

Note: Boxes only indicate an approximate market entry point for each program or model

The capitation models of the 1980s brought about significant changes in the nation's health system with the advent of the managed care era. In succession came such transformative new programs and systems as diagnosis-related group payments, other new Medicare payment models, the consumer movement with health savings and flexible savings accounts, and such other reimbursement reform models as bundled and global payments. A number of concepts underlie the changes in reimbursement that have occurred; and two worth noting in particular include:

♦ Risk-bearing: This concept has to do with placement of both risk and reward for the cost and quality of care delivered.348 As the managed care industry came into existence, HMOs and capitated payment models became its mainstay. Physicians in these models received set amounts based on the populations they promised to treat or the conditions of their patients. The potential for underutilization of needed services is a significant risk in these situations. A fee-for-service system lowers the risk of underutilization; however, because providers are rewarded for the volume of services

---
348 Goldsmith J. Analyzing Shifts in Economic Risks to Providers in Proposed Payment and Delivery System Reforms. *Health Aff (Millwood)*. 2010;29(7):1299-1304.

prescribed (pay-for-procedure), overutilization becomes another issue. In either case, performance in terms of quality of care is a lesser consideration. In this environment, concerns of medical practice based on volume rather than value may appear.

As the industry recognized advantages and disadvantages to patients and consumers with these models of reimbursement, partial capitation emerged as a new model. With partial capitation, the burden of risk is transferred shifts as providers receive less in up-front capitated payments in exchange for performance rewards. Medical homes and pay-for-performance are two of these initiatives. Consumer health plan products (such as health savings accounts and high-deductible health plans) shift the financial risk to the consumer. These products may also produce monetary savings at the expense of not having a qualified medical professional involved in the patient's healthcare decisions. The lessons learned from the use of these products and models led the industry to its operating environment of the late 2000s, which is more heavily focused on pay-for-performance and transfers risk to the organizations and professionals accountable for ensuring that quality care is delivered on the population and individual patient levels.

- *Productivity and reward*: Another concept underlying the present environment is that of productivity. One of the key drivers for organizations across all industries is the implementation of compensation systems that reward participants for strong performance and high-quality goods and services that yield greater value.[349] As the healthcare industry was confronted with the poor quality of care documented in the IOM's *To Err Is Human*, consumer awareness of problems in the U.S. healthcare system grew rapidly. This higher level of awareness, combined with the inexorable increase in the rate of growth of health costs, led to calls for change—specifically, improvements in quality and safety of care delivered by healthcare service providers; improved access to care; and demand to

---

[349] Cutler D. How Health Care Reform Must Bend the Cost Curve. *Health Aff (Millwood)*. 2010;29(6):1131-1135.

move away from the fee-for-service reimbursement system toward models that reward providers for delivering higher quality and value.

Financial Risk Sharing and Integration

Every CIN/ACO must contend with multiple issues in financial risk-sharing and strategy. We start with the assumption that a certain degree of financial risk is unavoidable for hospitals and physician practice organizations in a CIN/ACO. As we discussed in Chapter 2, the proposed qualification criteria for ACOs include the ability to take on greater degrees of risk based on capabilities and infrastructure in place to manage complexity and risk among ACO participants and patient populations. The agreements among ACO participants link higher levels of risk assumed to higher potential incentives. The incentives may be achieved by improving quality of care and population health for the entire panel of patients or certain disease conditions targeted for improvement under the ACO. Unless the practice or hospital has been optimized already to meet quality measures and productivity, the infrastructure needed to achieve the quality goals and incentives and reduce risk is through clinical integration.

For Medicare ACOs, DHHS will monitor risk sharing to ensure that ACOs do not underutilize care for at-risk patients. If any participant in a Medicare ACO program is found to avoid the provision of services to certain "at-risk beneficiaries," that participant will not only be placed under sanctions (including being put on probation or termination from the Medicare Shared Savings Program), but he or she may, also forfeit their mandatory 25% withholding of shared savings.[350]

An additional risk for Medicare ACOs is that of the risk scores assigned to Medicare beneficiaries based on their demographics and diagnosed conditions. The ACO's ability to effectively manage clinical risk associated with individual patients while simultaneously focusing on total population health management may be directly correlated to its incentive payments received. Two factors that affect such risk scores and incentive payments are accurate assessment of

---

[350] Fed. Reg. Vol. 76, No. 67. April 7, 2011. 425.12-14. Monitoring; Actions prior to termination; Termination, suspension, and repayment of Shared Savings. pp. 19648-19650.

beneficiary health status and the intensity of medical coding (i.e. the completeness of diagnostic codes assigned to beneficiaries). If an ACO increases coding intensity there is the potential for a favorable increase in the risk score associated with the beneficiary. In light of this possibility, CMS proposed that they would retain the option of auditing ACOs in this area for appropriate coding practices and risk adjustment methodologies.[351] This is an issue that ACO leaders must understand to safeguard against perceptions of inappropriate changes in risk scores or triggering CMS audits. Medical management and health information technology staff can help monitor this issue, which may also involve changes in the primary care and specialist provider mix.

CMS ACO: Exclusion from Participation

The Affordable Care Act specified situations in which a "provider of services or supplies" would not be allowed to participate in an ACO:[352]

1) Those participating in a model tested under the Innovation Center that involves shared savings or any other programs or demonstrations that involve shared savings.

2) Those participating in the "independence at home medical practice pilot program" under Section 1866-E of the Social Security Act.

The reason for these exclusions is to avoid mixing programs and potentially confounding the results. By excluding certain closely related programs and demonstrations, CMS can avoid having the benefits or detriments of one program spilling over to the other. The Proposed Rule also noted that as results of demonstration projects under the CMS Innovation Center are validated and made public, CMS will work to make available promising new developments from these new models for potential use by the shared savings program.[353]

---

[351] Fed. Reg. Vol. 76, No. 67. April 7, 2011. II(F)(4). Establishing an Expenditure Benchmark. pp. 19604-19606.
[352] H.R. 3590, Patient Protection and Affordable Care Act, §3022(b)(4). No duplication in participation in shared savings (2010).
[353] Fed. Reg. Vol. 76, No. 67. April 7, 2011. I(D)(1). Establishment of Center for Medicare and Medicaid Innovation (Innovation Center). pp. 19534-19535.

Legislative Scope and Impact

The Affordable Care Act is designed to have a profound financial impact on the United States. Different organizations have made different estimates of the long-term financial impact of the Affordable Care Act and its various programs. The Congressional Budget Office (CBO) and Joint Committee on Taxation (JCT) provided a pre-enactment assessment of the bill's long-term overall financial impact on the federal government's budget on March 20, 2010.

> CBO and JCT estimate that enacting both pieces of legislation—H.R. 3590 and the reconciliation proposal—would produce a net reduction in federal deficits of $143 billion over the 2010–2019 period as result of changes in direct spending and revenues.[354]

The Medicare ACO is anticipated to generate savings over the long term. Savings are expected to result from improvements in quality and care coordination. Benefits from these savings are to be split between CMS and participant organizations. Involvement as a Medicare ACO participant will put the organization at risk for some of the savings and benefit it if quality and financial performance meet certain standards. Chief financial officers and financial teams from potential Medicare ACO participant organizations will need to collaborate to address such matters as financial planning, risk modeling, medical coding operations, performance measurement, and determination of their impact.

Following much internal debate, CMS introduced two risk options for Medicare ACOs in the Proposed Rule. The first option is a "one-sided" risk model and the second is a "two-sided" risk model. The CMS Medicare ACO compensation model starts with the normal fee-for-service Parts A and B payments to individual providers for claims submitted to CMS. The second part of the model is the ACO shared savings program process, involving the two risk-bearing models.

---

[354] Congressional Budget Office. Letter to Nancy Pelosi, March 20, 2010. Estimated budgetary impact of the legislation, 2. Accessed online July 23, 2011, at http://www.cbo.gov/ftpdocs/113xx/doc11379/AmendReconProp.pdf.

The ***one-sided model*** is intended for organizations that are less mature in the infrastructure, systems, physician relations, and processes needed to run an ACO. The implication is that the one-sided model gives ACO participants a lower level of risk in the first and second-year performance periods. In exchange for not being responsible for losses, ACO participants also accept a lower percentage of shared savings (up to 50%) based on their quality performance scores plus a lower potential increase in their shared savings rate (up to 2.5%) for the inclusion of rural health clinics or federally qualified health centers in their network.

The ***two-sided risk model*** is intended for more mature organizations that have strong infrastructure, advanced health information technologies, DOJ/FTC-approved clinical integration programs, strong physician relations, and advanced quality improvement programs and processes in place to positively impact patient care. ACO participants adopting this model will start off the first performance period accepting a greater degree of risk that includes accepting responsibility for sharing in losses. But with this greater degree of risk comes greater potential for rewards with a higher percentage of earned shared savings (up to 60%) based on quality performance scoring plus a higher potential shared savings rate (up to 5.0%), based on the inclusion of rural health clinic or federally qualified health centers in their network.

Figure 42. CMS ACO Compensation Model Overview

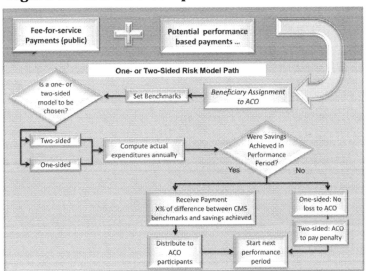

For organizations with advanced capabilities already providing coordinated and comprehensive care services across multiple care settings, the Medicare Innovation Center has introduced the Pioneer ACO Model as an alternative. This model is designed to produce best practices from leading organizations that choose to participate. Participants will have the opportunity for an even higher percentage of shared savings payments in exchange for accepting greater risk of shared losses. Organizations engaged at this level are believed to be better equipped to advance more rapidly to a population-based payment model as well as toward a multi-payer ACO model of care delivery.

Financial Elements of the CMS Shared Savings Model

Following is an outline of the financial elements of the Medicare Shared Savings Program. This description is not intended to cover every element and issue but provides some of the highlights. The final Proposed Rule will provide additional guidance on the methodology to be used for the first performance period.

Table 41. Financial Element Highlights of CMS ACO Shared Savings Program

Element	Key Points
CMS ACO agreement period	a. Minimum 3-year agreement between ACO and DHHS. Each ACO is evaluated in each year of the agreement period.
Beneficiary assignment	a. Beneficiaries are assigned to ACOs in which they are receiving a plurality of primary care physician services but they are not limited to seeing only those primary care physicians.
Setting benchmarks[355]	a. Estimate a benchmark for every agreement period for each ACO, making use of its most recent three years of fee-for-service data for Medicare Parts A and B beneficiaries.
	b. Benchmark to be updated on the basis of beneficiary characteristics and projected absolute amount of

---

[355] H.R. 3590, Patient Protection and Affordable Care Act, §3022(d)(1)(B)(ii). Determining benchmarks (2010).

Element	Key Points
	growth in national per capita expenditures for Parts A and B of the original fee-for-service program.
	c. Benchmarks to be reset at the start of each agreement period.
	d. Benchmarks must adhere to three technical adjustment impacts identified in the Proposed Rule.
1) Determine savings[356]	a. **One-sided Model**: Determine whether the ACO's fee-for-service Parts A and B beneficiaries (adjusted for beneficiary characteristics) estimated average per capita Medicare expenditures are below the specified benchmark.
	1. **Shared Savings:** Must be below the minimum savings rate (sliding scale) based on number of beneficiaries and minimum quality performance requirements.
	2. Passes the net savings threshold and is eligible for net 2% of benchmark in shared savings or may be eligible for **up to 7.5%** shared savings. Will receive a shared savings payment **up to 50%** based on quality performance.
	b. **Two-sided model**: Determine whether the ACO's fee-for-service Parts A and B beneficiaries (adjusted for beneficiary characteristics) estimated average per capita Medicare expenditures are below the specified benchmark.
	1. **Shared Savings:** Must be below the minimum savings rate of 2% based on number of beneficiaries and minimum quality performance requirements.
	2. Passes the net savings threshold and is eligible for net 2% of benchmark in shared savings or may be eligible for **up to 10%** shared savings. Will receive a shared savings payment **up to 60%** based on quality performance.
	3. **Shared Loss Rate**: based on the inverse of the ACO's final sharing rate.
	4. **Loss Recoupment Limits**: 5% in performance period 1, 7.5 % in performance period 2, 10% in

---

[356] H.R. 3590, Patient Protection and Affordable Care Act, §3022(d)(1)(B)(i). Determining savings (2010); Fed. Reg. Vol. 76, No. 67. April 7, 2011. 425.7. Payment and treatment of savings. pp. 19645-19647.

Element	Key Points
	performance period 3. *One-sided ACOs* in performance period 3 their loss recoupment limit is 5%.
Payments of shared savings to ACO[357]	a. When ACO meets requirements, a percentage (determined by DHHS) of the difference be*tween the bench*mark and the "estimated average per capita Medicare expenditures adjusted for beneficiary characteristics" for the agreement period will be paid to the ACO and remainder goes to CMS. b. DHHS will set a limit on the total shared savings that can be paid to any ACO.

Beneficiary assignment. At the end of each performance year CMS determines all beneficiaries who received services from a participating primary care physician within the ACO. Then a beneficiary is assigned to the ACO if they have received a plurality of their primary care services from the ACO physicians, based on the computation of allowed charges from those ACO primary care physicians. It is also important to note that primary care providers will be responsible for posting signs in their facilities to inform patients know, up front that the physicians are participating in the Medicare Shared Savings Program and that if the patients are seen by these primary care physicians they may be attributed to them.[358]

Setting Medicare ACO benchmarks. MedPAC noted in 2009 that when setting benchmarks for Medicare ACOs, CMS would have to account for geographic variations across the United States in spending at the beneficiary level. MedPAC also noted that the targets should be developed on the basis of "changes in spending" rather than the "level of spending," when accounting for the amount of resources used by any given ACO. These changes would also be tied to geographic variations and opportunities to achieve economies of scale in population-based health management. This kind of adjustment benefits larger practices and health systems more than smaller provider organizations.[359]

---

[357] H.R. 3590, Patient Protection and Affordable Care Act, §3022(d)(2). Payments for shared savings (2010); Fed. Reg. Vol. 76, No. 67. April 7, 2011. 425.7. Payment and treatment of savings. pp. 19645-19647.
[358] Fed. Reg. Vol. 76, No. 67. April 7, 2011. 425.6. Assignment of Medicare fee-for-service beneficiaries to ACOs. p. 19645.
[359] MedPAC Report to Congress: Improving Incentives in the Medicare Program. (June 2009). Chapter 2: Accountable Care Organizations. Accessed online August 27, 2011, at http://www.medpac.gov/chapters/Jun09_Ch02.pdf.

The Proposed Rule identified two options for establishing benchmarks.[360] In both options CMS trends prior years' experience forward. First, the past three years of Part A and Part B fee-for-service expenditures for a set of beneficiaries is determined. These expenditures are then trended forward using the national growth rates to arrive at a benchmark against which physician performance is measured. Option 1 uses beneficiaries who were previously patients of physicians in the ACO during the three years prior to the first performance period, and these beneficiaries used for calculating the benchmark may be different from those actually attributed to the ACO during the performance periods. Option 2 uses beneficiaries actually assigned to the ACO in the first performance period, and these beneficiaries may not have been previous patients of the physicians in the ACO. CMS proposed adoption of Option 1 in the Proposed Rule, although they believe either is legal and valid.

In additional, the following weights are applied in determining the benchmark for the three-year period to "ensure that the benchmark reflects more accurately the latest expenditure and health status of the ACO's assigned beneficiary population": BY3 (most recent year) at 60%, BY2 at 30%, and BY1 at 10%.[361] Three potential technical adjustments[362] to benchmarks were also discussed in the Proposed Rule.

- An indirect medical education (IME) adjustment and Medicare disproportionate share hospital (DSH) adjustment;
- Geographic payment adjustments;
- Incentive payments to ACOs and penalty payments made by ACOs participating in other CMS value-based purchasing initiatives.

For IME (payments received by teaching hospitals), DSH (payments received by hospitals that care for a higher percentage of low-income beneficiaries), and geographic payment adjustments, CMS proposed to not remove these incentives or payments from the computations of benchmarks in the first performance

---

[360] Fed. Reg. Vol. 76, No. 67. April 7, 2011. II(F)(3). Establishing an Expenditure Benchmark. pp. 19604-19606.
[361] Fed. Reg. Vol. 76, No. 67. April 7, 2011. 425.7.(b)(5). Payment and treatment of savings. p. 19646.
[362] Fed. Reg. Vol. 76, No. 67. April 7, 2011. II(F). Shared Savings Determination. Sections 5-7. pp. 19608-19609.

period for ACOs. CMS did, however, make a recommendation to remove value-based purchasing incentives from computations of both benchmarks and actual expenditures. There is a financial impact on ACO participants that are receiving incentive payments or paying penalties through their participation in the Physicians Quality Reporting System, CMS Meaningful Use of EHRs program, or the Electronic Prescribing (eRx) program. Including these incentive payments or penalties in the calculation of the ACO benchmarks or expenditures would result in artificially inflated or deflated financial evaluations. Thus CMS proposed to exclude these incentives and penalties to establish a fairer and more equitable financial evaluation of the performance of each ACO.[363] Given the significant impact these incentives and penalties have on physician practices and healthcare provider organizations, it will be important to monitor this issue.

Determining achievement of savings. To determine savings achieved by the ACO there will be an annual comparison of the benchmarks to the actual expenditures incurred, and the evaluation would be based on per capita Medicare expenditures adjusted for beneficiary characteristics. Determining actual expenditures also accounts for various CMS program incentive and penalty payments. Organizations should monitor the developments on inclusion or exclusion of these incentives and payments as they unfold in the final rule and future federal rule making.

To be effective, comparisons of benchmarks to actual performance must be prompt to allow course correction and true outcomes improvement. Health information technology systems must move toward real-time data gathering and analysis to identify gaps in care, variation from benchmarks, and challenges encountered across the ACO in meeting quality metrics and outcome improvements. This information must be made available to physicians and other ACO participant leaders to allow them to respond appropriately and change course. New tools and systems have been developed to provide predictive modeling capabilities, risk stratification and identification, and care/disease management support to give physician and healthcare leaders early

---

[363] Fed. Reg. Vol. 76, No. 67. April 7, 2011. II(F)(7). Technical Adjustments to the Benchmark: Impact of Bonus Payments and Penalties on Calculation of the Benchmark and Actual Expenditures. pp. 19609.

understanding of the impacts on the budget, and recognition of predicted savings to be realized through the shared savings program.

Payments for savings to ACO: Qualifying ACOs will continue to receive fee-for-service payments under Parts A and B, and shared savings distributions from CMS based on the ACO's quality performance, achievement of savings against benchmarks, and any additional increase based on inclusion of rural health clinics or federally qualified health centers. Participating physicians and other ACO participants will receive profits (or participate in losses if they are operating under the two-sided risk model) on the basis of contractual agreements with the ACO.

Organizations should monitor federal rule making processes not only for the final rule, but also for new developments that emerge as the program is implemented. As the industry evolves, government regulations will continue to change and new requirements will be put in place designed to improve the quality, cost, and access to care for Medicare patients.

Reimbursement and Compensation Reform

Shared savings programs are one of a number of payment reforms that have been introduced over the past decade. Various organizations have tested and implemented public and private ACOs and CINs across the United States. As noted in Chapter 1, payment reform started with the introduction of government-funded health care programs, and the recognition of the negative impact of such static payment rules as fee-for-service on the quality, accessibility, and affordability of care. Due to the complex nature of healthcare delivery systems, it has proven to be a multi-year process to design, pilot-test, and produce results and lessons learned from each new payment reform model. The latest payment policy to be introduced is the ACO, which builds on work done over the past fifteen years on clinically integrated networks. The ACO model is supported by three payment methodologies: bundled payments, global payments, and value-based purchasing.

Bundled Payments

One of the frequently discussed methods of payment reform is bundled payment. In one form of bundled payments, the payer provides a set amount for a particular episode of care, starting from the point of hospital admission for a specified procedure through discharge and possibly post-acute care requirements based on the terms set for the payment bundle (including an adjustment factor for severity of the case). This type of payment bundle may be determined by the physician and provider organization (such as hospital organizations), agreeing to a package of services for treating specific conditions that yields a single payment received and allotted on the basis of the agreement.[364] A number of organizations have tested and used payment bundling.

While academic medical centers (AMC) have not been discussed in detail, other observers have noted that these organizations may benefit greatly from ACO implementation and moving to a bundled payment approach in both care delivery and the education of future physicians.[365] In Paul Griner's article in the November 2010 issue of the *New England Journal of Medicine*, he pointed to a number of benefits and challenges for academic medical centers implementing bundled payment systems:

- Benefit: "Bundled payment is more consistent with AMCs' core values than is fee for service, and their teaching and service missions can benefit from its successful implementation—in part because it would encourage trainees to hone their physical exam skills."
- Benefit: "Bundled payment will be an incentive for hospital leaders to help their medical and nursing staffs reduce these inefficiencies by integrating their work more effectively. Among the results should be an improved learning environment for students of all the health professions."
- Challenge: "[The AMC] will need to address income disparities between primary care physicians and subspecialists";

---

[364] Evans J. Current state of bundled payments. *American Health and Drug Benefits*, August 2010. Accessed online July 23, 2011 at http://www.ahdbonline.com/sites/default/files/Evans_JulyAug2010.pdf.
[365] Griner P. Payment reform and the mission of academic medical centers. *N Engl J Med.* 2010;363(19):1784-1786.

- Challenge: The AMC will need to be more efficient––a skill not often found in such institutions––and "[It] will need to develop more centralized financial systems and management philosophies, recognizing the cultural transformation that may be required at some medical schools."

MedPAC recommended in 2009 that academic medical centers take a proactive stance for educating both students and residents on payment reform models and approaches.[366] Ensuring that medical students and residents obtain the skills necessary for leadership and financial acumen on these transformative issues is crucial for their future careers. Being equipped to operate in performance-based compensation environments will be vital to help them grow quickly into new roles—not only to provide excellent direct patient care but also to navigate and serve in multidisciplinary and cross-functional teams tackling the administrative and financial challenges faced by healthcare provider organizations.

Some noteworthy examples of projects involving bundled payment approaches include an ongoing CMS demonstration project and the Prometheus Payment Model. The Acute Care Episode (ACE) Demonstration is a CMS project testing bundled payments. The demonstration began in 2009 and presently involves four health systems in Texas, Oklahoma, New Mexico, and Colorado.[367] The demonstration tests the effectiveness of bundling Medicare Part A and B payments into a single payment for an episode of care on specific cardiovascular or orthopedic procedures meeting volume thresholds. In addition to competitively bid payment arrangements, providers (physicians, clinician care teams, and hospitals) are eligible for shared savings remuneration based on cost savings achieved on specified episodes of care. For this program CMS also provides patients with a 50% share of the savings realized by CMS for patients who undergo procedures at the participating sites. Participating organizations include:

---

[366] Medicare Payment Advisory Commission. Report to Congress: Improving incentives in the Medicare program, June 2009. Chapter 1: Medical education. Available at: www.medpac.gov/documents/Jun09_EntireReport.pdf, 18-19.
[367] Centers for Medicare and Medicaid Services. Acute care episode (ACE) demonstration project. Accessed online June 28, 2011, at: http://www.cms.gov/DemoProjectsEvalRpts/downloads/ACE_web_page.pdf.

- Hillcrest Medical Center, Tulsa, Oklahoma
- Baptist Health System, San Antonio, Texas
- Oklahoma Heart Hospital LLC, Oklahoma City, Oklahoma
- Lovelace Health System, Albuquerque, New Mexico

Each organization focuses on different procedures. The actual savings achieved at the episode-of-care level can be viewed at each facility for all procedures covered on the CMS website.[368]

Second is the Prometheus Payment Model developed in 2006 and funded by the Robert Wood Johnson Foundation.[369] The Prometheus model was set up to compensate provider organizations in two ways. First, the model calculated an evidence-informed case rate (ECR®)—that is, a patient-specific budget adjusted for the severity and complexity of the case. The ECR was translated into a bundled budget for all necessary interventions, accounting for the entire episode of care and services provided by the physicians, hospitals, laboratories, pharmacies, and post-acute care facilities and services. The Prometheus model also provides an allowance in addition to the ECR® to compensate for typically known potentially avoidable costs (PACs).

When care provider teams manage a full episode of care in an efficient and high-quality manner and avoid the occurrence of PACs they are rewarded by keeping a portion of the PAC allowance unused in the patient's episode. This bundled budget concept differs from bundled payments in that providers are still reimbursed on the basis of fee-for-service claims from payers; however, the budgets for the bundled services for specific types of episodes of care are compared to actual costs on a quarterly basis that includes a review of PACs that were avoided. When savings are achieved they result in bonuses for the provider teams and organizations involved. Four organizations are involved in piloting the Prometheus Model[370]; and they include:

---

[368] Centers for Medicare and Medicaid Services. Acute care episode (ACE) demonstration project. Accessed online June 28, 2011, at: http://www.cms.gov/DemoProjectsEvalRpts/downloads/ACE_web_page.pdf.
[369] de Brantes F, Rosenthal MB, Painter M. Building a bridge from fragmentation to accountability—the Prometheus Payment model. *N Engl J Med*. 2009;361(11):1033–1036.
[370] Robert Wood Johnson Foundation, Health Care Incentives Improvement Institute. Prometheus payment: On the frontlines of health care payment reform, July 2010. Accessed online August 27, 2011, at http://www.rwjf.org/files/research/66748.pdf.

- Health Partners of Minneapolis, MN
- Crozer-Keystone Health System, Philadelphia, PA
- Employers Coalition on Health, Rockford, IL
- Spectrum Health, Grand Rapids, MI

Global Payments

Global payment models are similar to the bundled payment model. They are already being widely used by many organizations, including integrated delivery networks, independent practice associations, and multispecialty physician groups. The primary difference between global payments and bundled payments is that a bundled payment is set for a specific episode of care, while global payments are not dictated by episodes treated by a physician or provider organization. The global payment model provides a physician or provider organization a single payment to cover all the costs of care for a person's treatment requirements during a specific period of time regardless of the number of inpatient episodes they experience.[371] Challenges in global payment systems were discussed in a study done by the Commonwealth Fund and published in February 2010. Global payments were described as "holding providers financially accountable, to a greater or lesser degree, for the total cost of care provided to the patient population assigned to them."[372] An excerpt from the report is provided in Appendix E, in which the authors also discuss the varying levels of risk that can be assumed under global payment models.

Global payments are also considered a form of capitated payments, which have decreased in recent years.[373] Organizations using variations of these payment models include Kaiser Permanente, MassHealth (Massachusetts

---

[371] Miller H. Pathways for physician success under healthcare payment and delivery reforms. Report for the American Medical Association, part C, June 2010. Comprehensive care payment, 26. Executive summary available at: http://www.ama-assn.org/ama1/pub/upload/mm/399/payment-pathways-summary.pdf.

[372] Robinow A. Commonwealth Fund Report, February 2010. The potential of global payment: insights from the field. Accessed online July 20, 2011 at http://www.commonwealthfund.org/~/media/Files/Publications/Fund%20Report/2010/Feb/1373_Robinow_potential_global_payment.pdf. pp. 3–5 and 13–14.

[373] Zuvekas SH, Cohen JW. Paying physicians by capitation: is the past now prologue? *Health Aff* (*Millwood*). 2010;29(9):1661–1666.

Medicaid Program[374]), the Veterans Health Administration, and Blue Cross/Blue Shield of Massachusetts (BCBSMA). Another organization, Northeast Health Systems Physician Hospital Organization, established a five-year alternative quality contract (AQC) program in 2010 (referenced at the end of Chapter 1) with a global payment model as the basis of its reimbursement strategy.[375]

Value-based Purchasing Programs

Value-based purchasing is considered by many as another phrase for pay-for-performance. According to CMS, "Value-based purchasing is a concept that links payment directly to the quality of care provided and is a strategy that can help transform the current payment system by rewarding providers for delivering high quality, efficient clinical care."[376] As such, value-based purchasing can include the Medicare Shared Savings (ACO) Program.

Section 3001 of the Affordable Care Act creates a hospital value-based purchasing program. This is the latest of a number of similar programs. In 2005 Congress passed the Deficit Reduction Act (DRA). Section 5001(b) of the DRA called for DHHS to develop a plan for a hospital value-based purchasing program.[377] That law as well as other efforts helped the development of a broader set of value-based purchasing programs. In 2009 CMS released "Roadmap for Implementing Value Driven Healthcare."[378] That report presented the CMS roadmap as a three- to five-year plan for multiple value-based purchasing program initiatives that would work in concert with ACOs and other incentive-oriented programs.

---

[374] Heit M, Piper K. Global payments to improve quality and efficiency in Medicaid: concepts and considerations. Boston, MA: Massachusetts Medicaid Policy Institute; November 2009. Accessed online July 20, 2011, at http://www.massmedicaid.org/~/media/MMPI/Files/20091116_GlobalPayments.pdf.

[375] *Becker's Hospital Review*, May 26, 2010. BCBS of Massachusetts, Northeast Health Systems sign 5-year global payment deal. Accessed online July 20, 2011, at http://www.beckershospitalreview.com/hospital-financial-and-business-news/bcbs-of-massachusetts-northeast-health-systems-sign-5-year-global-payment-deal.html.

[376] Fed. Reg. Vol. 76, No. 67. April 7, 2011. I(A). Introduction and Overview of Value-Based Purchasing. p. 19530

[377] Public Law 109–171, February 8, 2006. 2005 Deficit Reduction Act (DRA), §5001(b). Accessed online July 20, 2011, at http://www.gpo.gov:80/fdsys/pkg/PLAW-109publ171/pdf/PLAW-109publ171.pdf; Centers for Medicare and Medicaid Services. Issues paper, January 17, 2007. DHHS Medicare hospital value-based purchasing plan development. Accessed online July 20, 2011, at http://www.cms.gov/AcuteInpatientPPS/downloads/hospital_VBP_plan_issues_paper.pdf.

[378] Centers for Medicare and Medicaid Services. Roadmap for implementing value driven healthcare in the traditional Medicare fee-for-service program, January 2009. Accessed online July 20, 20111, at https://www.cms.gov/QualityInitiativesGenInfo/downloads/VBPRoadmap_OEA_1-16_508.pdf, p. 2.

The Affordable Care Act Section 3001 defines hospital value-based payments as incentives to hospitals that meet performance standards based on quality measures for a minimum number of cases for specific conditions and procedures within a given fiscal year. In addition to the hospital value-based purchasing program, the CMS roadmap provides plans for starting value-based purchasing programs for nursing homes,[379] home health care, and physician services related to the PQRS program.

The Affordable Care Act also contains Section 3007: Value-Based Payment Modifier under the Physician Fee Schedule.[380] This section requires the establishment of a value-based payment modifier that physicians or groups of physicians will be eligible for during specific performance periods. These payments will be based on performance measured against specific quality standards to be released by January 1, 2012. The rule making will take place in 2013 and reporting will begin in 2015.

Risk Shifting

Payment reform will have an impact on provider organizations, physicians, and payers potentially redesigning the health finance and delivery systems in fundamental ways. From the physician's perspective, payment reform requires an understanding of the risks and rewards, as well as knowing who bears the burden of risk between the stakeholders, including physicians, hospitals, and payers (including employer, government, and commercial plans). The diagram below illustrates a progression of payment models on the basis of financial risk.

---

[379] Centers for Medicare and Medicaid Services. Medicare demonstrations. Nursing home value-based purchasing program (2009). Accessed online July 20, 2011, at
http://www.cms.gov/DemoProjectsEvalRpts/MD/itemdetail.asp?filterType=none&filterByDID=-99&sortByDID=3&sortOrder=descending&itemID=CMS1198946&intNumPerPage=10.
[380] H.R. 3590, Patient Protection and Affordable Care Act, §3007. Value-based payment modifier under the physician fee schedule (2010).

Figure 43. Payment Model Reforms and Risk[381]

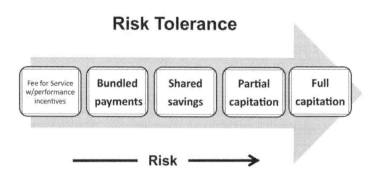

In this illustration, the shared savings programs (public and private) fall between other models in the risk tolerance continuum. Chapter 1 discussed the declining use of the full capitation contracts that were prevalent in the 1980s and 1990s. Physicians bore a greater burden of risk[382] with these contracts, which usually presented a commensurate potential for reward. At one end of the continuum is the fee-for-service system, which government and industry are moving away from in preference for some kind of value-based or pay-for-performance reimbursement.

When bundled payments are adopted, managing episodes of care and total population health become more important. The movement toward managing inter-episodes of care (also known as care coordination or transitional care) is an outgrowth of the need to better manage patients' overall health, and is associated with the evolution of CIN and ACO programs. Geisinger Health System's ProvenCare® program has demonstrated the value of improving "episode-based coordination of care," in which physicians and other stakeholders effectively collaborate to improve the clinical processes along the entire care continuum to "minimize avoidable complications" in coronary artery bypass graft surgeries. [383] The table below describes a three-level payment model with a central focus on increasing the level of risk and reward accepted by the healthcare provider and greater need to manage total population health in moving from Level 1 to Level 3.

[381] BDC Advisors presentation slide, January 2011.
[382] Welch P, Welch G. Fee-for-data: a strategy to open the HMO black box. *Health Aff* (*Millwood*). 1995;14(4):104-116.
[383] Goldsmith J. Analyzing shifts in economic risks to providers in proposed payment and delivery system reforms. *Health Aff* (*Millwood*). 2010;29(7):1299-1304.

Table 42. ACO Payment Models[384]

Level 1 Asymmetric shared savings	Level 2 Symmetric Model	Level 3 Partial Capitation Model
• Continue operating under current insurance contracts / coverage models (e.g. FFS)	• Payments can still be tied to current payment system, although ACO could receive revenue from payers and distribute funds to members (depending on ACO contracts)	• ACO receives mix of FFS and prospective fixed payment
• No risk of losses if spending exceeds targets	• At risk for losses if spending exceeds targets	• If successful at meeting budget and performance targets, greater financial benefits
• Most incremental approach with least barriers for entry	• Increased incentive for providers to decrease costs due to risk of losses	• If ACO exceeds budget, more risk means greater financial downside
• Attractive to new entities, risk-adverse providers, or entities with limited organizational capacity, range of covered services, or experience working with other providers	• Attractive to providers with some infrastructure or care coordination capability and demonstrated track record	• Only appropriate for providers with robust infrastructure, demonstrated track record in finances and quality and providing relatively full range of services

The NCQA is establishing an accreditation program for ACOs, and levels of risk may be an important consideration for ACO readiness assessment. Level 1 aligns with an ACO at a lower level of readiness to acceptable risk, which could mean that it also lacks the infrastructure to manage clinical or financial risk. Level 2, the symmetric model, gives ACO physicians greater opportunities for shared savings. Organizations interested in this level of risk/reward should have a stronger infrastructure and capabilities in place to accept greater accountability for care of the patient population in question. Level 3 represents a greater assumption of risk and reward, and could be an ACO at a higher level of capabilities, with more advanced systems and perhaps a clinically integrated network infrastructure.

---

[384] McClellan M, McKethan AN, Lewis JL, Roski J, Fisher ES. A national strategy to put accountable care into practice. *Health Aff (Millwood)*. 2010;29 (5):982-990: BDC Advisors presentation slide, January 2011.

While the FTC has specific requirements for clinically integrated networks, the way clinical integration is implemented can be different for ACOs because they typically have different objectives. The objectives of a CIN is to collectively negotiate physician payment rates with payers, while the ACO typically becomes a payer, negotiating global premium and shared savings rates with patients, or with groups of patients owned by a payer (government, employer, health plan, etc). The benefits of a clinical integration program have been studied and validated, and it should be seriously considered by any organizations participating in the Medicare ACO program. Whether or not an organization has an immediate goal of becoming an ACO, establishing a strong CIN program helps set the foundation for future participation in shared savings and similar programs, and builds the healthcare provider organization's capacity to understand quality and cost, improve margins, and accept and manage higher levels of risk necessary under newer reimbursement models and scenarios progressing from Level 1 to Level 3.

Each ACO will ultimately determine its level of risk sharing, based on its ability to tolerate risk as influenced by the strength of its infrastructure and capabilities. As the industry continues to advance the various pay-for-performance models, physicians will continue to see decreases in their fee-for-service payments but and have increasing opportunities to earn additional compensation by demonstrating positive patient outcomes, meeting quality standards, and demonstrating improvement in performance as reported to public and private payer organizations.

Health care reform has spawned the development and testing of these new payment models; as a result the financial environment for physicians, hospitals, and other providers of healthcare services will continue to evolve. Academic medical centers and physician training programs will help to prepare current and future physicians for the new compensation models they will confront.[385]

---

[385] Griner P. Payment Reform and the Mission of Academic Medical Centers. *N Engl J Med*. 2010 4;363(19):1784-6.

Other Financial Topics

Two other financial topics of interest are 1) the effect of medical care ratios on CINs and ACOs; and 2) funding opportunities to support ACO development.

Medical Care Ratios

As noted in Chapter 1, Section 2718 of the Affordable Care Act imposed new regulations on the operations of health insurance companies. That section mandates that 80–85% of the premium revenues collected by insurance companies go toward payment for clinical services and direct patient care. The law is intended to require insurance companies to better manage administrative costs by putting a cap on these expenses. The National Association of Insurance Commissioners collaborated with DHHS in developing the details for calculating the medical care ratio because such calculations are a highly complex issue and require substantial vetting by industry stakeholders to arrive at a consensus. The final rule on the medical care ratio was approved and released by DHHS on November 22, 2010 and took effect on January 1, 2011.

A few highlights of the rule include:

- *Establishing greater transparency and accountability*. Beginning in 2011, the law requires insurance companies to publicly report their spending of premium dollars. This information will provide consumers with information, clearly accounting for the amount that goes toward actual medical care and activities to improve health versus the amount spent on administrative expenses like marketing, sales, member services, administration, claims processing, physician relations, advertising, underwriting, and executive salaries and bonuses.

- *Ensuring Americans receive value for their premium dollars.* Beginning in 2011, the law requires insurance companies in the individual and small-group markets to spend at least 80 percent of the premium dollars collected on clinical services and direct patient care. Insurance companies in the large-group market must spend at least 85 percent of premium dollars on medical care and quality improvement activities.

◆ *Providing consumer rebates.* Insurance companies that do not meet the medical care ratio standard because they had less paid out for medical care than required by law will be required to provide rebates to their customers. Insurers will be required to make the first round of rebates to customers in 2012. Regardless of whether the rebate is provided to enrollees directly or indirectly through their employers, each enrollee must receive a rebate proportional to the premium amount paid by that enrollee.[386]

As the healthcare finance system faces such changes as these, those involved in health policy decisions impacting ACOs, medical homes and CINs will need to ensure that changes to reimbursement policy or rules for private insurance payers remain flexible and provide appropriate incentives to support the transformation occurring on the physician and hospital side of the industry. The medical care ratio rule may encourage the industry to move away from the fee-for-service system toward pay-for-performance, bundled payments, shared savings, and value-based purchasing models for reimbursing medical homes, ACOs and CINs. Alternatively, these changes could reduce the funding available in the system by giving rebates to consumers, forcing health plans to run leaner, and eliminating potential funding sources for such innovative physician and hospital programs, as ACOs and CINs. To ensure the viability of these innovative programs, it will be important for providers to receive reimbursement for initiatives that may include fees for care coordination, incentives for quality improvement, and reimbursement for investments in health information technology needed to help drive these initiatives for the CIN, ACO and primary care's medical home transformation. It remains to be seen whether funds currently available for innovation go toward healthcare delivery, or back to the consumer.

---

[386] Healthcare.gov. News release, November 22, 2010. Medical loss ratio: getting your money's worth on health insurance. Accessed online July 27, 2011, at http://www.healthcare.gov/news/factsheets/medical_loss_ratio.html.

In certain areas of the country the reimbursement fee structure remains largely fee-for-service, and providers have an economic incentive to maintain their current structure. It is in more competitive markets or highly penetrated managed care markets where systems have already moved to some degree of at-risk contracts that participants have an incentive to change. In the other areas, moving too quickly could mean putting the organization at a financial disadvantage. What is happening in the market, however, is that moving too late to secure the participants necessary to form some kind of integrated organization will put an organization at a distinct disadvantage as others move first.

The bottom line is that if the economic engine that keeps a hospital's margin healthy is acute care inpatient revenues, then reducing a large segment of that business without a different funding vehicle could in fact lead to the extinction of the parent entity. Payers, including the government, employers, and health plans, have decided health reforms are needed to make that reduction so "the writing is on the wall." Clayton Christensen makes this point in a variety of ways. To survive in this new world means to seek out and establish new funding sources not only through *sustaining innovations* but also through *disruptive innovations*. Engaging payers and other participants early in the process to assure funding resources to cover high-acuity losses will be important in this payment transition period.

Funding Opportunities for Clinical Transformation

As physician practices and other provider organizations grapple with the capital requirements for covering the multiyear expenditures needed to establish clinical and cultural transformations associated with CINs and ACOs, many require new sources of funding. Part of the answer to this challenge will involve the initial determination of the organization positioned as head of the ACO or CIN.

CMS recognizes the financial challenges faced by healthcare organizations and burdens of implementing new programs. The CMS Innovation Center is assessing the potential to test payment programs to aid physician practices and ACO participants with the financial burdens associated with transformation to an ACO model. Although it is currently being explored and structured, the concept under evaluation would "pre-pay a portion of future savings to aid the ACO participants with funds for investing in needed infrastructure to fully engage in the ACO program."[387] Organizations working on ACOs with private payers may find the challenge to lie more in deciding whether the infrastructure requirements are to be funded by the larger hospitals; by integrated delivery networks that have larger resource pools in place (e.g. health information technology, staff, finances, and the like); or by private payer organizations that also have the financial resources to provide support for the infrastructure development needed by small physician groups.

One successful model currently being used by a large health plan is allocation of financial responsibility according to the risk/reward ratio--the more you contribute, the more revenue you realize. As partnerships are negotiated across the industry, decisions on the best way to finance these transformation initiatives will be made, and new structure will be created that address the local market and its economic realities.

The incentives, compensation systems, and financial support needed to establish infrastructure may be a reason for payers to work together closely to ensure uniformity in the establishment of CINs and ACOs and to ensure that incentives are large enough to engage stakeholders and offset the loss of inpatient fee-for-service payments. Examples of positive results from coordination and teamwork are already being realized in cases like the demonstration projects noted in Chapter 1 with the Dartmouth-Brookings Collaborative, the Premier ACO Collaborative, and the BCBSMA AQC project and in the Prometheus Model project noted earlier in this chapter.

---

[387] Center for Medicare and Medicaid Services Innovation. Areas of Focus. Advanced Payment Initiative. Accessed online July 1, 2011, at http://innovations.cms.gov/areas-of-focus/seamless-and-coordinated-care-models/advance-payment/.

Future of Payment Reforms

The next generation of payment and reimbursement models is crystallizing through the efforts of countless physicians, hospitals, health insurance plans, researchers, policy analysts, and healthcare executives across the country. A high-level functional stream roadmap to remind us of key points and highlights is provided at the end of this chapter. Here a second conceptual map is also introduced. The model of the learning health system is introduced to give perspective on the complex issue of payment system reform. Second is a continuation of the series of functional stream maps provided throughout this book.

Learning Organizations

The concept of a learning organization is applicable to the healthcare industry. In the area of payment reform an abundance of new payment models and incentive programs have been piloted and demonstrated for years, with results providing feedback to leaders and policy decision makers.

The IOM's 2001 *Crossing the Quality Chasm* report[388] discussed the concept of learning organizations. In 2007 the IOM also held a Learning Healthcare System Workshop,[389] which engaged some of the principals who introduced the concept in 2001. Given the complexity of the financial issues and time required to design, test, implement, collect data, and analyze incentive programs, the learning system concept provides a philosophy as well as a model to convey the evolution of the healthcare industry and mark the best path forward. This concept is similar to continuous quality improvement, and is designed to strengthen performance in concert with improvements in quality, access, and cost of care. The learning system model illustrated below is a possible path—which could have many variations—for the evolution of a CIN/ACO in its financial reimbursement model maturation.

---

[388] Institute of Medicine, Committee on Quality of Health Care in America. Building organizational support for change: stages of organizational development. In: *Crossing the Quality Chasm: A New Health System for the 21st Century*. Washington, DC: National Academies Press; 2001. pp. 112–117.

[389] Institute of Medicine roundtable on evidence-based medicine. Workshop on the learning healthcare system, October 2007. Accessed July 22, 2011, at: http://books.nap.edu/openbook.php?record_id=11903&page=R1.

Figure 44. The Learning System: Payment Reform Progression

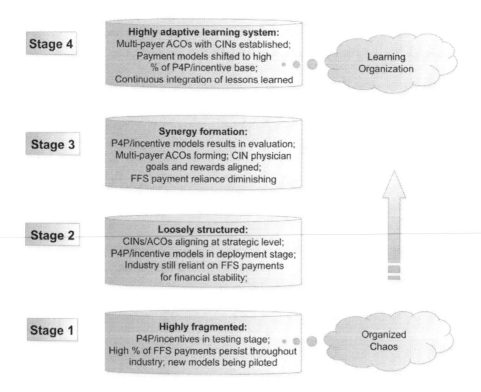

Stage 4 — Highly adaptive learning system: Multi-payer ACOs with CINs established; Payment models shifted to high % of P4P/incentive base; Continuous integration of lessons learned — Learning Organization

Stage 3 — Synergy formation: P4P/incentive models results in evaluation; Multi-payer ACOs forming; CIN physician goals and rewards aligned; FFS payment reliance diminishing

Stage 2 — Loosely structured: CINs/ACOs aligning at strategic level; P4P/incentive models in deployment stage; Industry still reliant on FFS payments for financial stability;

Stage 1 — Highly fragmented: P4P/incentives in testing stage; High % of FFS payments persist throughout industry; new models being piloted — Organized Chaos

The four-stage model is based on the "Stages of Evolution of the Design of Health Organizations" provided by the IOM in 2001.[390] Any number of factors could be presented or applied to the various stages along with application of the ACO qualification criteria from Fisher and colleagues discussed in Chapter 2. This application of the model focuses on the transition away from fee-for-service payments toward an increasingly higher percentage of incentive and pay-for-performance payments for physician and provider compensation. It also features the evolution of the system toward better-organized and clinically integrated multi-payer models. The IOM, CMS Innovation Center, and others are collectively providing policy leadership for progress along this path. In addition, such private sector stakeholders as trade associations and commercial health insurance plans are collaborating with physicians and hospitals to introduce new collaborative

---

[390] Institute of Medicine. Stages of Organizational Development. In: *Crossing the Quality Chasm.* pp. 112–117.

care models that are proving highly effective. As results of CIN/ACO implementations and new payment approaches translate into lessons learned, and best practices emerge, the industry will continue to advance toward Stage 4 as a highly adaptive learning system.

The Financial Roadmap

CIN/ACO initiatives require strong governance, financial, and administrative models as they mature. Roadmap 6 identifies five functional streams of importance to the operations of a CIN/ACO to ensure that appropriate fiduciary actions and responsibilities for and by all stakeholders involved in these new models of care delivery. Physician leaders should partner with senior financial leaders, including CFOs, practice administrators and others. This partnering is important to set the strategic agenda for reimbursement and physician compensation policies and processes as well as financial and contracting relationships for all participants. Understanding the risk tolerance of the organization charged with leading the establishment of the CIN or ACO is a critical function requiring the engagement of physician executives and administrators early in planning and decision-making. An organization at an early point in its establishment of infrastructure may be more inclined to focus efforts on establishing a CIN as a precursor to pursuing establishment of an ACO. A greater tolerance of risk and commensurate greater rewards, can be anticipated as ACOs mature and deal more effectively with the complexities associated with delivering higher value healthcare services while retaining accountability and responsibility for the results.

Figure 45. Roadmap 6: Navigating the Financial Issues

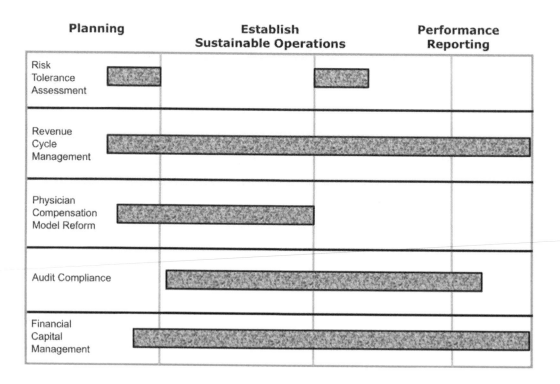

Risk tolerance assessment can be viewed as a continuous monitoring activity: but in this roadmap illustration it is considered a functional evaluation at the point of critical executive decision-making. Hence the diagram shows assessing risk and reward in the early planning stages, and then again after some period of sustained operations.

Second, and key to the longevity of every healthcare organization, is the need to proactively engage in revenue cycle management. The CIN and or ACO will have additional responsibility for risk management, and must have a strong financial team to manage the flow of reimbursements, physician/staff compensations, and expenses associated with the day-to-day operations of the organization. This management will also require visibility into quality and performance objectives; an understanding of whether or objectives are being met; and the ability to respond and change course when necessary. Physician leaders and other key executives in leadership will need to see monthly and sometimes weekly or daily updates on this critical function to ensure that funds are flowing properly through the organization's financial system, as these senior teams are ultimately responsible for the financial administration of the CIN/ACO.

Physician compensation is the third functional stream identified on the financial roadmap. Physicians are the lifeblood of these entities because they are responsible for attracting patients/beneficiaries to hospital facilities and outpatient centers for needed inpatient or outpatient services. Compensation models are changing along with reimbursement models and physicians who are better equipped to understand data about their practices, how they are performing, and whether they are meeting quality metrics and continuous improvement goals, will be better prepared to assume greater degrees of financial risk and rewards. They will also be better positioned to engage more actively in these new models of care finance and delivery. As the industry shifts away from the fee-for-service reimbursement, the physician workforce is adjusting its financial compensation plans to better align with pay-for-performance realities adopted throughout the industry.

Fourth in the financial management of healthcare organizations is auditing. Audits are a frequently occurring activity needed to ensure the integrity of organizations. Both internal compliance staff and external parties, including CMS, public accounting firms, state health departments, the Internal Revenue Service and other parties conduct periodic audits.

The last functional stream is financial capital management. New resources and the capital to finance them are necessary to establish new care delivery models. While capital management is listed on the map, it is not least in importance. Without appropriately management of this function a CIN or ACO will not have the ability to secure and maintain needed resources and infrastructure. Many healthcare provider organizations were negatively affected by the economic and financial downturn of the past decade. As organizations work their way back to financial health, if they wish to participate in the new health delivery models, allocation of funds necessary to start and sustain new operations will be crucial.

DISCLAIMER: The material in this chapter regarding the Medicare Shared Savings Program and associated financial rules is not intended to be *all-inclusive or final*. The intent is to raise awareness of many technical and financial issues, recognizing that final details will become available through final and additional federal rule making.

INFOCUS: Challenges Ahead

There are a number of financial challenges and risks to be navigated in establishing and operating CINs and ACOs. Many can be mitigated by engagement of appropriate stakeholders and careful planning. Healthcare service provider organizations have the challenge of evaluating and determining the reimbursement models to be adopted by their organizations including the risks and rewards associated with different configurations. As the industry continues to move toward a pay-for-performance and value-driven culture, fee-for-service reimbursements will continue to decline, resulting in a shift in payment methods and accommodation by physicians and hospital organizations as they work toward the design and implementation of such new models of finance and delivery, such as CINs and ACOs. As the Congressional Budget Office increases its forecasted deficit reduction from provisions in the Affordable Care Act (by nearly $70B over 10-years in one recent estimate) there may be opportunities to reduce these financial challenges. Much will depend on how physicians, hospitals, and other health system stakeholders act, and whether Congress believes it is getting value for the funds spent; and whether additional funding should go towards the healthcare system or other pressing government programs.

Another challenge presented by the Affordable Care Act is the new health insurance exchanges. As insurance exchanges open in 2014 and the nation's insured population increases, there may be an influx of new patients coming into primary care practices and hospital organizations. There are substantial workforce challenges in managing the increased workload. The operational burden of higher demand for services, including the new focus on quality and value that is becoming a central theme, will prove to be equally challenging. The formation of CINs and ACOs, with their repositioning of accountability and risk while increasing the potential reward, will serve as one way to deal with the new environment and help mitigate such challenges.

Establishing meaningful and realistic financial objectives that account for the transition in risk will be essential for physicians and hospitals to improve the quality of care and get paid appropriately. Organizations that embrace a collaborative governance approach will be better positioned to report performance to leadership and take corrective actions that improve population-based care and benefit from financial reforms.

Table 43. Chapter 9 Challenges and Risks

Challenges	Risks
Developing a transition plan for increasing risk tolerance and understanding commensurate rewards in the CIN/ACO while working in a largely indemnity oriented market.	Moving too early without new funding sources may result in the inability to underwrite loss of inpatient revenues, while moving too late may result in losing competitive advantage in the market.
Development of total cost-of-care actuarial and accounting capabilities that account for performance measures.	Inadequate infrastructure to track and monitor outcomes measures and performance may result in suboptimal insights for physicians and CIN/ACO leadership about the organization's financial performance and outcomes.
Instituting curriculum redesign in AMCs to ensure future physicians receive proper training on payment and compensation model reforms.	Inadequate changes to physician training will result in future physicians not being aware of forthcoming reforms that impact their future compensation and payment for services.
Sharing of risk and distribution of shared gains/losses among participating physicians and participants in a Medicare ACO.	Unintended consequences from shared savings programs that result in negative impact to quality of patient care services.

Potential Mitigation Strategies

√ Understand both risks and rewards, and allocate the rewards according to risk assumed.

√ Begin to pilot-test shared risk initiatives to develop core competencies.

√ Begin to explore total cost of care accounting vehicles.

√ Engage financial modeling expertise to forecast financial impacts on all stakeholders based on changes needed in pay-for-performance, clinical integration, and ACO programs.

√ Plan for early launch of payer relationship strategy discussions to move toward multi-payer ACO models at an accelerated pace.

√ AMCs apply MedPAC's recommendation to strengthen future physicians skills in care delivery and organizational leadership under reformed payment systems.

Chapter 10. Over the Horizon

The chief condition on which, life, health and vigor, is action. It is by action that an organism develops its faculties, increases its energy, and attains the fulfillment of its destiny.

Colin Powell
12th Chairman of the Joint Chiefs of Staff
65th U.S. Secretary of State

Where We Stand

Sustainable advances in the healthcare system in the United States will require many changes. CINs and ACOs are part of the new fabric of care delivery organizations that will help improve healthcare finance and delivery. New information technology solutions along with changes in the workforce and regulatory reforms will bring the system to a new plateau of excellence in quality healthcare services.

Many challenges remain, however, and these will have to be overcome in order to achieve sustainability. The federal government has already put in motion insurance market reforms in the Affordable Care Act; however, we have not addressed the issue of how our nation's health system will accommodate the needs of expanded insurance coverage for 40 to 45 million Americans.[391] Many efforts have been made to improve the healthcare system have been attempted since the IOM report, *To Err Is Human* was released in 1999. These initiatives include implementation of new health information technologies: improvement in quality management techniques and tools; the growth of consumerism and pay-for-performance models; transformation of primary care; and transition to accountability for the delivery of high quality and affordable healthcare services. The physician's traditional Hippocratic Oath[392] includes a commitment to care for those in need. In the United States the system is failing to adequately provide

---

[391] Holahan J. The 2007–09 Recession and Health Insurance Coverage. *Health Aff (Millwood) 2010;*30(1):1–8.
[392] Loewy EH. Oaths for Physicians – Necessary Protection or Elaborate Hoax? *MedGenMed.* 2007 Jan 10;9(1):7.

adequate care for many in need of healthcare services.[393] ACOs, clinical integration programs, and other new models of healthcare finance and delivery will bring opportunities to improve quality and outcomes, reduce medical errors and adverse events,[394] and effect change for the benefit of all segments of the population. With these changes will come new ways to evaluate performance and a new focus on comparative effectiveness research for health services, therapeutic products, and care delivery models.

These issues and others have led to a paradigm shift, giving rise to CINs, ACOs and other innovations. Other changes in publicly funded programs under the Public Health Service Act (as outlined in Title X of the Affordable Care Act), such as strengthening public health services as well as preventive health and wellness programs, increased funding for training of new healthcare workers, and improving the nation's Indian Health Service programs will also help.

Throughout this book we have covered many issues, including the history of the industry, explanations of the reasons for change, and major initiatives in the past decade to improve the health system. CINs, ACOs, and patient-centered medical homes now serve as central topic of discussion as they are being promoted as vehicles for the next stage of care transformation.

The importance of physician leadership and the continued growth of the next generation of physician leaders cannot be overstated. As the industry shifts to models of care in which the burdens and benefits of risk are increasingly carried by physicians and hospital providers, there will be a growing need for more physician leaders who can collaborate with nursing administrators and other experts to envision changes, set strategic objectives, and execute plans to achieve greater quality, affordability, and accessibility as outlined in CMS's Three Part Aim and the IOM's six aims of higher quality healthcare.

---

[393] Institute of Medicine, Committee on Quality of Health Care in America. Executive Summary. In: *To Err Is Human*. Washington, DC: National Academies Press; 2000. pp. 1-3.
[394] Landrigan CP, Parry GJ, Bones CB, Hackbarth AD, Goldmann DA, Sharek PJ. Temporal Trends in Rates of Patient Harm Resulting from Medical Care. *N Engl J Med*. 2010; 363(22): 2124-2134; Wilson D. Mistakes Chronicled on Medicare Patients. *New York Times*. November 11, 2010. .Accessed online July 20, 2011, at http://www.nytimes.com/2010/11/16/business/16medicare.html; Adverse Events in Hospitals: National Incidence Among Medicare Beneficiaries..*Department of Health and Human Services Office of Inspector General Report*. November 2010. Accessed online July 20, 2011, at http://oig.DHHS.gov/oei/reports/oei-06-09-00090.pdf.

The landscape of antitrust law and regulatory issues has also been discussed here. It is critical to understand these rules and regulations to ensure that joint venture agreements and operating plans are properly developed and implemented. Health information technology, quality improvement, and financial perspectives were all discussed, as they are critical issues for the development of these new models of care delivery.

A number of ACO initiatives (public as well as private) along with clinical integration programs and medical homes have been started across the country. In building on these efforts, most ACOs should change over time to a multi-payer focus. ACOs established as health system and physician organizations licensed to sell health insurance products, they have already achieved multi-payer status. These ACOs have developed the infrastructure to go beyond a clinically integrated network and become a true ACO health plan with the capability to negotiate payment terms with all-comers––including consumers looking for a provider-owned insurance product; other hospitals and physicians interested in becoming part of their network; and other insurance entities who need the ACO network to deliver care.

As such government-funded ACOs, as the Medicare Shared Savings Program and the Pioneer ACO Model catch up with innovations taking place in the private sector, cross- fertilization of new ideas and business models is likely to occur. For example, a single payer is an important step for a single-payer Medicare ACO in leveraging resources to maximize value and achieve economies of scale to reduce the overall cost of care for all segments of the population, whereas commercial ACO health plans already benefit from such economies. Opportunities to capitalize on the benefits of commercial ACO health plan efforts should be expedited to maximize returns on investments—and most importantly to close the healthcare quality gap in the communities served.

Future Economic Impact

The economic effects of health reforms in the Affordable Care Act include both reductions in expenditures for health services and increases in the cost of doing business for physicians and hospitals. The March 2010 final estimate from the Congressional Budget Office on budget deficit and revenue impacts of the Affordable Care Act projected a total $143B in reduced spending and decreased budget deficit over the ten-year period from 2010 to 2019.[395] The regulatory impact analysis section of the Proposed Rule a detailed analysis of the estimated start-up investment costs for participation in the Medicare Shared Savings Program and the net savings for the federal government in calendar years 2012 through 2014. This analysis factored in a number of assumptions and uncertainties mentioned in Chapter 3. CMS estimated the number of ACO start-ups to fall between 75 and 150. Their estimated costs and projected benefits are summarized below:

Table 44. Summary of Estimated Start-up Costs and Projected Financial Benefits from Participation in Medicare Shared Savings Program (Calendar Years 2012 through 2014)[396]

Category	Projected Cost	Projected Benefit
Estimated start-up operating expenditures	$131.6M to $263.3M	
Estimated savings distributions		$170M to $960M
Estimated net savings		$510M

It should be noted that these estimates do not account for ACOs or shared savings initiatives between private payers and health care provider organizations separate from the CMS program. Nor do the estimates take into account the costs or economic and efficiency benefits to be realized from new CINs started either independently of ACOs or developed as part of an ACO infrastructure.

As private sector and government-sponsored (i.e. Medicare) shared savings programs are implemented, the effects on participating organizations should be evaluated against the impact of other financial incentive programs as discussed

---

[395] Congressional Budget Office (CBO) Letter to the Honorable Nancy Pelosi regarding the CBO and Joint Committee on Taxation estimate of the direct spending and revenue effects of an amendment in the nature of a substitute to H.R. 4872, the Reconciliation Act of 2010. March 20, 2010. Accessed online July 20, 2011, at http://www.cbo.gov/ftpdocs/113xx/doc11379/AmendReconProp.pdf.
[396] Fed. Reg. Vol. 76, No. 67. April 7, 2011. V(F). Regulatory Impact Analysis; Conclusion. p. 19640.

in Chapter 9. Healthcare organizations are embarking on major organizational changes and transformation initiatives in response to turbulent and competitive reimbursement environment. Many complex changes may have to be undertaken to prepare for the launching of new care delivery models. In the future, comparative effectiveness evaluations of the micro- and macroeconomic effects along with population-level health outcomes will be needed to inform legislators, policy makers, and academics of the effects of these paradigm shifts. While the transition will not be easy and there will be numerous factors to manage, there is a path to success through these innovative programs to improve health outcomes for patients and the financial stability of physicians and hospitals. We have striven to cover these pathways to success in the previous chapters.

Strategic focus

There is a wide range of issues to analyze and manage over the course of launching a public or private ACOs or CINs. Strategic planning is essential at multiple points in the process, not just the beginning. Effective environmental scanning is essential to keep physicians and other leaders abreast of critical issues that will affect the organization's planning process and tactical activity. It is important to be aware of both micro and macro issues, as either may affect the success of your plans. One can view the scanning process through a set of lenses, as illustrated below.

Figure 47. Strategic Lenses for CIN/ACO Strategy Review

| Economic | Societal | Political | Clinical |

Economic Perspectives	Societal Perspectives	Political Perspectives	Clinical Perspectives
Supply drivers-healthcare workers	Cultural Considerations	Pending reform legislation	Population health
Public demand for services	Uninsured care	Congressional allies	Emergent conditions
Antitrust issues	Aging population care	Election impact	New interventions
Market influencers	Pediatric care	Grassroots movements	Delivery system reform

Analysis of Emerging Trends and Innovations Under Each Lens

Insights gained from an environmental scanning process should serve as background information in support of planning as well as due diligence for physician leaders, legal counsel and other members of a CIN or ACO's governance team. Each of these four lenses provides a different but interrelated perspective to consider in setting and correcting course for the organizations they lead.

Economic Perspectives. There are a number of issues to consider in evaluating the economic impact of various changes required to advance an ACO or CIN. The public demand for healthcare services changes in regions and local markets over time. Demand for health services depends on population growth or loss, shifting demographics, and even government regulations (e.g. certificates of need). The ways in which hospitals, physician practices, insurers and safety net organizations collaborate effectively to deliver healthcare services will vary depending on the market realities of each region. In addition, the need for, and ability to collaborate will be dictated in part by antitrust and regulatory laws.

The supply of healthcare workers, ranging from physicians and nurses to pharmacists, physician assistants, and others clinicians, is expected to grow but nonetheless to be insufficient to meet the growing needs of the general population, especially with the aging of the baby boomer generation. The short supply of healthcare workers combined with the aging of the population will have a dramatic economic impact on national, regional and local collaboration strategies. Monitoring of local market competition by physicians and hospital organizations should be an essential component of any CIN or ACO strategy. Other factors can also influence markets, such as changing population demographics, safety net organizations, and the health of local economies, all of which should be taken into account in evaluating the potential economic effects on CINs and ACOs.

Societal Perspectives. Given the forecasted reduction of the uninsured population due to insurance reforms in the Affordable Care Act, there is a projected increase in demand for healthcare services that will affect physicians, hospitals, and other healthcare service providers. The effects of the baby boomer generation have been discussed and should also be considered by CIN and ACO leaders. Strategic issues under this lens also involve consideration of health disparities.

Political Perspectives. Health policy, politics, and legislation at local, state, and federal levels will impact CINs and ACOs as they are established and mature. New policies will drive changes in care delivery, and many changes will result from the reforms under the Affordable Care Act. Changes in elected and appointed leadership in healthcare agencies at federal and state levels will have additional effects. National priorities shift over time and resources dedicated to healthcare by federal and state government officials are reevaluated when power and authority change at the national level.

Many issues in the political arena start with grassroots movements. The power of organized citizens across the country, especially in recent years with healthcare reform efforts leading to passage of the Affordable Care Act, is part of the fabric of America. Without the opportunity for empowerment and freedom of speech, change would come more slowly and in many areas be impossible.[397]

Clinical Perspective. The fourth lens for CINs, ACOs and their leadership is the clinical perspective. These new models of care focus on improving the health of the population they serve. Being cognizant of emergent clinical conditions that affect the health of a population, and preparing to take action should be a strategic priority. These emergent conditions may be shaped by different demographics, in different regions of the country, natural disasters, changing economies or seasonal weather among other factors. Nonetheless, each can take their toll on the health of a population and strain the healthcare system in the region. Opportunities to implement new interventions can come through innovations in health services, public health programming to support chronic problems in communities, or new technologies that offer promise to solving problematic health conditions. These interventions can provide new insights for the strategic objectives of CINs and ACOs.

Examining situations through these four perspectives can be part of the strategic planning process for a CIN or ACO. The insights and knowledge gained will support physician and administrative leaders' needs for information to evaluate strengths, weaknesses, opportunities, and threats; provide direction in dealing with government regulators and politicians; and provide a perspective on the spectrum of issues affecting the startup of these new healthcare organizations.

Planning for the Community

As CINs and ACOs are formed through various joint agreements, partnerships, and other collaborations, it will be important for their leaders to work with government agencies at local and state levels to improve population-based health management. Many physicians and clinical leaders are already engaged at various levels in public health matters. These groups examine health disparities,

---

[397] Pertschuk M. Grassroots Health. *PreemptionWatch.org*. November 19, 2010. Accessed online July 20, 2011, at http://www.preemptionwatch.org/2010/11/grassroots-health/; Iglehart JK. Visions for Change in U.S. Health Care —The Players and the Possibilities. *N Engl J Med*. 2009;360(3):205-207.

changes in population health outcomes, patient safety, and other issues. Matters that affect CIN/ACO implementation include:

- ♦ Existing public health and community services that can be used in patient care, and in some cases state and local governments will require coordination with these services;

- ♦ New models for care delivery and payment reform that are piloted, tested and implemented under CMS Innovation Center programs;

- ♦ The conversion to ICD-10 in 2013, which that will increase the granularity of healthcare data, enriching them it for clinical decisions and research, and providing additional information for total population health improvement;

- ♦ Other new public health programs from the Affordable Care act to be launched on national and local levels;

The formation of CINs and ACOs may increase industry consolidation and impact collaboration within markets. These new models of care delivery bring the potential of lowered barriers to collaboration to improve population health and health surveillance capabilities. One model originally introduced in 2000 and redesigned in 2010, offers a framework for community health action planning.[398] Figure 48 illustrates this planning model and other elements that CIN/ACO leaders can implement to drive improvements in regional population health management.

---

[398] Fawcett S, Schultz J, Watson-Thompson J, Fox M, Bremby R. Building multisectoral partnerships for population health and health equity. *Prev Chronic Dis*. 2010;7(6). Accessed online July 20, 2011, at http://www.cdc.gov/pcd/issues/2010/nov/10_0079.htm ; Institute of Medicine. *The Future of the Public's Health in the 21st Century*. Chapter 4. Community, Figure 4-1 Framework for Collaborative Community Action On Health. Washington, DC. National Academies Press; 2002. Accessed online July 20, 2011, at http://books.nap.edu/openbook.php?record_id=10548&page=186.

Figure 48. Framework for Community / Population Health Planning and Management

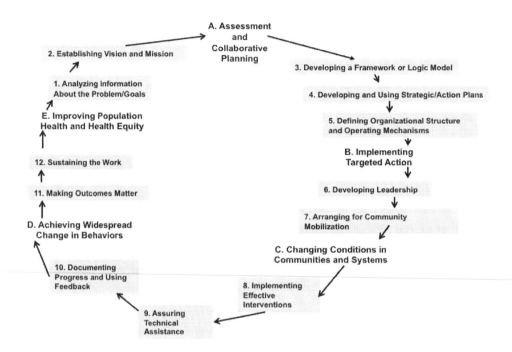

Elements A through E are the original elements of the framework. In the transition from a volume-driven compensation system to one that rewards value and quality of care, coordinating with community services will support strategic objectives for improving health outcomes. The implementation and evolution of community-level planning models, in which CINs and ACOs serve as part of larger systems, will help to achieve true more effective population-based health management and support organizational transformation in care delivery. A number of organizations referenced throughout this book have set the pace for this type of involvement, including the Geisinger Health System, the Mayo Clinic, Advocate Physician Partners, and Kaiser Permanente.

Elements 1 through 12 provide an added layer of actions proposed by Fawcett and colleagues. Although the actions are sequentially numbered, each can be taken independently. Atul Gawande, a professor of health policy and management has written on the value of using checklists to improve safety,[399] similar to "documenting progress and using feedback" to improve community health. "Developing leadership" is an essential need for any healthcare organization in the twenty-first century. Physician leadership in particular is critical because physicians are charged with greater responsibility in accountable care organizations and are natural leaders of clinically integrated networks. "Sustaining the work" includes evaluating how well an organization maintains its progress in the transformation of the organization.[400] When sustainability is planned as part of for in organizational transformation, the value of change is demonstrated not only in terms of economic impact and improved quality for patients but also in maintaining high quality and value for all citizens in the future.

The potential benefits for communities, CINs and ACOs in initiating a community-wide planning process include early identification of health risks for patient populations in their geographic region; outreach and recruitment of physician and clinical leaders; and implementation of systems for evaluating performance and providing feedback to CIN/ACO leaders from community stakeholders and the patients served. These efforts will ultimately lead to continuous quality improvement and delivery of higher-quality care throughout the communities served.

The Learning Organization: Advancing the Care Delivery Model

Advancing and evolving the finance and delivery of healthcare will take time, energy, and resources. The current U.S. healthcare system has reached a point of fragmentation but is transitioning to a new era of improved quality and accountability. Transition can be facilitated by utilization of the learning organization model as discussed throughout this book, CINs and ACOs can be a significant part of this transformation. Their implementation should improve quality and access to care, streamline care transitions for patients and caregivers, and help improve health outcomes. Recalling the four-stage model of progression

---

[399] Gawande A. Chapter 2. The Checklist. *In: The Checklist Manifesto. How to Get Things Right*. New York, NY: Metropolitan Books, 2009. pp. 35-47.
[400] Weiner B. A theory of organizational readiness for change. *Implementation Science*. 2009;4(67).

illustrated in Chapter 9, we can see movement toward achieving a higher level of accountability and results.

Figure 49. CIN/ACO: Evolving as a Learning Organization

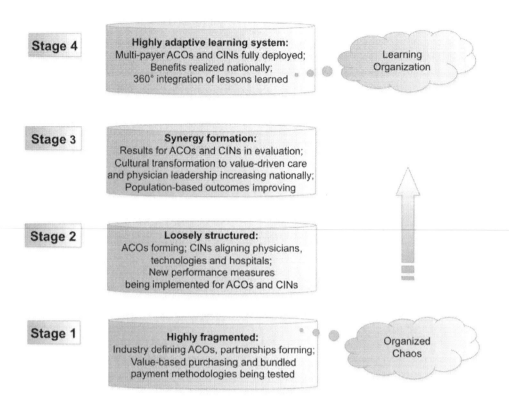

The stages of this model illustrate a hypothetical progression from a fragmented state of operation (Stage 1) to that of a highly efficient and adaptive learning system (Stage 4).   CINs and ACOs must incorporate value-based purchasing practices as part of their evolution.[401] Initiatives undertaken to reach Stage 4 also bring opportunities to increase interconnectivity among all care delivery stakeholders. A few points on each stage include:

Stage 1. The first stage is characterized as fragmented and decentralized. The industry is beginning the journey of redefining its path, however, it is testing new models of care delivery (e.g. ACOs) and methods of payment, as it moves away from traditional fee-for-service. Important elements in Stage 1 are the

---

[401] H.R. 3590, Patient Protection and Affordable Care Act, §3022(b)(2)(G). ACO requirements (2010).

formation of new joint arrangements needed to formalize the implementation of CINs as precursors of ACOs, the introduction of learning organization systems and frameworks,[402] and the adoption of tools that assist clinicians in adhering to evidence-based decision making,[403] at the individual patient and population levels.

Stage 2. In the second stage of development, CINs and ACOs appear in their operational state, and opportunities emerge to evaluate the new models of care implemented in different configurations with different targeted patient populations. CINs focus on strengthening integration of physicians, technologies, and hospitals. As ACOs continue to strengthen, the industry starts to see improved levels of care coordination and clinical outcomes. Application of advanced clinical decision support tools to improve use of evidence-based medicine continues to grow with improved health information technology to support physician and clinician workflow.

Stage 3. The synergy formation stage. One of the most important elements at this point in the industry transformation, and at the local CIN/ACO level will be the lowering of barriers to progress that limited healthcare operations for decades. Physician leadership of CINs and ACOs continues to grow in influence. The effects of utilization-restricting managed care are less apparent as the infrastructure has shifted to "pay-for-performance" and a value-based culture. Another change is the move toward stronger population-based health management––one of the visions of the Healthy People 2020[404] goals.

Stage 4. Organizations and the industry as a whole reach the learning organization level at Stage 4. CINs and ACOs will have developed the infrastructure, processes, and staff to support vertically and horizontally integrated systems, and both public and private sector payers cooperate in multi-payer approaches to maximize shared savings and achieve economies of scale while improving quality of care and lowering cost across the country.

---

[402] Crites GE, McNamara MC, Akl EA, Richardson SW, Umscheid CA, Nishikawa J. Evidence in the learning organization. *Health Research Policy and Systems*. 2009;7(4).

[403] Kilicoglu H, Demner-Fushman D, Rindflesch TC, Wilczynski NL, Haynes RB. Towards Automatic Recognition of Scientifically Rigorous Clinical Research Evidence. *JAMA*. 2009;16(1):25–31. Accessed online July 21, 2011, at http://www.ncbi.nlm.nih.gov/pmc/articles/PMC2605595/pdf/25.S1067502708001874.main.pdf.

[404] Healthy People 2020 Initiative's Framework. Accessed online July 21, 2011, at http://www.healthypeople.gov/2020/Consortium/HP2020Framework.pdf.

Legislative Outlook

Healthcare reforms at the federal government level are bringing about widespread change in the United States. Starting with the Balanced Budget Act of 1996, the Beneficiary Improvement and Protection Act of 2000, the Medicare Modernization Act in 2003, ARRA in 2009, and the Affordable Care Act in 2010, the industry has witnessed enactment of many reforms. While elements of the Affordable Care Act are the subject of debate and legal challenge, the act has introduced new programs, to support the evolution of the nation's healthcare infrastructure and safety net operations with new models of care delivery, new programs for training the workforce, and a new entity for improving the affordability, access and quality of care delivered.

As CINs and ACOs start to produce results, they can be analyzed to determine the value delivered in terms of lowered cost and higher quality of care. As these new models are evaluated, the legislation that created these initiatives will also be evaluated for its effects on budget and costs. Policy and legislative changes are certain to continue as the industry identifies what works and what doesn't, the models are refined, and Congress continues to evaluate and change the finance and delivery of care.

Another policy consideration for ACOs is patient-centered care. Patient-centeredness[405] is a criterion for Medicare ACOs.[406] Key elements of this policy include improving patient communication, meeting each patient's unique needs, granting patients access to their medical records, integrating care with community resources, and instituting mechanisms for coordination of care. In addition, patient-centeredness is thought to contribute to the effectiveness of medical home initiatives and ACOs in several ways: [407]

---

[405] H.R. 3590, Patient Protection and Affordable Care Act, §30222(b)(2)(H). Requirements for ACOs (2010).
[406] Fed. Reg. Vol. 76, No. 67. April 7, 2011. II(B)(10). Patient Centeredness Criteria. pp. 19547–19548.
[407] Epstein RM, Fiscella K, Lesser CS, Stange KC. Why The Nation Needs A Policy Push On Patient-Centered Health Care. *Health Aff (Millwood)*. 2010;29(8):1489–1495.

- *Communications*: education of clinicians on best practices and communication techniques that mitigate health disparities, and technology enablers that improve health communications with patients;

- *Measures of effectiveness*: evaluating new interventions, technologies, clinical processes, and interactions with patients and families that directly affect patient relationships.

The field of comparative effectiveness research holds the promise in examining the effectiveness of different medical interventions, and providing physicians and other caregivers information on evidence-based medicine and advanced clinical decision support. With the Patient-Centered Outcomes Research Institute,[408] there may also be efforts to assess the effectiveness of ACOs in comparison to other models of healthcare finance and delivery. On a related note, the Proposed Rule identified the importance of comparing results from services across multiple ACOs, recognizing that different models may work better and competition fosters improvement.[409]

As ACO policies evolve and the movement matures, new legislation will invariably be considered by Congress. Such topics as quality monitoring and measurement, performance reporting, payment reform, and others will emerge during the process of Congressional oversight and deliberation that will affect the evolution and refinement of ACOs.

Next Generation

While this book has focused on the formation of clinically integrated networks and their evolution into accountable care organizations, the reader needs to recognize that this too, in its currently proposed form, will have a product life cycle that evolves as shown through the learning organization model. Shared savings will work when there are savings to be captured for the benefit of CIN/ACO participants and their patient populations served. If you take these

---

[408] H.R. 3590, Patient Protection and Affordable Care Act, §6301(b). Establishment of Patient-Centered Outcomes Research Institute (2010).
[409] Fed. Reg. Vol. 76, No. 67. April 7, 2011. I.(4)(b). Competition and Quality of Care. p. 19630.

models to maturity, at some point, the industry will eventually experience diminishing returns such that the economic engine that once fueled a CIN/ACO will have been extinguished. So what would the next phase in this evolutionary process look like?

Many argue that internalizing some or all of the insurance risk will be an evolutionary step that needs to be taken. Commercial insurers recognize the changes coming in the industry and are starting to seek new and innovative ways to partner with providers in light of the oncoming transformation. Of course, this too may have a finite life cycle as we look for other ways in which to curtail the health care spend rate and growth in cost for the United States. Limiting brokerage fees, networks going direct to employers and potentially going direct to consumers are all potential next steps as we continually move along this health care reform journey. While no one can predict precisely where this journey will end, it seems worthy of consideration as we plan and develop these new models of care delivery.

Figure 50. Potential Pathway for CIN/ACO Industry Transformation

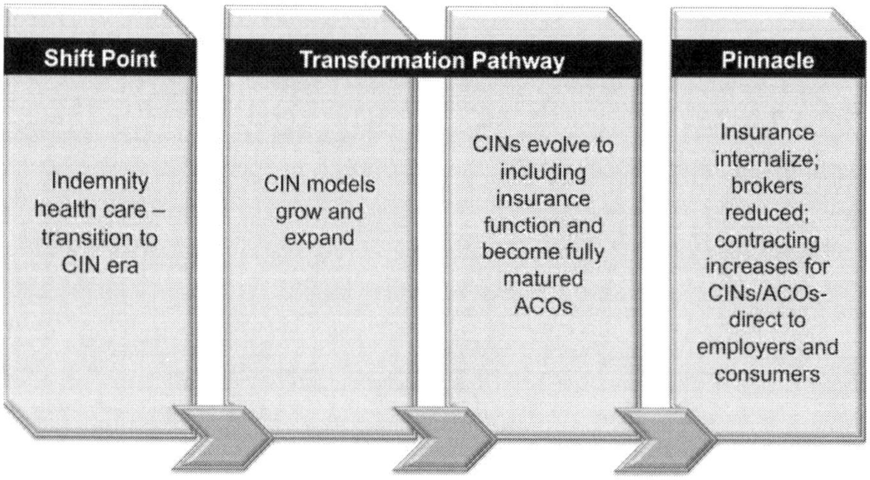

Shift Point	Transformation Pathway		Pinnacle
Indemnity health care – transition to CIN era	CIN models grow and expand	CINs evolve to including insurance function and become fully matured ACOs	Insurance internalize; brokers reduced; contracting increases for CINs/ACOs- direct to employers and consumers

Figure 50 illustrates a potential pathway for this concept. Not bound to any given time horizon, it is provided in our closing comments for reflective thought on the potential future evolution of clinically integrated networks on the way to accountable care.

In Conclusion

The Proposed Rule initially defined requirements for participation in the new Medicare Shared Savings Program. The Final Rule will answer some but not all questions raised by the industry about the establishment and operation of these organizations. Private sector ACOs will continue to advance, potentially setting the benchmark for viable operation of ACOs. Private sector ACO health plans could provide important insights as the federal government works toward a multi-payer model to take advantage of common infrastructure, common quality measures, and economies of scale. CINs and medical home principles are part of the ACO infrastructure. Integration of primary and specialty care into hospital systems for the formation of integrated delivery networks may bring the end of cottage-industry physician practices; however in this era of accountable care the benefits of improved patient care from the economies of scale in large organizations are considerable and will continue to grow.

From a policy perspective, CMS' focus on the Three Part Aim is related to the Healthy People 2020 goal to *Achieve health equity, eliminate disparities, and improve the health of all groups*[410] and the IOM's six aims for improvement in healthcare. These strategic initiatives are important for Medicare ACOs to understand and should be an important part of strategy for all accountable care organizations.

Five ACO models were identified earlier along with the CIN model. Which model works best in a specific situation depends on many factors. As results are published from studies evaluating both the economic impact and improvement in clinical quality and outcomes from these new models, opportunities for learning organizations to implement continuous quality improvement will increase in the coming years. The introduction of new processes, technologies, and health interventions should be embraced by ACOs and CINs to further the opportunities to improve quality and lower the cost of care. Given the rapid adoption of health information technology, further assessments of the impact on care coordination,

---

[410] Healthy People 2020 Framework. Overarching Goals. Accessed online July 21, 2011, at http://www.healthypeople.gov/2020/Consortium/HP2020Framework.pdf.

medical errors, and quality of care should be made to support application of new technologies in CIN and ACO operations.

A collection of models has been provided throughout the book, some original and some credited to the work of others, as well as roadmaps at the end of several chapters. These roadmaps are only intended only to stimulate critical thinking and support strategic planning in the launch of a CIN or ACO. Each set of organizations will bring different strengths and capabilities that physician leaders and others in governance groups must evaluate to identify the best options and set the course of action for the stakeholders, consumers, and patients served.

Hospitals and hospital systems must redefine themselves as they increasingly face major changes in reimbursement and delivery of care. In the new paradigm, in which value is more important than volume, medical specialists will assist their primary care colleagues in coordinating care and keeping patients healthy, and primary care physicians will look to their specialist colleagues for definitive therapies that make the most clinical and financial sense for their patients. As performance is reimbursed more than procedures, as Clayton Christensen observed, hospitalizations will become more often regarded as outpatient treatment failures and quality measures will define performance standards. By improving communication through information technology, keeping patient-centered quality as the guiding standard, and enabling physicians to lead, we are on the cusp of real change.

Bibliography

Akobeng, AK, Understanding Randomised Controlled Trials. *Arch Dis Child.* 2005;90(8):840–4.

American Academy of Family Physicians (AAFP). AAFP Accountable Care Organization Task Force Report October 2009. Leawood, KS: AAFP, 2009.

American Health Information Management Association (AHIMA). e-HIM Workgroup on the Transition to ICD-10-CM/PCS. Planning organizational transition to ICD-10-CM/PCS. *Journal of AHIMA.* 2009;80(10):72–77.

American Hospital Association (AHA) Committee on Research. *Accountable Care Organizations: Research Synthesis Report.* Chicago, IL: AHA, 2010.

Ash JS, Sittig DF, Poon EG, Guappone K, Campbell E, Dykstra RH. The extent and importance of unintended consequences related to computerized provider order entry. *J Am Med Inform Assoc.* 2007;14(4):415–423.

Barrett JS, Mondick JT, Narayan M, Vijayakumar K, Vijayakumar S. Integration of modeling and simulation into hospital-based decision support systems guiding pediatric pharmacotherapy. *BMC Med Inform Decis Mak.* 2008;8(6).

Berenson R. Shared savings program for accountable care organizations: a bridge to nowhere? *Am J Manag Care.* 2010;16(10):721–726.

Bertakis KD, Azari R. Patient-Centered Care is Associated with Decreased Health Care Utilization. *J Am Board Fam Med.* 2001 May-Jun;24(3):229–39.

Berwick DM. A primer on leading the improvement of systems. *BMJ.* 1996;312:619–622.

Besanko D, Dranove D, Shanley M, Schaefer S. (2004). Competitors and competition. In: *Economics of Strategy.* 3rd ed. Hoboken, NJ; John Wiley and Sons, Inc., 218–223.

Blumenthal D, Tavenner M. The "meaningful use" regulation for electronic health records. *N Engl J Med.* 2010;363(6):501–504.

BodenheimerT, Wagner EH, Grumbach K. Improving primary care for patients with chronic illness: the chronic care model, Part 2. *JAMA.* 2002;288(15):1909–1914.

Boland P, Polakoff P, Schwab T. Accountable care organizations hold promise, but will they achieve cost and quality targets? *Manag Care.* 2010;19(10):12–16.

de Brantes F, Rosenthal MB, Painter M. Building a bridge from fragmentation to accountability—the Prometheus Payment model. *N Engl J Med.* 2009;361(11):1033–1036.

Burke T, Rosenbaum S. Accountable care organizations: implications for antitrust policy. Princeton, NJ: Robert Wood Johnson Foundation, 2010.

Campbell EM, Sittig DF, Ash JS, Guappone K, Dykstra RH. Types of unintended consequences related to computerized provider order entry. *J Am Med Inform Assoc* 2006;13(5):547–556.

Casalino LA, Devers KJ, Lake TK, Reed M, Stoddard JJ. Benefits of and barriers to large medical group practice in the U.S. *Arch Intern Med.* 2003;163(16):1958–64.

Center for Healthcare Research & Transformation (CHRT). *Health Care Cost Drivers: Chronic Disease, Comorbidity, and Health Risk Factors in the U.S. and Michigan.* Ann Arbor, MI: CHRT, 2010.

Centers for Medicare and Medicaid Services (CMS). *Roadmap for Implementing Value Driven Healthcare in the Traditional Medicare Fee-for-Service Program.* Baltimore, MD: CMS, 2009.

Chassin MR, Loeb JM, Schmaltz SP, Wachter RM. Accountability measures—using measurement to promote quality improvement. *N Engl J Med.* 2010 Aug 12;363(7):683–8.

Chaudry J, Jain A, McKenzie S, Schwartz RW. Physician leadership: the competencies of change. *J Surg Educ.* 2008;65(3):213–220.

Christensen C, Grossman J, Hwang J. *The Innovator's Prescription: A Disruptive Solution for Healthcare.* New York, NY: McGraw-Hill; 2009.

Collins J. *Good to Great: Why Some Companies Make the Leap and Others Don't.* New York, NY: Harper Business, 2001.

Concato J, Lawler EV, Lew RA, Gaziano JM, Aslan M, Huang GD. Observational Methods in Comparative Effectiveness Research, *Am J Med.* 2010;123(12 Suppl 1):e16–e23.

Crites GE, McNamara MC, Akl EA, Richardson SW, Umscheid CA, Nishikawa J. Evidence in the learning organization. *Health Research Policy and Systems.* 2009;7(4).

Cutler D. How Health Care Reform Must Bend the Cost Curve. *Health Aff (Millwood).* 2010;29(6):1131–1135.

Daniels R. *Nursing Fundamentals: Caring & Clinical Decision Making*, Clifton Park, NY: Thomson Learning, 2004.

David A, Baxley L. Education of Students and Residents in Patient Centered Medical Home (PCMH): Preparing the Way. *Ann Fam Med.* 2011 May-Jun;9(3):274-5.

DelliFraine JL, Langabeer JR 2nd, Nembhard IM. Assessing the evidence of Six Sigma and Lean in the health care industry. *Qual Manag Health Care.* 2010 Jul-Sep;19(3):211–25.

Devers K, Berenson R. Can accountable care organizations improve the value of health care by solving the cost and quality quandaries? Princeton, NJ: Robert Wood Johnson Foundation, 2009.

Donabedian A. Evaluating the quality of medical care. *Milbank Quarterly* 2005;83(4):691–729. Reprinted from *Milbank Memorial Fund Quarterly* 1966;44(3):166–203.

Epstein RM, Fiscella K, Lesser CS, Stange KC. Why the Nation Needs a Policy Push on Patient-Centered Health Care. *Health Aff (Millwood).* 2010;29(8):1489–1495.

Etheredge L. Creating a High-Performance System for Comparative Effectiveness Research *Health Aff (Millwood).* 2010. 29(10):1761–1767.

Falk I, Rorem R, Ring M. A summary of the findings. In: *The Costs of Medical Care: A Summary of Investigations on the Economic Aspects of the Prevention and Care of Illness.* Chicago, IL: University of Chicago Press, 1933.

Fawcett S, Schultz J, Watson-Thompson J, Fox M, Bremby R. Building multisectoral partnerships for population health and health equity. *Prev Chronic Dis.* 2010;7(6).

Federal Trade Commission and Department of Justice. *Improving Health Care: A Dose of Competition.* Washington, DC: Federal Trade Commission, 2004.

Fields D, Leshen E, Patel K. Analysis and commentary. Driving quality gains and cost savings through adoption of medical homes. *Health Aff (Millwood).* 2010;29(5):819–826.

Fisher ES, McClellan MB, Bertko J, et al. Fostering accountable health care: moving forward in Medicare. *Health Aff (Millwood)* 2009;28(2):w219–w231.

Fisher ES, Shortell SM. Accountable care organizations: accountable for what, to whom, and how. *JAMA.* 2010 20;304(15):1715–6.

Fisher ES, Staiger DO, Bynum JP, Gottlieb DJ. Accountable care organizations: the extended medical staff. *Health Aff (Millwood).* 2007 ;26(1):w44–w57.

Ford EW, Menachemi N, Peterson LT, Huerta TR. Resistance is futile: but it is slowing the pace of EHR adoption nonetheless. *J Am Med Inform Assoc.* 2009;16(3):274–281.

Fraschetti R, Sugarman M. Successful Hospital-Physician Integration. *Trustee.* 2009;62(7):11–2, 17–8.

Gawande A. *The Checklist Manifesto. How to Get Things Right.* New York, NY: Metropolitan Books, 2009.

Gittell J, Seidner R, Wimbush J. A Relational Model of How High-Performance Work Systems Work. *Organization Science.* 2010;21(2):490–506.

Glasser J., Salzberg C. Information Technology for Accountable Care Organizations. *Hospitals & Health Networks*, September 2010.

Goldsmith J. Analyzing Shifts In Economic Risks To Providers In Proposed Payment And Delivery System Reforms. *Health Aff (Millwood).* 2010;29(7):1299–1304.

Gosfield AG. The stark truth about the Stark law. Part I. *Fam Pract Manag.* 2003;10(10):27–33.

Gray BH, Gusmano MK, Collins SR. AHCPR and the Changing Politics of Health Services Research. *Health Aff (Millwood),* 2003 Jan-Jun;Suppl Web Exclusives:W3-283–307.

Greaney T. Thirty years of solicitude: antitrust law and physician cartels. *Houston Journal of Health Law and Policy.* 2007;72:189–226.

Greenes, R.A., ed. *Clinical Decision Support, the Road Ahead.* Maryland Heights, MO: Academic Press, 2007.

Griner P. Payment Reform and the Mission of Academic Medical Centers. *N Engl J Med.* 2010 4;363(19):1784–6.

Guterman S, Davis K, Stremikis K, Drake H. Innovation In Medicare and Medicaid Will Be Central to Health Reform's Success. *Health Aff (Millwood).* 2010;29(6):1188–1193.

Health Care Incentives Improvement Institute (HCI3). *Prometheus Payment: On the Frontlines of Health Care Payment Reform.* Newtown, CT: HCI3, 2010.

Heit M., Piper K. *Global Payments to Improve Quality and Efficiency in Medicaid: Concepts and Considerations.* Boston, MA: Massachusetts Medicaid Policy Institute, 2009.

Hellinger FJ. Antitrust enforcement in the healthcare industry: the expanding scope of state activity. *Health Serv Res.* 1998;33(5 Pt 2):1477–1494.

Hester J Jr. Designing Vermont's pay-for-population health system. *Prev Chronic Dis.* 2010;7(6):1–6.

Holahan J. The 2007–09 Recession and Health Insurance Coverage. *Health Aff (Millwood) 2010;*30(1):1–8.

Horwitz RI, Viscoli CM, Clemens JD, Sadock RT. Developing improved observational methods for evaluating therapeutic effectiveness. *Am J Med.* 1990;89:630–638.

Iglehart JK. Visions for Change in U.S. Health Care—The Players and the Possibilities. *N Engl J Med.* 2009;360(3):205–207.

Institute of Medicine, Committee on Assuring the Health of the Public in the 21st Century. *The Future of the Public's Health in the 21st Century.* Washington, DC. National Academies Press, 2002.

Institute of Medicine. Committee on Comparative Effectiveness Research Prioritization. *Initial National Priorities for Comparative Effectiveness Research.* Washington, DC: National Academies Press, 2009.

Institute of Medicine, Committee on Quality of Health Care in America. *Crossing the Quality Chasm: A New Health System for the 21st Century.* Washington, DC: National Academies Press, 2001.

Institute of Medicine, Committee on Quality of Health Care in America. *To Err Is Human.* Washington, DC: National Academies Press; 2000.

Institute of Medicine, Committee on Redesigning Health Insurance Performance Measures, Payments, and Performance Improvement Programs. *Rewarding Provider Performance: Aligning Incentives in Medicare.* Washington, DC: National Academies Press, 2006.

Institute of Medicine, Roundtable on Evidence Based Medicine. *Workshop on the Learning Healthcare System.* Washington, DC: National Academies Press, 2007.

Jacobs P, Rapoport J. Regulation and antitrust policy in health care. In: *The Economics of Health and Medical Care,* 5th ed. Sudbury, MA: Jones and Bartlett Publishers, 2004.

Jarousse LA. Leadership in the Era of Reform. *H&HN Mag*azine, November 2010.

Jarousse LA. On the Agenda. *Trustee.* 2011 Feb;64(2).

Javitt JC, Rebitzer JB, Reisman L. Information technology and medical missteps: Evidence from a randomized trial. *J Health Econ* 2008;27(3):585–602.

Javitt JC, Steinberg G, Locke T, Couch JB, Jacques J, Juster I, Reisman L. Using a Claims Data-based, Sentinel System to Improve Compliance with Clinical Guidelines: Results of a Randomized Prospective Study. *Am J Manag Care.* 2005 Feb;11(2):93–102.

Jha AK, DesRoches CM, Campbell EG, et al. Use of electronic health records in U.S. hospitals. *N Engl J Med.* 2009;360(16):1628–1638.

The Joint Commission, *Safely Implementing Health Information and Converging Technologies*, Sentinel Event Alert #42. Oak Brook, IL: Joint Commission Resources, 2008.

Juster IA. Technology-Driven Interactive Care Management Identifies and Resolves More Clinical Issues than a Claims-Based Alerting System. *Dis Manag* 2005;8(3):188–97.

Katayama AC, Coyne SE, Moskol KL. Another round of Stark law changes coming your way as early as October 1, 2008. *WMJ.* 2008;107(6):305–306.

Kawamoto K, Houlihan CA, Balas EA, Lobach DF. Improving clinical practice using clinical decision support systems: a systematic review of trials to identify features critical to success. *BMJ.* 2005;2;330(7494):765.

Kerr EA, Krein SL, Vijan S, Hofer TP, Hayward RA. Avoiding pitfalls in chronic disease quality measurement: a case for the next generation of technical quality measures. *Am J Manag Care.* 2001;7(11):1033–1043.

Kilicoglu H, Demner-Fushman D, Rindflesch TC, Wilczynski NL, Haynes RB. Towards Automatic Recognition of Scientifically Rigorous Clinical Research Evidence. *JAMA.* 2009;16(1):25–31.

Kocher R, Ezekiel EJ, DeParle NA. The Affordable Care Act and the future of clinical medicine: the opportunities and challenges. *Ann Intern Med.* 2010;153(8):536–539.

Kocher R, Sahni NR. Physicians versus hospitals as leaders of accountable care organizations. *N Engl J Med.* 2010;363(27):2579–2582.

Kongstvedt, P.R., ed. *Essentials of Managed Health Care*, 5th ed. Sudbury, MA: Jones and Bartlett Publishers, 2007.

Konschak C, Jarrell L. *Consumer-centric Healthcare: Opportunities and Challenges for Providers.* Chicago, IL: Health Administration Press, 2010.

Kotter J, Rathgeber H. *Our Iceberg Is Melting.* New York, NY: St. Martin's Press, 2005.

Kotter J, Schlesinger L. Choosing strategies for change. *Harvard Business Review.* 1979;57(2):106–114.

Landrigan CP, Parry GJ, Bones CB, Hackbarth AD, Goldmann DA, Sharek PJ. Temporal Trends in Rates of Patient Harm Resulting from Medical Care. *N Engl J Med.* 2010;363(22):2124–2134.

LeTourneau B. Communicate for change. *J Healthc Manag.* 2004;49(6):354–357.

Loewy EH. Oaths for Physicians—Necessary Protection or Elaborate Hoax? *MedGenMed.* 2007 Jan 10;9(1):7.

Luft HS. Becoming accountable—opportunities and obstacles for ACOs. *N Engl J Med.* 2010;363(15):1389–1391.

McClellan M, McKethan AN, Lewis JL, Roski J, Fisher ES. A national strategy to put accountable care into practice. *Health Aff (Millwood).* 2010;29(5):982–990.

McDonald KM, Sundaram V, Bravat DM, et al. *Closing the Quality Gap: A Critical Analysis of Quality Improvement Strategies.* Rockville, MD: Agency for Healthcare Research and Quality; 2007.

McIntyre D, Rogers L, Heier E. Overview, history, and objectives of performance measurement. *Healthcare Finance Review.* 2001;22(3):7–21.

Medicare Payment Advisory Commission (MedPAC). *Report to Congress: Improving Incentives in the Medicare Program*, Chapter 2: Accountable Care Organizations. Washington, DC: MedPAC, 2009.

Miller J. Aetna Manages Cancer Care. *Managed Healthcare Executive.* July 2011;21(7):18–21.

Miller H. *Pathways for Physician Success under Healthcare Payment and Delivery Reforms.* Chicago, IL: American Medical Association and the Center for Healthcare Quality and Payment Reform, 2010.

Mirabito AM, Berry LL. Lessons that patient-centered medical homes can learn from the mistakes of HMOs. *Ann Intern Med.* 2010;152(3):182–185.

Molpus J. The Leap to Accountable Care Organizations. *HealthLeaders Media Intelligence*, April 2011. Survey results, p. 15.

Moore, J.F. *The Death of Competition: Leadership & Strategy in the Age of Business Ecosystems.* New York, NY: Harper Business, 1996.

Morrisey MA, Alexander J, Burns LR, Johnson V. Managed care and physician/hospital integration. *Health Aff (Millwood).* 1996;15:62–73.

Navathe A. and Conway P. Optimizing Health Information Technology's Role in Enabling Comparative Effectiveness Research. *Am J Manag Care.* 2010;16(12):SP44-SP47.

Office of Inspector General, U.S. Department of Health and Human Services (DHHS). General Report: Adverse Events in Hospitals: National Incidence among Medicare Beneficiaries. Washington, DC: DHHS, 2010.

Paulus RA, Davis K, Steele GD. Continuous innovation in health care: implications of the Geisinger experience. *Health Aff (Millwood).* 2008;27(5):1235–1245.

Physicians Foundation. *2010 Physician Survey on Impact of Healthcare Reform.* Irving, TX: Merritt Hawkins, 2010.

Pisapia J, Reyes-Guerra D, Coukos-Semmel E. Developing the leader's strategic mindset: establishing the measures. *Leadership Review.* 2005;5:41–68.

Pourshadi KM. Putting Patient-Centered Care into Perspective. *HealthLeaders Media.* May 2, 2011.

President's Council of Advisors on Science and Technology (PCAST). Report to the President realizing the full potential of health IT to improve healthcare for Americans: The path forward. Washington, DC: PCAST, 2010.

Raskovich A, Miller NH. Cumulative innovation and competition policy. Washington, DC: Department of Justice Economic Analysis Group, 2010.

Raths D. Is ICD-10 a Quality Initiative? Innovators will use ICD-10 to further their business models and clinical capabilities. *Healthc Inform.* 2010;27(9):24–28.

Rittenhouse DR, Shortell SM, Fisher ES. Primary care and accountable care—two essential elements of delivery-system reform. *N Engl J Med.* 2009;361(24):2301–2303.

Robinow A. *The Potential of Global Payment: Insights from the Field.* New York, NY: Commonwealth Fund, 2010.

Robinson JC. Applying value-based insurance design to high-cost health services. *Health Aff (Millwood).* 2010;29 (11):2009–16.

Schroeder R. Just-in-time systems and lean thinking. In: *Operations Management: Contemporary Concepts and Cases,* 3rd ed. New York, NY: McGraw-Hill Irwin, 2007.

Schwartz RW, Tumblin TF. The power of servant leadership to transform health care organizations for the 21st-century economy. *Arch Surg.* 2002;137(12):1419–1427.

Senge P. *The Fifth Discipline: The Art and Practice of the Learning Organization.* New York: Knopf Doubleday Publishing Group, 1990, 2006.

Serio CD, Epperly T. Physician leadership: a new model for a new generation. *Fam Pract Manag.* 2006;13(2):51–54.

Shortell S. Challenges and Opportunities for Population Health Partnerships. *Preventing Chronic Disease.* 2010;7(6):1–2.

Shortell SM, Casalino LP, Fisher ES. How the center for medicare and medicaid innovation should test accountable care organizations. *Health Aff (Millwood).* 2010;29(7):1293–1298.

Sinaiko AD, Rosenthal MB. Patients' role in accountable care organizations. *N Engl J Med.* 2010;363(27):2583–2585.

Sisko AM, Truffer CJ, Keehan SP, Poisal JA, Clemens MK, Madison AJ. National health spending projections: the estimated impact of reform through 2019. *Health Aff (Millwood).* 2010;29(10): 1933–1941.

Smithson K, Baker S. Medical Staff Organizations: A Persistent Anomaly. *Health Aff (Millwood).* 2006;26(1):w76–w79.

Starr P. The Social Origins of Professional Sovereignty. In: *The Social Transformation of American Medicine.* New York, NY: Harper Collins, 1982.

Steele GD, Haynes JA, Davis DE, et al. How Geisinger's advanced medical home model argues the case for rapid-cycle innovation. *Health Aff (Millwood).* 2010;29(11):2047–2053.

Steindel SJ. International classification of diseases, 10th edition, clinical modification and procedure coding system: descriptive overview of the next generation HIPAA code sets. *J Am Med Inform Assoc.* 2010;17(3):274–282.

Stoller JK. Developing physician-leaders: a call to action. *J Gen Intern Med.* 2009;24(7):876–878.

Suc J, Prokosch HU, Ganslandt T. Applicability of Lewin's change management model in a hospital setting. *Methods Inf Med.* 2009;48(5):419-428.

Taylor M. The ABCs of ACOs. Accountable care organizations unite hospitals and other providers in caring for the community. *Trustee.* 2010;63(6):12–14.

Thorpe K, Ogden L. The Foundation That Health Reform Lays for Improved Payment, Care Coordination, and Prevention. *Health Aff (Millwood).* 2010;29(6):1183–1187.

Tunis SR, Stryer DB, Clancy CM. Practical clinical trials: increasing the value of clinical research for decision making in clinical and health policy. *JAMA.* 2003 Sep 24;290(12):1624-32.

Vermont Health Care Reform Task Force. *Report of the Health Care Reform Readiness Task Force.* Williston, VT: Department of Vermont Health Access, 2010.

Vest J, Gamm L. A critical review of the research literature on Six Sigma, Lean and StuderGroup's Hardwiring Excellence in the U.S.: the need to demonstrate and communicate the effectiveness of transformation strategies in healthcare. *Implementation Science.* 2009;4(35):1–9.

Weiner B. A theory of organizational readiness for change. *Implementation Science.* 2009;4(67).

Weiner JP, Kfuri T, Chan K, Fowles JB. e-Iatrogenesis: the most critical unintended consequence of CPOE and other HIT. *J Am Med Inform Assoc.* 2007;14(3):387–388.

Wilensky GR. The Policies and Politics of Creating a Comparative Clinical Effectiveness Research Center. *Health Aff (Millwood),* 2009;28(4):w719–w729.

Xirasagar S, Samuels ME, Curtin TF. Management training of physician executives, their leadership style, and care management performance: an empirical study. *Am J Manag Care.* 2006;12(2):101–108.

Zuvekas SH, Cohen JW. Paying physicians by capitation: is the past now prologue? Health *Aff (Millwood).* 2010;29(9):1661–1666.

Glossary and Acronyms

Accountable care organization- Collaborations between physicians, hospitals, and other providers of clinical services that will be clinically and financially accountable for healthcare delivery for designated patient populations in a defined geographic market. The ACO is physician led with a focus on population-based care management and providing services to patients under both public and private payer programs.

Anticompetitive effect- business practices and actions that attempt to or have the potential for reducing competition in a geographic market leading to illegal restraint of trade and antitrust law violations.

Bundled payment- making a single payment for both the services provided by the hospital and the services provided by physicians during an inpatient stay for a particular diagnosis or treatment.[411]

Clinically integrated network- collections of physicians and hospitals working together as an integrated unit to achieve economies of scale in care delivery, enable joint contracting with insurers, and launch programs designed to increase the quality and coordination of patient care while reducing the cost of that care.

Comparative effectiveness research- any work that compares different medical devices, drugs, and treatment methods to determine which are more effective at treating a disease or condition.

Disruptive innovation- "A process by which a product or service takes root initially in simple applications at the bottom of a market and then relentlessly moves 'up market', eventually displacing established competitors."[412]

Ecosystem- "An economic community supported by a foundation of interacting organizations and individuals—the organisms of the business world. The economic community produces goods and services of value to customers, who are themselves members of the ecosystem. The member organisms also include suppliers, lead producers, competitors, and other stakeholders. Over time, they co-evolve their capabilities and roles, and tend to align themselves with the directions set by one or more central companies. Those companies holding leadership roles may change over time, but the function of ecosystem leader is valued by the community because it enables members to move toward shared

---

[411] Harold Miller. June 2010. Pathways for Physician Success Under Healthcare Payment and Delivery Reforms. Report for the American Medical Association (AMA). Part C. Comprehensive Care Payment. Page 26.
[412] Definition of disruptive innovation from website of Clayton Christensen. Accessed online July 29, 2011 at http://claytonchristensen.com/disruptive_innovation.html.

visions to align their investments, and to find mutually supportive roles."[413]

Electronic medical record- A health information technology system that includes a clinical data repository, clinical decision support (CDS), controlled medical vocabulary, computerized provider order entry, pharmacy order entry, and clinical documentation applications. These systems warehouse patient's personal health data for both inpatient and outpatient environments in use by physicians and clinicians to document, monitor, and manage health care delivery.

Electronic health record- This is a record in electronic format capable of being shared across multiple care settings. They may include data in on each patient's demographics, medical history, medications and allergies, laboratory test results, radiology results, vital signs, and billing information. Electronic health records are intended to feed into health information exchanges and the eventual National Health Information Network (NHIN).

Emotional intelligence- How leaders handle themselves and their relationships.

Fee-for-service payment- Payments for unbundled individual services (e.g. office visit, procedure, test, etc) payable to physicians or provider organizations from public or private payer organizations.

Global payment- Form of payment that provides a physician or provider organization a single payment to cover all the costs of care for a patient's treatment requirements during a "specific period of time" regardless of the number of inpatient episodes they experience.[414]

Health system- "Set of institutions and actors that affect people's health, such as organizations that care, health plans, educational systems, and city and county governments."[415]

Monopoly extension- Action of a firm that captures greater surplus from the market and promotes innovation and welfare growth rates.

Monopoly extraction- Actions of the firm that lengthens incumbent tenure, inhibits innovation and welfare growth rates when net intertemporal cost of innovation is negative.

---

[413] Moore, J. (1996). *The Death of Competition: Leadership & Strategy in the Age of Business Ecosystems*. New York: HarperBusiness. Pg. 26.
[414] Harold Miller. June 2010. Pathways for Physician Success Under Healthcare Payment and Delivery Reforms. Report for the American Medical Association (AMA). Part C. Comprehensive Care Payment. Page 26.
[415] Kottke T., Isham G. (July 2010). Measuring Health Care Access and Quality to Improve Health in Populations. *Preventing Chronic Disease*. 7(4): 1-8. Accessed online July 28, 2011, at http://www.cdc.gov/pcd/issues/2010/jul/09_0243.htm.

Quality benchmarks- Clinical quality process or health outcome goals established by CMS or private payers for ACOs to achieve within a specified time period and for a specified beneficiary population in order to qualify for shared savings payments.

Systems thinking- Attaining an understanding of the interrelationships of complex entities and how the individual components can affect the functionality of the whole and serves as part of the foundation for the Learning Organization theory.[416]

Value-based purchasing- Types of payments made as incentive payments for hospitals that meet performance standards based on specified quality measures tracked against specific conditions and measures in a given fiscal year.

Vision setting- The ability to describe the future for the organization and convey it in a meaningful way.

---

[416] Senge P. The fifth discipline: the art and practice of the learning organization. Knopf Doubleday Publishing Group:/New York, NY, 1990, 2006.

Acronyms

Acronym	Meaning
ACO	Accountable care organization
CAH	Critical access hospital
CER	Comparative effectiveness research
CIN	Clinically integrated network
CIP	Clinical integration program
CMS	Center for Medicare and Medicaid services
CMPL	Civil monetary penalties law
EHR	Electronic health record
FFS	Fee-for-service payment system
FQHC	Federally qualified health center
GDP	Gross domestic product
HEDIS	Healthcare effectiveness data and information set
HIPAA	Health Insurance Portability and Accountability Act of 1996
HIT	Health information technology
IDN	Integrated delivery network
IOM	Institute of Medicine
IPA	Independent practice association
MedPAC	Medicare payment advisory council
MSPG	Multi-specialty physician group
MSR	Minimum savings rate
NHE	National health expenditure
NICE	National Institute for Health and Clinical Excellence
P4P	Pay-for-performance payment system
PCMH	Patient-centered medical home
PCORI	Patient-centered outcomes research institute
PCT	Pragmatic randomized clinical trials

Acronyms, cont.

Acronym	Meaning
PHI	Protected health information
PHO	Physician hospital organization
PQRI	Physician quality reporting initiative
PQRS	Physician quality reporting system
RCT	Randomized controlled trial
RHC	Rural health centers
TJC	The joint commission
VBP	Value-based purchasing

Appendix A: CMS Board of Trustees Report (Excerpt)

2010 Annual Report of the Boards of Trustees of the Federal Hospital Insurance and Federal Supplementary Medical Insurance Trust Funds. August 5, 2010
Excerpt from Section II. Overview. Short Range Results

"The financial status of the HI trust fund is substantially improved by the lower expenditures and additional tax revenues instituted by the Affordable Care Act. These changes are estimated to postpone the exhaustion of HI trust fund assets from 2017 under the prior law to 2029 under current law and to 2028 under the alternative scenario. **Despite this significant improvement, however, the fund is still not adequately financed over the next 10 years. HI expenditures have exceeded income annually since 2008 and are projected to continue doing so under current law through 2013.**

The SMI trust fund is adequately financed over the next 10 years and beyond because premium and general revenue income for Parts B and D are reset each year to match expected costs. However, further Congressional overrides of scheduled physician fee reductions, together with an existing "hold-harmless" provision restricting premium increases for most beneficiaries, could jeopardize Part B solvency and require unusual measures to avoid asset depletion. In particular, without legislation, **Part B premiums payable in 2011 and 2012 by new enrollees, high-income enrollees, and State Medicaid programs (on behalf of low-income enrollees) will probably have to be raised significantly above normal requirements to offset the loss of revenues caused by the hold-harmless provision, raising serious equity issues.**

Part B costs have been increasing rapidly, having averaged 8.3 percent annual growth over the last 5 years, and are likely to continue doing so. Under current law, an average annual growth rate of 4.8 percent is projected for the next 5years. This rate is unrealistically constrained due to multiple years of physician fee reductions that would occur under current law, including a scheduled reduction of 23 percent for December of 2010. If Congress continues to override these reductions, as they have for 2003 through November of 2010, the Part B growth rate would instead average roughly 8 percent. For Part D, the average annual increase in expenditures is estimated to be 9.4 percent through 2019. **The U.S. economy is projected to grow at an average annual rate of 5.1 percent during this period, significantly more slowly than Part D and the probable growth rate for Part B.**"

Note: HI = Hospital Insurance; SMI = Supplemental Insurance

Appendix B: Affordable Care Act Section 3502

2010 Patient Protection and Affordable Care Act. Section 3502: Establishing Community Health Teams to Support the Patient-Centered Medical Home. Subsection (c). Requirements for the Health Teams.

"(c) REQUIREMENTS FOR HEALTH TEAMS.—A health team established pursuant to a grant or contract under subsection (a) shall—

(1) establish contractual agreements with primary care providers to provide support services;

(2) support patient-centered medical homes, defined as a mode of care that includes—

(A) personal physicians;

(B) whole person orientation;

(C) coordinated and integrated care;

(D) safe and high-quality care through evidence informed medicine, appropriate use of health information technology, and continuous quality improvements;

(E) expanded access to care; and

(F) payment that recognizes added value from additional components of patient-centered care;

(3) collaborate with local primary care providers and existing State and community based resources to coordinate disease prevention, chronic disease management, transitioning between health care providers and settings and case management for patients, including children, with priority given to those amenable to prevention and with chronic diseases or conditions identified by the Secretary;

(4) in collaboration with local health care providers, develop and implement interdisciplinary, inter-professional care plans that integrate clinical and community preventive and health promotion services for patients, including children, with a priority given to those amenable to prevention and with chronic diseases or conditions identified by the Secretary;

(5) incorporate health care providers, patients, caregivers, and authorized representatives in program design and oversight;

(6) provide support necessary for local primary care providers to—

(A) coordinate and provide access to high-quality health care services;

(B) coordinate and provide access to preventive and health promotion services;

(C) provide access to appropriate specialty care and inpatient services;

(D) provide quality-driven, cost-effective, culturally appropriate, and patient- and family-centered health care;

(E) provide access to pharmacist-delivered medication management services, including medication reconciliation;

(F) provide coordination of the appropriate use of complementary and alternative (CAM) services to those who request such services;

(G) promote effective strategies for treatment planning, monitoring health outcomes and resource use, sharing information, treatment decision support, and organizing care to avoid duplication of service and other medical management approaches intended to improve quality and value of health care services;

(H) provide local access to the continuum of health care services in the most appropriate setting, including access to individuals that implement the care plans of patients and coordinate care, such as integrative health care practitioners;

(I) collect and report data that permits evaluation of the success of the collaborative effort on patient outcomes, including collection of data on patient experience of care, and identification of areas for improvement; and

(J) establish a coordinated system of early identification and referral for children at risk for developmental or behavioral problems such as through the use of infolines, health information technology, or other means as determined by the Secretary;

(7) provide 24-hour care management and support during transitions in care settings including—

(A) a transitional care program that provides onsite visits from the care coordinator, assists with the development of discharge plans and medication reconciliation upon admission to and discharge from the hospitals, nursing home, or other institution setting;

(B) discharge planning and counseling support to providers, patients, caregivers, and authorized representatives;

(C) assuring that post-discharge care plans include medication management, as appropriate;

(D) referrals for mental and behavioral health services, which may include the use of infolines; and

(E) transitional health care needs from adolescence to adulthood;

(8) serve as a liaison to community prevention and treatment programs;

(9) demonstrate a capacity to implement and maintain health information technology that meets the requirements of certified EHR technology (as defined in section 3000 of the Public Health Service Act (42 U.S.C. 300jj)) to facilitate coordination among members of the applicable care team and affiliated primary care practices; and

(10) where applicable, report to the Secretary information on quality measures used under section 399JJ of the Public Health Service Act."

Appendix C: Case Studies

Case Studies: December 2010 Report on Medicare Physician Group Practice Demonstration (Report Excerpt)
Available at:
http://www.cms.gov/DemoProjectsEvalRpts/downloads/PGP_Fact_Sheet.pdf

"Physician Group Practices

CMS selected ten physician groups on a competitive basis to participate in the demonstration. The groups were selected based on technical review panel findings, organizational structure, operational feasibility, geographic location, and demonstration implementation strategy. Multi- specialty physician groups with well-developed clinical and management information systems were encouraged to apply since they were likely to have the ability to put in place the infrastructure necessary to be successful under the demonstration.

The demonstration allows CMS to test new incentives in diverse clinical and organizational environments including freestanding multi-specialty physician group practices, faculty group practices, physician groups that are part of integrated health care systems, and physician network organizations. The demonstration has fostered a nation-wide learning collaborative among the groups who voluntarily participate in this demonstration as a result of their leadership in their communities and profession. CMS is working with the groups to identify successful health care redesign and care management models developed for the demonstration that can be replicated and spread across the health care system.

The ten physician groups represent 5,000 physicians and 220,000 Medicare fee-for-service beneficiaries. The physician groups participating in the demonstration are:
Billings Clinic, Billings, Montana Dartmouth-Hitchcock Clinic, Bedford, New Hampshire The Everett Clinic, Everett, Washington Forsyth Medical Group, Winston-Salem, North Carolina Geisinger Health System, Danville, Pennsylvania Marshfield Clinic, Marshfield, Wisconsin Middlesex Health System, Middletown, Connecticut Park Nicollet Health Services, St. Louis Park, Minnesota St. John's Health System, Springfield, Missouri University of Michigan Faculty Group Practice, Ann Arbor, Michigan

Performance Results

Performance Year 1 Results -- At the end of the first performance year, all 10 of the participating physician groups improved the clinical management of diabetes patients by achieving benchmark or target performance on at least 7 out of 10 diabetes clinical quality measures. Two of the physician groups -- Forsyth Medical Group and St. John's Health System -- achieved benchmark quality performance on all 10-quality measures.

In performance year one, two physician groups shared in savings for improving the overall efficiency of care they furnish their patients. The two physician groups, Marshfield Clinic and the University of Michigan Faculty Group Practice, earned $7.3 million in performance payments for improving the quality and cost efficiency of care as their share of a total of $9.5 million in Medicare savings.

Performance Year 2 Results -- At the end of the second performance year, all 10 of the participating physician groups continued to improve the quality of care for chronically ill patients by achieving benchmark or target performance on at least 25 out of 27 quality markers for patients with diabetes, coronary artery disease and congestive heart failure. Five of the physician groups -- Forsyth Medical Group, Geisinger Clinic, Marshfield Clinic, St. John's Health System, and the University of Michigan Faculty Group Practice -- achieved benchmark quality performance on all 27 quality measures.

In performance year two, four physician groups shared in savings for improving the overall efficiency of care they furnish their patients. The four physician groups, Dartmouth-Hitchcock Clinic, The Everett Clinic, Marshfield Clinic, and the University of Michigan Faculty Group Practice, earned $13.8 million in performance payments for improving the quality and cost efficiency of care as their share of a total of $17.4 million in Medicare savings.

Performance Year 3 Results -- At the end of the third performance year, all 10 of the participating physician groups continued to improve the quality of care for patients with chronic illness or who require preventive care by achieving benchmark or target performance on at least 28 out of 32 quality markers for patients with diabetes, coronary artery disease, congestive heart failure, hypertension, and cancer screening. Two of the physician groups -- Geisinger Clinic and Park Nicollet Health Services -- achieved benchmark quality performance on all 32-quality measures.

Over the first three years of the demonstration, physician groups increased their quality scores an average of 10 percentage points on the diabetes, 11 percentage points on the congestive heart failure measures, 6 percentage points on the coronary artery disease measures, 10 percentage points on the cancer screening measures, and 1 percentage point on the hypertension measures.

In addition to achieving benchmark performance for quality, five physician groups shared in savings under the demonstration's performance payment methodology. The five physician groups, Dartmouth-Hitchcock Clinic, Geisinger Clinic, Marshfield Clinic, St. John's Health System, and the University of Michigan Faculty Group Practice, earned $25.3 million in performance payments for improving the quality and cost efficiency of care as their share of a total of $32.3 million in Medicare savings.

Performance Year 4 Results – At the end of the fourth year of performance evaluation, all ten of the physician groups achieved benchmark performance on at least 29 of the 32 measures. Three groups – Geisinger Clinic, Marshfield Clinic, and Park Nicollet Health Services achieved benchmark performance on all 32 performance measures and all ten of the groups achieved benchmark performance on the ten heart failure and seven coronary artery disease measures.

The PGPs have increased their quality scores from baseline to performance year 4 an average of 10 percentage points on the diabetes measures, 13 percentage points on the heart failure measures, 6 percentage points on the coronary artery disease measures, 9 percentage points on the cancer screening measures, and 3 percentage points on the hypertension measures.

In addition to the quality performance, five physician groups -- Dartmouth-Hitchcock Clinic, Geisinger Clinic, Marshfield Clinic, St. John's Health System, University of Michigan -- earned incentive payments based on the estimated savings in Medicare expenditures for the patient population they serve. The groups received performance payments totaling $31.7 million as their share of the $38.7 million of savings generated for the Medicare Trust Funds in performance year 4.

Care Management Strategies
One of the unique features of this demonstration is that physician groups have the flexibility to redesign care processes, invest in care management initiatives, and target patient populations that can benefit from more effective and efficient delivery of care. This helps Medicare beneficiaries maintain their health and avoid further illness and admissions to the hospital. The following provides an overview of the quality and efficiency innovations underway at each demonstration site.

Billings Clinic focuses on providing evidence-based care, including preventive services, at the time of each patient visit. This is accomplished by the creation of a summary that identifies gaps in care and redesigning workflow for nursing and support staff. An example is the improved management of patients with diabetes through the use of a diabetes patient registry, electronic medical record modules, a team of diabetes experts/educators offering a patient friendly report card, and a pharmacy driven insulin protocol for glycemic control in the inpatient setting. As a result of these efforts focused on diabetes care, a majority of the clinic's eligible physicians have been recognized through NCQA's Diabetes Physician Recognition Program for excellence in diabetes care. The Clinic also continues efforts to: (1) redesign heart failure care by leveraging an RN-directed telephonic computerized patient monitoring system; (2) decrease medication errors by using electronic prescribing and reconciling medications at every care opportunity; (3) expand the palliative care team; and (4) develop a community crisis center to benefit dual eligible patients with mental health related events. For more information, contact: F. Douglas Carr, M.D. at dcarr@billingsclinic.org.

Dartmouth-Hitchcock Clinic focuses on improving quality while reducing costs through implementation of evidence-based care initiatives. The clinic uses recognized experts to educate physicians and support staff in understanding evidence-based care guidelines. Electronic tools and reports including disease registries, dashboard reports to track progress on quality measures, and electronic medical record enhancements are used by the physicians and staff at the point of patient contact to proactively identify patients with gaps in chronic disease care and focus on preventive care. Evidence-based care implementation also requires changing workflow processes and roles for support staff. For example, in the primary care departments, the physician and nurse work together to provide a patient centered approach to care highlighted by patient and family involvement in developing and implementing the plan of care. Care is coordinated by nurses who target interventions to high-risk patients using motivational education on disease and personal health care through in-office visits and/or post hospital discharge phone calls. For more information, contact: Barbara Walters, D.O. at Barbara.A.Walters@Hitchcock.org.

The Everett Clinic is improving health care delivery to seniors by: (1) providing electronic patient reports to primary care physicians to use in addressing issues with diabetes, heart disease, hypertension, and mammogram and colonoscopy screening results; (2) coaching hospitalized patients and caretakers to guide them through complicated care processes during hospital stays and upon discharge; (3) having physicians follow-up with patients within ten days of hospital discharge to address any unsolved or new health problems; (4) partnering with local providers to deploy new palliative care programs in physicians' offices to improve end-of-life care for approximately 800 patients; (5)

making delivery of primary care services more efficient and patient-friendly by removing non-value-added steps ("lean principles"); and (6) implementing evidence based guidelines to improve appropriateness for ordering radiology imaging tests. For more information, contact: James Lee, M.D. at Jlee@everettclinic.com.

Forsyth Medical Group focuses on care coordination at transitions of care to promote safe, patient-centered services. Concentration on the frail elderly, high-risk diseases and poly-pharmacy issues identifies those patients at greatest risk for readmission and adverse events associated with multiple therapies. COMPASS Disease Management Navigators and Safe Med Pharmacists collaborate with inpatient services and systems to identify these at risk populations. Programs target inpatient discharges to assess the patient's understanding and adherence to discharge instructions and to navigate the patient back to the primary care provider for follow-up care. The Chronic Care Model transitions to a Patient Centered Medical Home with this emphasis on care coordination and self-management education for chronic conditions. Physician champions promote programs targeted to improve quality measures and patient outcomes. Educational materials continue to reach a broad range of patients with chronic disease and the scope of education was broadened to include end of life care, fall risk assessment and prevention and medication reconciliation and safety. The COMPASS Disease Management Program grew in both services offered to patients and contacts by nurse disease managers with an expanded emphasis on preventive care and intervening with patients with pre-disease for diabetes and peripheral arterial disease. For more information, contact: Nan Holland, R.N. at nlholland@novanthealth.org.

Geisinger Clinic focuses on: (1) A unique implementation of the Medical Home model of care including patient-centered, team based care across the continuum, practice-integrated case management, fully revamped payment incentives, and the proactive identification of high risk patients; (2) Transitions of care coordination and case management including medication reconciliation, enhanced access for early post discharge follow-up, self-management Action plans for chronic care exacerbation management, telephonic and/or device-based remote monitoring and associated order execution for beneficiaries with congestive heart failure; (3) Using its electronic health record to identify and systematically resolve care gaps to ensure comprehensive prevention and treatment of all medical conditions; (4) Automating identification, notification and scheduling of pneumococcal and influenza immunization services; and (5) Redesigned systems of care monitored by performance on "all or none" evidence-based bundles for diabetes, coronary artery disease, chronic kidney disease and adult prevention. For more information, contact: Ronald A. Paulus, M.D. at: rapaulus@geisinger.edu.

Marshfield Clinic is participating in the demonstration as a reflection of its mission to serve patients through accessible, high quality health care, research and education. The clinic expanded a number of on-going successful initiatives and accelerated the development and adoption of others including enhancements to its electronic health record to systematically expand a support structure to implement care management and coordination. Specifically, the clinic expanded its anticoagulation care management program across the entire system and developed a heart failure care management program with the goal of improving clinical care, improving quality of life and decreasing costs and hospitalizations. In addition, the clinic continues to promote use of its nurse advice line, develop clinical practice guidelines and monitor population-based clinical performance through clinical dashboards. For more information, contact: Theodore A. Praxel, M.D. at praxel.theodore@marshfieldclinic.org.

Middlesex Health System is participating in the project as a network of physicians affiliated with a community hospital. Interventions focus on processes to improve electronic linkages and communications among all providers for each patient and demonstrate quality and safety across the continuum of care. Building on a long history of close collaboration between the hospital, its medical staff and a commitment to the mission of community health improvement, the Hospital commissioned a community health assessment to identify service gaps and secure an understanding of the current and projected health needs of the service area. Services such as an inpatient COPD pathway and enhanced outpatient care for COPD patients were deployed to close existing service gaps. Care Management programs and support services designed to educate and promote patient self- management skills around chronic diseases such as heart failure, diabetes, asthma and Nurse Navigators for cancer patients are offered. Efforts to ensure appropriate immunizations, cancer screenings, support groups, smoking cessation program availability, medication safety, innovative palliative care, and use of tele-monitoring technology are also utilized. For more information, contact: Arthur McDowell, M.D. at Arthur_McDowell_MD@midhosp.org.

Park Nicollet Health Services started an inpatient palliative care program and continues to enhance their care of patients with diabetes and heart failure. An innovative telephone monitoring program was instituted for high-risk heart failure patients. Over 560 patients with heart failure have been enrolled into an automated telephonic program to improve their quality of life. Each patient makes a daily call to provide weight and symptom reports, allowing nurse case managers at the clinic to spot early signs of deterioration and intervene in their heart failure management. Electronic patient registries are the cornerstone of management for patients with chronic disease and have been combined with Park Nicollet's existing electronic medical record. As a result, patient information can be reviewed by the physician care team prior to upcoming appointments for unmet health care needs. Another improvement was initiating same-day lab testing prior to the visit for many of these chronic disease patients. Using these steps, along with pre-visit planning, significantly increased time for important face-to-face interaction with the provider when crucial decisions need to be made about treatment. For more information, contact: Mark Skubic at Mark.Skubic@ParkNicollet.com.

St. John's Health System developed a comprehensive patient registry to respond to the demonstration's quality improvement incentives. The registry is designed to track patient information, identify gaps in care, and ensure that appropriate and timely care is provided. A key element of the patient registry is the visit planner that is designed to complement physicians' established clinical work-flow process. It provides a "to do" list for physicians prior to each patient visit, with reminders for needed tests or interventions. The visit planner consists of a one-page summary for each patient showing key demographic and clinical data, including test dates and results. An exception list highlights tests or interventions for which the patient is due and provides physicians with reports on areas where patient care can be improved. The provider/clinic manger uses the decentralized reporting feature to generate un-blinded outcome reports from the registry at both the individual provider and clinic levels. In addition, a case manager was deployed in the emergency department to collaborate with the health system and community services to provide transition planning. A heart failure team has been designated to drive the coordination of heart failure care, provider education, and increase outcome success. Special groups are being convened to focus on diabetic retinal eye exams, mammography and colorectal cancer screenings. For more information, contact: James T. Rogers, M.D. at James.Rogers@Mercy.net or Donna Smith at Donna.Smith@Mercy.net.

University of Michigan Faculty Group Practice focus on improving transitional care and complex care coordination for Medicare patients. The group's transitional care call-back program contacts Medicare patients discharged from the emergency department and acute care hospital to address gaps in care during the transition between care settings. This program also provides short-term care coordination with linkages to visiting nurse and community services and coordination with primary care and specialty clinics. The group also developed a complex care coordination program with social workers and nurses who work with physicians to assist patients who have multiple risks, high costs and complex health status. In the hospital setting, the group developed a pharmacy facilitated discharge program for patients with high-risk medications and a palliative care consult service to work with patients and families to ease end of life transitions. In the second year of the project, these services were joined by a sub-acute service that brings geriatric faculty into local sub-acute facilities and an expanded geriatric inpatient consult service that provides expertise in geriatric medicine and transitional care. The group also has a heart failure nurse telemanagement program that coordinates with its heart failure clinics. The group's quality program uses patient registries with relevant quality indicators and individual physician/provider feedback on the quality of care for their patients. For more information, contact: Caroline S. Blaum, M.D. at cblaum@umich.edu.

For More Information
The demonstration started April 1, 2005 and the fifth performance year ended March 31, 2010. As included in The Affordable Care Act, we are currently working on a transitional demonstration while the Medicare Shared Savings Program is being developed.
For additional information, visit the Physician Group Practice webpage at:
http://www.cms.DHHS.gov/DemoProjectsEvalRpts/MD"

Appendix D: Joint Principles of PCMH

Joint Principles of the Patient-Centered Medical Home[417]	
Personal Physician	Each patient has an ongoing relationship with a personal physician trained to provide first contact, continuous and comprehensive care.
Physician directed medical practice	The personal physician leads a team of individuals at the prActice level who collectively take responsibility for the ongoing care of patients.
Whole person orientation	The personal physician is responsible for providing for all the patient's health care needs or taking responsibility for appropriately arranging care with other qualified professionals. This includes care for all stages of life; acute care, chronic care, preventive services, and end of life care.
Care is coordinated and/or integrated	--across all elements of the complex health care system (e.g., subspecialty care, hospitals, home health agencies, nursing homes) and the patient's community (e.g., family, public and private community-based services). Care is facilitated by registries, information technology, health information exchange, and other means to assure that patients get the indicated care when and where they need and want it in a culturally and linguistically appropriate manner.
Quality and Safety	<ul><li>Practices advocate for their patients to support the attainment of optimal, patient-centered outcomes that are defined by a care planning process driven by a compassionate, robust partnership between physicians, patients, and the patient's family.</li><li>Evidence-based medicine and clinical decision-support tools guide decision making.</li><li>Physicians in the practice accept accountability for continuous quality improvement through voluntary engagement in performance measurement and improvement.</li><li>Patients Actively participate in decision-making and feedback is sought to ensure patients' expectations are being met.</li><li>Information technology is utilized appropriately to support optimal patient care, performance measurement, patient education, and enhanced communication.</li><li>Practices go through a voluntary recognition process by an appropriate non-governmental entity to demonstrate that they have the capabilities to provide patient centered services consistent with the medical home model.</li><li>Patients and families participate in quality improvement Activities at the practice level.</li></ul>

---

[417] Seven principles and descriptions come from the Patient-Centered Primary Care Collaborative. Accessed online August 17, 2011, at http://www.pcpcc.net/joint-principles.

Joint Principles of the Patient-Centered Medical Home[417]	
Enhanced Access	Care is available through systems such as open scheduling, expanded hours and new options for communication between patients, their personal physician, and practice staff.
Payment	It appropriately recognizes the added value provided to patients who have a patient-centered medical home. The payment structure should be based on the following framework: • It should reflect the value of physician and non-physician staff patient-centered care management work that falls outside of the face-to-face visit. • It should pay for services associated with coordination of care both within a given practice and between consultants, ancillary providers, and community resources. • It should support adoption and use of health information technology for quality improvement. • It should support provision of enhanced communication access such as secure e-mail and telephone consultation. • It should recognize the value of physician work associated with remote monitoring of clinical data using technology. • It should allow for separate fee-for-service payments for face-to-face visits. (Payments for care management services that fall outside of the face-to-face visit, as described above, should not result in a reduction in the payments for face-to-face visits). • It should recognize case mix differences in the patient population being treated within the practice. • It should allow physicians to share in savings from reduced hospitalizations associated with physician-guided care management in the office setting. • It should allow for additional payments for achieving measurable and continuous quality improvements.

Appendix E: Commonwealth Fund Study
Excerpt from Commonwealth Fund Study on The Potential of Global Payment: Insights From the Field (February 2010)

"Global payment comes in many shapes and sizes, but has the common characteristic of holding providers financially accountable, to a greater or lesser degree, for the total cost of care provided to the patient population assigned to them. One critical element, according to the experts, is that financial incentives to manage patient resource use must exceed economic incentives to provide too much or too little care.

Global payment models vary based on the amount of risk assumed by the provider organization and the methods used to limit risks. Risks can be limited based on what services are included in the global payment and what, if any, adjustments are considered when evaluating provider performance. Risks can be limited based on what services are included in the global payment and what, if any, adjustments are considered when evaluating provider performance.

Sidebar: Capitation Problems Addressed in Next Generation Global Payment Models
- Incentive to skimp on care
- Incentive to skim risk
- No accountability for quality
- Limited ability to manage risk
- Limited data
- Patient and provider dissatisfaction with "gatekeeping"
- Lack of provider financial reserves
- Provider reluctance to assume risk

The potential cost exposure for professional services is minimal relative to the highly variable cost generated by the small percentage of patients who are hospitalized. Alternatively, provider organizations can be at risk for all covered services, but the risk amount may be limited to the approximate amount the provider would have received for those patients if they were paid on a fee-for-service basis.

Global payments are funded and administered in a wide variety of ways. Particularly with very large integrated provider organizations, an agreed-upon amount of money per member rep- resenting the total budget available to care for all needed services for patients under the provider's care is prospectively deposited by the payer in a provider-owned account. Any costs incurred outside the contracted provider organization are then drawn from this account either by the payer or the provider organization.

Alternatively, when the provider is at risk only for a subset of covered services for their patient population, a slice of the expected total cost per member is prospectively allocated into a provider-owned account or into a dedicated account held by the payer. Claims for services that are performed by providers that are not part of the provider organization are typically drawn from this account and the balance is available to the provider to compensate for the services they have rendered within their system.

Each payer–provider global payment arrangement considers multiple methodological variations. Typically, no two arrangements are the same for providers contracting with multiple plans and for payers contracting with multiple providers. Plans and providers report variations in global payment arrangements including:

- Which patients are included (e.g., Medicare, Medicaid, commercial)
- Which products are included (e.g., fully insured, self-insured, HMO, PPO)
- How to determine which patients are under the provider's care (e.g., patients specify and lock in provider, patients are attributed to providers based on de facto provider use)
- Which covered services are included (e.g., all covered services, all services except pharmacy, all services except mental health, professional services only, primary care services only, etc.)
- Methodology and technology used for risk adjustment
- Methodology used for adjustment for catastrophic claims
- How risk is limited based on performance levels around a target, (e.g., in some types of arrangements providers can be at risk for +/− 10% of what their fee-for-service payments would have been, with the payer retaining the balance of the risk)
- How providers outside the globally paid organization are contracted and paid
- Level of fee-for-service payments or withholds made prior to reconciliation
- Timing and data sharing for reconciliation payments

A full range of provider structures are operating successfully under global payment.

Large, integrated delivery systems are able to work well under global payment. However, since the vast majority of physicians in the U.S. are not part of such structures, conventional wisdom suggests that global payment can at best be applied only to a small subset of providers or that all providers will ultimately need to become part of such a system. The provider leaders interviewed for this project represented a wide range of organizational sizes and types. Very large, hospital-dominated systems; large multispecialty clinics with and without hospital ownership; mid-sized primary care practices; and IPAs representing very small primary care practices all have found ways to be successful in global payment programs. Some successful IPAs have expanded or are in the process of expanding geographically into new, previously unorganized markets. They are finding that the information and clinical support infrastructures they have refined over the years can be leveraged across a broader physician base."[418]

---

[418] Robinow A. The Potential of Global Payment: Insights From the Field. *Commonwealth Fund Report*. 2010. pp. 3-5: What is Global Payment? (Excerpt), pp. 13-14: Provider structures using global payments. Accessed online September 09, 2011, at http://www.commonwealthfund.org/~/media/Files/Publications/Fund%20Report/2010/Feb/1373_Robinow_potential_global_pay ment.pdf.

Appendix F: Challenges, Risks, and Mitigation Strategies
Compilation of Challenges, Risks and Mitigation Strategies for All Chapters

Appendix F: Chapter 2 Challenges and Risks

Challenges	Risks
Implementing an integrated performance reporting system.	Revenue lost in transition to new reimbursement models.
Achieving consensus across ACO participant medical homes on clinical guidelines.	Without consensus on clinical guidelines, unintended adverse consequences may be experienced in patient care services due to a lack of standardization during the shift to population-based disease condition management.
Aligning advanced medical home objectives with ACO qualification level criteria.	Lost opportunity to further solidify the linkage between primary care and hospital organizations.
Attribution of patients to specific providers in ACOs.419	Loss of required beneficiaries and inability to hold an ACO accountable for a patient's care received outside their region.420
Having sufficient resources to manage large-scale complexity, overcome tradition, and change activities required for a multiyear ACO implementation.	Emergence of barriers and silos; slower rates of adoption; and loss of efficiency and achieving economies of scale for all ACO participants.
Managing the impact on revenue cycle for hospitals when chronic disease management has been optimized but payment methods have not caught up.	Negative economic impact on consumers related to potentially higher out-of-pocket expenses and increased cost of navigating the care system.

---

[419] Luft HS. Becoming accountable—opportunities and obstacles for ACOs. *N Engl J Med.* 2010;363(15):1389-1391.
[420] Luft HS. Becoming accountable—opportunities and obstacles for ACOs. *N Engl J Med.* 2010;363(15):1389-1391.

Potential Mitigation Strategies
√ **Impact on patient care**: Use of predictive modeling tools[421] for identification of chronically illness population segments, and drilling down to individual patients for targeted prevention efforts.
√ **Impact on patient care:** Implement ambulatory care and disease management programs[44] to meet the patient's needs following inpatient treatment, and interventions, and between physician office visits.
√ **Lack of investment 1:** Engaging resources to establish financial plans that identify options for securing needed investments to cover capital, training, and expenses of the formation, ramp-up, and transition periods.
√ **Lack of investment 2:** Encouraging physicians in need of capital infusion to consider partnering with health systems and such large entities as health plans.
√ **Mitigating financial impact**: Physicians and providers negotiate rapid-cycle implementation of new payment methods to compensate for new and improved models of healthcare services.
√ **Organizational transformation**: Utilize change management and process improvement methodologies to minimize risk and facilitate adoption.

---

[421] Boland P, Polakoff P, Schwab T. Accountable care organizations hold promise, but will they achieve cost and quality targets? *Manag Care*. 2010;19(10):12-6, 19.

Appendix F: Chapter 3 Challenges and Risks

Challenges	Risks
Engaging physicians to develop and participate in a network initiative and gaining their "buy-in."	Hospital systems may develop networks in isolation or from the top down and fail to maintain a sufficient number of providers to adequately manage the patient population.
Determining whether an ACO will be physician practice-led or hospital-led.	Selection of a suboptimal leadership model that doesn't maximize improvement in quality and cost of care.
Establishing a strong clinical integration program that meets the Medicare ACO requirement for participants.	Hospitals that create true cooperation and interdependence and move from a focus on inpatient to outpatient services may lose revenue in the near term.[422]
Securing seed funding for an ACO startup.	Lack of investment will strain CIN/ACO participant's ability to secure necessary infrastructure, processes, and talent.
Securing competent leadership to ensure the success of the CIN and/or ACO and mitigate risk of failure.	Continued fragmentation and lack of synergy across the ecosystem resulting in setbacks and inability to achieve goals.

Potential Mitigation Strategies

√ **Engaging Physicians**. Provider organizations should consider bolstering their physician network development initiatives to strengthen early physician engagement in the development and management of the CIN or ACO.

√ **Who Drives the Bus.** Regardless of whether the ACO is led by a physician practice or hospital, its stakeholders should elect the board of directors from participant organizations and it should establish a shared governance approach.

√ **Collaboration**. CIN and ACO participants should collaborate with payers early in planning an ACO startup to ensure alignment with risk sharing models, contracts and incentives to mitigate loss of revenue during the transition period.

√ **Funding.** Leaders should proactively seek grant opportunities for startup funds through the CMS Innovation Center and other entities sponsoring ACO demonstration projects.

---

[422] Kocher R, Sahni NR. Physicians versus hospitals as leaders of accountable care organizations. *N Engl J Med.* 2010;363(27):2579–2582.

Appendix F: Chapter 4 Challenges and Risks

Challenges	Risks
Securing an adequate physician and nursing professional workforce to meet patient demand for healthcare services.	Shortage of clinical professionals to care for a larger patient population and inability to meet new quality and productivity requirements.
Funding the determinants of innovation (development, ownership, diffusion) to maintain a pipeline of operational improvements.	Stalling the growth of the CIN or ACO and not being able to meet an ever increasingly greater demand for improvement in healthcare service quality.
Transitioning physician network operations from a traditional supplier focus to a partnership focus in relation to integrated delivery networks and physician-hospital organizations.	Continued and presence of barriers to collaboration and trust that affect movement toward the two-sided risk model.
Third-party payers may not wish to work with a developing CIN or ACO.	CIN/ACO administrative functions hampered due to lack of such expertise as underwriting and data mining in deriving population level health statistics.

Potential Mitigation Strategies

√ Engage the physicians early in the process and give them the resources to lead the process. Developing a formal communication plan with slide decks, collaterals, and other venues are worth the time and energy.

√ Clearly define the near term technologies needs and research vendors that can meet those narrowly defined needs. Avoid "world hunger" approaches to technology in the near term as you get your initiative underway.

√ Engage third party payers early enough to gauge their willingness to work with the CIN/ACO and to open dialog about clinical interventions that would bring the greatest value to your mutual patients.

√ Strive for an innovative approach and think "outside the box" to find novel arrangements that allow "win-win" situations for the stakeholders involved.

Appendix F: Chapter 5 Challenges and Risks

Challenges	Risks
Ensuring that clinical operations across CIN/ACO participants demonstrate the indicia of clinical integration established by the FTC.	If indicia of clinical integration are not met, the FTC or DOJ can rule against the formation of a CIN and or ACO and unwind the makings of the network.
Moving quickly enough to remain competitive in a market amidst the changing landscape of federal safe harbors and state antitrust laws.	Loss of opportunities to form the best non-exclusive joint ventures for the benefit of the local patient and beneficiary population.
Maintaining tax-exempt status of a Medicare ACO and keeping service lines that generate unrelated business income at arms length from the ACO.	Loss of tax-exempt status would result in significant federal and state tax burdens on shared savings distributions.
Maintaining government affairs resources to ensure regulatory compliance and monitor the changing landscape of regulations for the Shared Savings Program, HITECH Act, HIPAA, and other laws.	Lack of insights for CIN and ACO leaders on regulatory matters and risk of loss of competitive balance in geographic markets with the potential of creating anticompetitive practices.

Potential Mitigation Strategies

√ Conduct an antitrust and regulatory readiness assessment that includes the areas of clinical, legal, financial, and administrative operations.

√ Engage legal counsel with expertise in antitrust matters, IRS Code implications, and state regulatory issues pertinent to CIN/ACO legal and contractual arrangements.

√ Monitor changes in federal and state laws and regulations as they are released.

√ Develop a strategy for clinically integrated networks that are needed to meet the formative requirements for the Medicare ACO.

√ Develop an antitrust and regulatory action plan to ensure compliance across the framework of federal and state antitrust laws and regulations.

Appendix F: Chapter 6 Challenges and Risks

Challenges	Risks
Aggregation of patient health information from disparate systems at different levels of maturity.	Inefficient interfaces between EMRs and other health information technology across CIN/ACO participants. Creates potential for patient data corruption and breakdown in data transfer with patient transitions.
Selecting and implementing a CDRS to meet the business intelligence needs of CINs and ACOs.	Implementing CDRS in an environment in which true integration and HIE does not truly exist is a large challenge for the industry.
Enabling the HIE deployment framework to benefit all CIN/ACO participants.	Occurrence of technology incompatibilities; inability to stratify risk across participants; and insufficient clinical decision support that negatively impacts quality of patient care.
Meeting Stage 2 and 3 criteria (yet to be defined) for CMS Meaningful Use of EHRs program.	May put future incentive payments to eligible providers and hospitals at risk.
Instituting coordinated network-wide ICD-10 conversion plans.	Not planning sufficiently for ICD-10 conversion could result in negative impact to CIN/ACO revenue cycle and disrupt continuity of care.

Appendix F: Chapter 6 Challenges and Risks, cont.

Potential Mitigation Strategies
√ Knowing the customer and focusing on physician workflow and clinical decision support needs.
√ Ensuring effective project implementation of semantic terminology and conversions.
√ For CDRS carefully define the near term reporting needs and limit the scope of work to definable elements that will reap the greatest value to the CIN/ACO.
√ Establishing cross-functional committees to manage HIE implementations.
√ Ensuring that all health data elements and disparate systems are accounted for in HIE required interfaces.
√ Engaging an HIE oversight council with C-level executives who make key decisions to mitigate strategic risks and set priorities to establish the HIE deployment framework.

Appendix F: Chapter 7 Challenges and Risks

Challenges	Risks
Factoring in local variations in populations, patient conditions and service utilization for comparative performance measurement and reporting.	Having incomplete and potentially inaccurate comparisons of ACOs and CINs clinical outcomes performance.
Meeting reporting requirements for multiple programs whose measures are not yet harmonized.	Conflicting Meaningful Use, HEDIS, PQRS, and other measures may create burdensome workloads and unnecessary stress on physician practices thus increasing the potential for variations inaccuracies in reported clinical and financial results.
Fully evaluating patient and caregiver experience and linking responses to specific episodes of care.	Not capturing sufficient data to evaluate the qualitative perception of patients on the care received and of physicians or nurses on the care delivered.
Ensuring sufficient training is put in place and attended by physicians and clinicians on the transition from ICD-9 to ICD-10.	Not factoring in ICD-10 transition to quality measure trends post 2013 may result in inaccuracies in evaluating CIN/ACO performance on health outcomes.
Focusing on reporting of static, regulatory required metrics, rather than identifying the underlying root cause and forgetting to make continuous quality improvements.	Meeting all quality metrics, but having no improvement in quality or reductions on cost, thereby missing out on shared savings or other incentives.

Chapter 7 Challenges and Risks, cont.

Potential Mitigation Strategies
√ Support requests for input to federal rule making processes with meaningful and well-constructed ideas to assist legislators in crafting new or refined laws.
√ Implement advanced clinical decision support tools that are integrated with harmonized performance reporting. Engage physicians in quality metric development and performance improvement teams to identify opportunities to improve processes, reduce waste, and achieve cost savings that effect transformation around the structure of care, process of care, and health outcomes at the population level.
√ Upgrade the quality management team with sufficient resources so that team members can not only monitor and report but can also measure and improve structure, process, and outcomes.

Appendix F: Chapter 8 Challenges and Risks

Challenges	Risks
Understanding the need for clinical decision support in a CIN/ACO, and how best to use CER results.	Making coverage and clinical decisions without adequate, supporting research findings. Continue "business as usual" without investing in effective decision support.
Ensuring that clinical decision support uses CER to improve evidence-based care.	Decision making without adequate or advanced clinical decision support (i.e., using evidence-based medicine, at the point of care, based on patient-specific requirements).
Understanding capital and actuarial requirements of the ACO, and making decisions based on the best medicine and quality care, rather than educated guesses.	Not doing the right thing for the CIN/ACO and patient due to peer or salesman pressure.
Giving sufficient time and effort to pharmacy and therapeutics (P&T) and Quality Committee work to determine the best clinical pathways to fulfill financial (ACO health plan), clinical (physician), and patient obligations.	Use of incomplete information on various treatment modalities leading to incorrect decisions that violate Hippocratic or fiduciary duties.
Finding appropriate advanced clinical decision support service, whether internally generated or outsourced.	Using existing CER models but learning too late that they do not apply to your patient population.

Appendix F: Chapter 8 Challenges and Risks, cont.

Potential Mitigation Strategies
√ Identify appropriate sources of information to make informed coverage and clinical decisions.
√ Build off lessons learned and best practice from various sources, including AHRQ, CMS, and experienced private sector organizations, including non-profit groups and health insurance payers.
√ Maintain vibrant and effective P&T and quality committee processes.
√ Keep track of new developments in government, and private sector comparative effectiveness research. Look for ways to leverage all resources, to reduce the cost of clinical decision support and coverage determinations.

Appendix F: Chapter 9 Challenges and Risks

Challenges	Risks
Developing a transition plan for increasing risk tolerance and understanding commensurate rewards in the CIN/ACO while working in a largely indemnity oriented market.	Moving too early without new funding sources may result in the inability to underwrite loss of inpatient revenues, while moving too late may result in losing competitive advantage in the market.
Development of total cost-of-care actuarial and accounting capabilities that account for performance measures.	Inadequate infrastructure to track and monitor outcomes measures and performance may result in suboptimal insights for physicians and CIN/ACO leadership about the organization's financial performance and outcomes.
Instituting curriculum redesign in AMCs to ensure future physicians receive proper training on payment and compensation model reforms.	Inadequate changes to physician training will result in future physicians not being aware of forthcoming reforms that impact their future compensation and payment for services.
Sharing of risk and distribution of shared gains/losses among participating physicians and participants in a Medicare ACO.	Unintended consequences from shared savings programs that result in negative impact to quality of patient care services.

Potential Mitigation Strategies

√ Understand both risks and rewards, and allocate the rewards according to risk assumed.

√ Begin to pilot-test shared risk initiatives to develop core competencies.

√ Begin to explore total cost of care accounting vehicles.

√ Engage financial modeling expertise to forecast financial impacts on all stakeholders based on changes needed in pay-for-performance, clinical integration, and ACO programs.

√ Plan for early launch of payer relationship strategy discussions to move toward multi-payer ACO models at an accelerated pace.

√ AMCs apply MedPAC's recommendation to strengthen future physicians skills in care delivery and organizational leadership under reformed payment systems.

Appendix G: 33 Final Quality Measures

The following table is a list of the 33 final quality measures for the first performance period of the CMS Shared Savings Program.[423]

No.	Domain	Measure Title and Description	NQF Measure #/Measure Steward
AIM: Better Care for Individuals			
1.	Patient/Care Giver Experience	Clinician/Group CAHPS: Getting Timely Care, Appointments and Information	NQF #5, AHRQ
2.	Patient/Care Giver Experience	Clinician/Group CAHPS: How Well Your Doctors Communicate	NQF #5, AHRQ
3.	Patient/Care Giver Experience	Clinician/Group CAHPS: Access to Specialists	NQF #5, AHRQ
4.	Patient/Care Giver Experience	Clinician/Group CAHPS: Patients' Rating of Doctor	NQF #5, AHRQ
5.	Patient/Care Giver Experience	Clinician/Group CAHPS: Health Promotion and Education	NQF #5, AHRQ
6.	Patient/Care Giver Experience	Clinician/Group CAHPS: Shared Decision Making	NQF #5, AHRQ
7.	Patient/Care Giver Experience	Medicare Advantage CAHPS: Health Status/Functional Status	NQF #6, AHRQ
8.	Care Coordination/ Patient Safety	Risk-Standardized, All Condition Readmission:	NQF #TBD CMS
9.	Care Coordination/ Patient Safety	Ambulatory Sensitive Conditions Admissions: Chronic obstructive pulmonary disease	NQF #275 AHRQ
10.	Care Coordination/ Patient Safety	Ambulatory Sensitive Conditions Admissions: Congestive Heart Failure	NQF #277 AHRQ
11.	Care Coordination/ Patient Safety	Percentage of PCPs who Successfully Qualify for an EHR Incentive Payment	CMS
12.	Care Coordination/ Patient Safety	Medication Reconciliation: Reconciliation After Discharge from an Inpatient Facility	NQF #97 AMAPCPI/ NCQA

[423] Centers for Medicare & Medicaid Services. *Medicare Shared Savings Program: Accountable Care Organizations.* October 2011. 42 CFR Part 425. [CMS-1345-F]. Section II.F.2. Measures to Assess the Quality of Care Furnished by an ACO. pp. 324-26. Accessed online October 21, 2011 at http://www.ofr.gov/inspection.aspx.

Appendix G: 33 Final Quality Measures, cont.

No.	Domain	Measure Title and Description	Measure Type
13.	Care Coordination/ Patient Safety	Falls: Screening for Fall Risk .	NQF #101 NCQA
AIM: Better Health for Populations			
14.	Preventive Health	Influenza Immunization:	NQF #41 AMA-PCPI
15.	Preventive Health	Pneumococcal Vaccination	NQF #43 NCQA
16.	Preventive Health	Adult Weight Screening and Follow-up	NQF #421 CMS
17.	Preventive Health	Tobacco Use Assessment and Tobacco Cessation Intervention	NQF #28 AMA-PCPI
18.	Preventive Health	Depression Screening	NQF #418 CMS
19.	Preventive Health	Colorectal Cancer Screening	NQF #34 NCQA
20.	Preventive Health	Mammography Screening	NQF #31 NCQA
21.	Preventive Health	Proportion of Adults 18+ who had their Blood Pressure Measured within the preceding 2 years	CMS
22.	At-Risk Population- Diabetes	Diabetes Composite (All or Nothing Scoring): Hemoglobin A1c Control (<8 percent)	NQF #0729 MN Community Measurement
23.	At Risk Population Diabetes	Diabetes Composite (All or Nothing Scoring): Low Density Lipoprotein (<100)	NQF #0729 MN Community Measurement
24.	At Risk Population Diabetes	Diabetes Composite (All or Nothing Scoring): Blood Pressure <140/90	NQF #0729 MN Community Measurement
25.	At Risk Population Diabetes	Diabetes Composite (All or Nothing Scoring): Tobacco Non-Use	NQF #0729 MN Community Measurement
26.	At Risk Population Diabetes	Diabetes Composite (All or Nothing Scoring): Aspirin Use	NQF #0729 MN Community Measurement
27.	At Risk Population Diabetes	Diabetes Mellitus: Hemoglobin A1c Poor Control (>9 percent)	NQF #59 NCQA
28.	At Risk Population Hypertension	Hypertension (HTN): Blood Pressure Control	NQF #18 NCQA
29.	At Risk Population — Ischemic Vascular Disease	Ischemic Vascular Disease (IVD): Complete Lipid Profile and LDL Control<mg/dl	NQF #75 NCQA
30.	At Risk Population — Ischemic Vascular Disease	Ischemic Vascular Disease (IVD): Use of Aspirin or Another Antithrombotic	NQF #68 NCQA

Appendix G: 33 Final Quality Measures, cont.

No.	Domain	Measure Title and Description	NQF Measure #/ Measure Steward
31	At Risk Population Heart Failure	Heart Failure: Beta-Blocker Therapy for Left Ventricular Systolic Dysfunction (LVSD) Percentage of patients aged 18 years and older with a diagnosis of heart failure who also have LVSD (LVEF <40%) and who were prescribed beta-blocker therapy.	NQF #83 AMA-PCPI
32.	At Risk Population — Coronary Artery Disease	Coronary Artery Disease (CAD) Composite: All or Nothing Scoring: Drug Therapy for Lowering LDL-Cholesterol	NQF #74 CMS (composite) / AMA-PCPI (individual component)
33.	At Risk Population — Coronary Artery Disease	Coronary Artery Disease (CAD) Composite: All or Nothing Scoring: Angiotensin-Converting Enzyme (ACE) Inhibitor or Angiotensin Receptor Blocker (ARB) Therapy for Patients with CAD and Diabetes and/or Left Ventricular Systolic Dysfunction (LVSD)	NQF # 66 CMS (composite) / AMA-PCPI (individual component)

Appendix H: Organizations in the National Priorities Partnership

AARP	AFL-CIO	AHRQ*
Aligning Forces for Quality	Alliance for Home Health Quality and Innovation	Alliance for Pediatric Quality
America's Health Insurance Plans	American Board of Medical Specialties	American Health Care Association
American Medical Association	American Medical Informatics Association	American Nurses Association
AQA	Association of State and Territorial Health Officials	Certification Commission for Health Information Technology
CDC*	CMS*	Consumers Union
HRSA*	HIMSS	Hospice and Palliative Care Coalition
Hospital Quality Alliance	IHI	IOM
Johnson & Johnson Health Care Systems	The Joint Commission	Leapfrog Group
National Association of Community Health Centers	National Association of State Medicaid Directors	National Business Group on Health
NCQA	National Governors Association	National Hispanic Medical Association
National Initiative for Children's Healthcare Quality	NIH*	National Partnership for Women & Families
NQF	Network for Regional Healthcare Improvement	Nursing Alliance for Quality Care
Pacific Business Group on Health	Partnership for Prevention	Patient Centered Primary Care Collaborative
Pharmacy Quality Alliance	Physician Consortium for Performance Improvement	Planetree
Quality Alliance Steering Committee	U.S. Chamber of Commerce	Veterans Health Administration*

* Indicates non-voting members of the partnership

Index

A

Academic medical center, 280
Accountability, 48
Accountable care organization, 327
See also ACO, 3
Accountable Care Organization Learning
Network, 33
ACO, 13, 30, 42, 48, 55, 67, 75, 81, 92, 96, 101,
106, 107, 108, 112, 114, 121, 123, 135, 141,
144, 146, 152, 159, 162, 172, 182, 190, 193,
197, 198, 207, 211, 214, 215, 220, 228, 270,
278, 279, 290, 291, 294, 297, 302, 304, 308,
311, 313, 315, 317
Alignment, 78
assumptions and uncertainties, 86
Benchmark, 276, 278
Clinical perspective, 308
Design principles, 14, 46
Economic impact, 306
functional stream, 36
Governance, 73, 97
Health information technology, 95
Legal structures, 87
Multipayer ACO, 35
Payer relations, 105
Physician relations, 99
Projected financial benefit, 304
Strategic planning, 305
Virtual models, 70
Administrative operations, 106
Advocate Health, 71
Advocate Physician Partners, 98, 130
Advocate Physician Partners 2011 Value Report,
130
Aetna, 34
Afforable Care Act
Section 3014, 212

Affordable Care Act, 9, 87, 150, 156, 236, 265,
271, 298, 307, 314
Section 1101, 26
Section 2706, 22, 28, 33
Section 3001, 29, 284
Section 3013, 208
Section 3015, 208, 212
Section 3021, 28
Section 3022, 20, 162, 206
Section 3502, 55, 178
Section2718, 289
Agency for Health Care Research and Quality, 239

Agency for Healthcare Research and Quality
See also AHRQ, 214
AHRQ, 214
Alignment strategies, 78
Alternative Quality Contract Program, 35, 284
American Academy of Family Physicians, 41
American Academy of Family Physicians Task
Force, 50
American Academy of Pediatrics, 40, 41
American College of Physicians, 41
American Medical Association, 67, 73, 119, 215
American Osteopathic Association, 41
American Recovery and Reinvestment Act
See also ARRA, 19
Analytics, 197
Anticompetitive actions, 132
Anticompetitive effect, 123, 327
Anti-Kickback Statute, 144, 145, 147
Antitrust, 118
Antitrust action plan, 158, 161, 350
Antitrust review, 105
Antitrust safety zone, 123, 132
AQC, 284
Arizona v. Maricopa County Medical Society, 131
ARRA, 19, 163, 236, 314

B

Baby boomer, 9, 307
Balanced Budget Act of 1996, 314
BCBSMA, 283
Beacon Community Cooperative Agreement
Program, 192
Beneficiary assignment, 276
Beneficiary Improvement and Protection Act of
2000, 314
Beneficiary volume, 147
Berwick, Donald, 21, 62, 210
Billings Clinic, 31
Blue Cross and Blue Shield, 248
Blue Cross Blue Shield of Massachusetts, 283
See BCHSMA, 35
Brookings Institute, 34
Budget and finance, 103
Bundled payment, 279, 290, 327
Bush, George, 163
Business acumen, 64
Business associate, 151

C

Carilion Clinic, 34
CDRS, 196
Center for Disease Control and Prevention, 239
Center for Medicare and Medicaid Services
    See also CMS, 5
CER, 233
    Claims data, 254
Certificate of Need, 155
Change management, 57, 62, 80, 82, 347
Christensen, Clayton, 139, 291, 318
CHRISTUS Health, 174
Chronic Care Model, 40
CIN, 3, 13, 42, 55, 67, 81, 88, 92, 96, 101, 106,
    108, 112, 114, 123, 126, 141, 144, 146, 152,
    159, 172, 182, 190, 211, 214, 220, 270, 279,
    290, 292, 297, 308, 311, 313, 317
Claims data, 96
Clayton Act, 120, 121
Cleveland Clinic, 70
Clinical data reporting system
    See also CDRS, 196
Clinical decision support, 197, 198, 256, 313
    See also CDS, 167
Clinical integration, 68, 76, 123, 128, 138, 140,
    162, 193
    FTC criteria, 19
Clinical quality and outcomes, 101
Clinical quality measures, 220
Clinical reporting system, 203
Clinically integrated network, 59, 104, 327
    See also CIN, 3
CMS Acute Care Episode (ACE) Demonstration,
    281
CMS Innovation Center, 28, 36, 109, 271, 294,
    309
CMS meaningful use, 86, 97, 148, 156, 157, 163,
    167, 207, 219, 228, 256, 266, 278
Collins, James, 65
Committee on the Costs of Medical Care, 11
Committee on the Quality of Health Care in
    America, 3
Communication, 64, 80
Community health relations, 111
Community health teams, 28
Comparative effectiveness, 305, 315
Comparative effectiveness research, 233, 327
Compensation models, 297
Computerized physician order entry, 167
Computerized provider order entry, 166
Congressional Budget Office, 272, 298, 304
Consumer Assessment of Healthcare Providers
    and Systems, 214
    See CAHPS, 220
Consumer-directed health plans, 6, 7
Coordination of care, 95
Cottage industry, 99

Covered entity, 151
Critical access hospital, 23, 138
Cross-functional practices, 79
Cross-functional teaming, 78
Crossing The Quality Chasm, 40, 64, 293
Crosson, Jay, 171
Cultural realignment, 85
Cushing, Harvey Williams, 40

D

Dartmouth Institute, 34
Dartmouth-Hitchcock Clinic, 31
Deficit Reduction Act, 284
Department of Defense, 239
Department of Health and Human Services
    See also DHHS, 20
Department of Justice
    See also DOJ, 88
Department of Veterans Affairs, 239
Determinants of innovation, 109
DHHS, 20, 77, 144, 150, 151, 209, 212, 270, 284,
    289
Diagnosis related group, 2, 29
Disease management program, 57, 347
Disruptive innovation, 139, 140, 291, 327
Disruptive value network, 139
DMAIC, 226
DOJ, 110, 120, 121, 125
Donabedian, Avedis, 201, 211, 224
Dzau, Victor, 109

E

Economic impact, 131, 305
Ecosystem, 327
EHR, 177, 193, 219, 220
E-iatrogenesis, 166
Einstein, Albert, 3
Electronic health records, 47, 328
Electronic medical record, 328
Electronic Prescribing Initiative, 157
Emotional intelligence, 64, 328
EMR, 79, 95, 97, 162, 163, 165, 166, 167, 177,
    179, 186, 198
EMR Adoption Model, 164
EMR Safe harbor, 149
EMR-based workflow, 181
Evanston Northwestern Health System, 131
Exclusive physician network, 132
Extended Hospital Medical Staff, 59, 60

F

Fawcett, Stephen, 310
FDA, 236, 245
Federal Trade Commission, 88
    See also FTC, 12

W

Waiver, 122, 123, 144
Waiver authority, 150

Williams, Ronald, 233
Woodcock, Janet, 261
World Health Organization, 205

Made in the USA
Lexington, KY
30 May 2012